Tranquilizer Use and Well-Being

A Longitudinal Study of Social and Psychological Effects

Robert D. Caplan
Antonia Abbey
David J. Abramis
Frank M. Andrews
Terry L. Conway
John R. P. French, Jr.

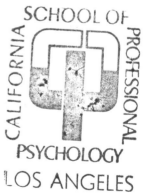

Survey Research Center
Institute for Social Research
The University of Michigan

1984

ISR Code No. 9019

R.D. Caplan, Principal Investigator; other investigators in
alphabetical order. F.M. Andrews and J.R.P. French, Jr.,
Co-Principal Investigators.

Library of Congress Cataloging in Publication Data:

Tranquilizer use and well-being.

  (Research report series / Institute for Social Research)
  Includes bibliographical references.
  1. Tranquilizing drugs. 2. Diazepam. 3. Drug
utilization--Social aspects--Michigan--Detroit Metropolitan
Area--Longitudinal studies. 4. Drug utilization--
Michigan--Detroit Metropolitan Area--Psychological
aspects--Longitudinal studies. 5. Health surveys--
Michigan--Detroit Metropolitan Area. I. Caplan, Robert D.
II. Series: Research report series (University of
Michigan. Institute for Social Research) [DNLM:
1. Diazepam. 2. Stress, Psychological--drug therapy.
3. Substance Dependence--psychology. 4. Quality of Life.
QV 77.9 T772]
RM333.T73 1984   616.86'3   84-9116
ISBN 0-87944-296-4 (pbk.)

Published in 1984 by:

The Institute for Social Research
The University of Michigan, Ann Arbor, Michigan

6   5   4   3   2   1

Manufactured in the United States of America

FOREWORD AND ACKNOWLEDGMENTS

When the idea of conducting a study of the social effects of the minor tranquilizer Valium was first proposed to us it seemed attractive because it provided two opportunities. One was the opportunity to contribute to theory and knowledge regarding social-psychological processes relating to stress and its effects on well-being. Another was the opportunity to examine an important social issue, and thereby contribute to the discussion of the effects of minor tranquilizer use in our society.

Because the study deals with social issues and health care, it may be of interest to a number of segments of our society. They include patients, physicians, pharmacists, pharmaceutical manufacturers, counselors, and legislators. This realization has made project members aware of the likelihood that the study would not go unnoticed, whatever its findings. In the course of designing and carrying out this study, we have interacted with most of the above-mentioned groups in order to understand their concerns and perspectives.

Each of the above groups may have a particular focus on the social effects of Valium. This is expected because each enters the process of health care at a different stage and plays a different role. This study cannot address all of the questions that each group requires to carry out its role in the health care process of our society. Nevertheless, it is hoped that the basic questions that were examined are of general interest. The following acknowledgements are a short currency for the help of more than 800 people and many organizations that made this study possible.

v

To begin, we would like to thank the Ethics Committee of the Wayne County Medical Society for its review of the study's purpose and of its procedures for ensuring confidentiality and anonymity.

The Michigan Board of Pharmacy provided the legal authorization enabling this study to draw potential respondents from pharmacy records, with the final approval of the participating pharmacists. This study was the first to have such access under Michigan law. We are grateful to the Board for the time and effort it took to carefully consider the merits of this study.

We also extend thanks to the many respondents and pharmacists who cooperated with this study. As participants, they remain anonymous.

During early stages of the study, small pilot tests of various interview components were made. These tests were not necessarily carried out with persons receiving a prescription for Valium. As a contributor to the pilot phase, Gary Gregg is thanked for some detailed, exploratory, case study interviewing that he conducted. William Bogard, M.D., a practicing psychiatrist who treats anxious patients, also helped by meeting with us to discuss early drafts of the interview schedule. We are also indebted to Robert Carpenter, M.D., who, as Director of the Outpatient Clinic for the University of Michigan Hospital, allowed us to pilot test various measures at that site. Similarly, we thank Robert Cubberly, M.D., for arranging for us to do additional pilot testing of measures at Metropolitan Tuxedo Hospital. We also want to thank the staffs at Providence Hospital (in Oak Park, Michigan), Group Health Service (Saginaw, Michigan), and Bon Secours (in St. Clair Shores, Michigan), for allowing us to conduct pilot tests with their outpatients. None of these sites was involved in the final data collection for the study. Nevertheless, their help during early stages of design was very important.

Technical advice on the coding of medications was obtained from a number of persons including Donald Green, M.D., of Hoffmann-La Roche. Professors Eddie Boyd, Duane Kirking, and Leslie Shimp of The University of Michigan School of Pharmacy

vi

are especially thanked for their considerable contribution. They developed a detailed set of codes of stimulant and depressant actions of the many medications mentioned by respondents in this study.

Steven Heeringa of the Survey Research Center developed the frame for sampling pharmacies for the study. Jeanne Keresztesi of the Survey Research Center's Field Section coordinated all of the interviewing operations. The excellent response rate, the high morale among those she supervised, and the smooth operation of a complex data collection are due in large part to her expertise and effort. The high quality of the data and the high response rates are also due to the field supervisors and the approximately 40 interviewers who performed at the highest professional standards.

There are many other staff at the Institute for Social Research who played a role in the study. Coders, under the supervision of Joan Scheffler, transferred the interview data to machine readable format with the degree of accuracy that has typified the Coding Section of the Survey Research Center. The research assistants, Linda Betleski, Bradford Parks, Linda Burns, put in many hours on a variety of tasks including the tabulating of results from numerous computer runs, text work in building the codebooks and typing of the final report and other related documentation, and in a wide variety of other project tasks. The data analysts, Pam O'Connor, Jeanne Kuo, Alice Yan, and Pauline Nagara, handled an often burgeoning queue of analysis tasks, frequently under the pressures of tight deadlines. Mary Jo Griewahn was the project secretary and coordinator of clerical support for the project. We are grateful to all of these persons for the skill of their work and the quality of their output.

Throughout this study, the research team has benefited greatly from intellectually stimulating, task-oriented interchanges with Edward Kaim and Harry Diakoff of Kaim Associates.

The study was generated in significant part by the initiative of Robert Jones of Hoffmann-La Roche, the manufacturer of Valium. He was aware that research was needed to inform the debate about the social effects of Valium and of other minor tranquilizers. It was this awareness, in large part, that led to subsequent meetings between the University of Michigan's Institute for Social Research and Hoffmann-La Roche and to the latter's decision to launch such a study. Thereafter, Robert Jones, along with Kaim Associates met with the project on a nearly-quarterly basis, so that all major decisions on design and analysis strategy could be reviewed jointly.

This study was underwritten by a contract from Hoffmann-La Roche. The contract guarantees us the freedom to search for answers as objectively as possible and to report them without restriction to the scientific community and to other public domains. The sponsor has demonstrated repeatedly throughout the study its commitment to an objective, independent, scientific exploration.

In keeping with the guarantee of an independent study, the interpretations and opinions expressed in this report are our own. Whether or not they come to represent those of the sponsor, the scientific community, and other individuals or groups must await the expression of opinions from each of these parties. The purpose of making these findings public is so they can be discussed and evaluated by the larger society. This step is an important and necessary component of the scientific process.

TABLE OF CONTENTS

Foreword and Acknowledgments   v

Overview   1

Chapter 1 SOCIAL EFFECTS OF MINOR TRANQUILIZERS:
OVERVIEW   6

    Social and Anxiolytic Effects   6

    Social Significance of this Study   7

        Prevalence   7

        Public attitudes   8

        Effects and use   8

    Population Studies of Benzodiazepine
    Effectiveness   9

    Clinical Studies of Benzodiazepine Effectiveness .   10

    What this Study Can and Cannot Examine   11

Chapter 2 BASIC THEORETICAL MODEL   13

    Stressors   17

        Objective vs. Subjective Stressors   18

        Role Ambiguity   19

        Role Conflict   19

        Misfit on Control   20

        Poor Health as a Stressor   22

        Life Events   22

    Strains   23

        Anxiety, Anger, and Depression   23

        Somatic Complaints   24

    Coping, Defense, and Affect Management   24

        Coping and Defense   24

        Main Effects of Coping, Defense,
        and Affect Management   26

        Moderator Effects   26

Outcomes of Stressors, Coping and Defense, and
Strains: Quality of Performance and Quality of
Life   27

    Quality of Performance   27

Quality of Life   29

    Social Support and Social Conflict   30

        Social Support   30

        Social Conflict   34

Main and Conditioning Effects   34

        Social Support and Anxiolytic Therapy   36

The Well-being of Others   36

Summary   37

Chapter 3 METHOD   39

Rationale   39

Procedures Considered but Rejected   40

    Recruitment Via Clinics and Private Practice   40

    Recruitment at Pharmacies   42

Respondent Recruitment Procedures   44

Pilot Testing of Procedures Used in the Study . .   45

    Procedures Used   45

    Implications of These Procedures   46

Procedures of Data Collection   47

    Interviewer Training   47

        General training   47

        Pilot tests   48

        Prestudy briefing   48

    Quality Control   49

    Interviewer Morale   49

    Contact with Potential Respondents   50

    Interview Setting and Procedures   51

Acceptance and Refusal Rates   53

    Acceptance Rate at Time 1   53

    Continuance Rate at Follow-up Interviews . .   55

Continuation Rates for Subgroups of Respondents .   56

Interview Design   61

Procedures of Coding   64

Procedures of Data Management   66

Descriptive Characteristics of Respondents   68

    Focal respondents   68

        Comparisons with 1979 U.S. Census data .   68

        Descriptive characteristics of Valium
        users and nonusers   69

        Quality of life evaluations compared to
        national samples   70

    Significant others   74

Chapter 4   THE MEASURES   78

On the Nature of Scales and Indices   78

Criteria for Selection and Design of Scales Used
in this Study   80

    Conceptual Relevance   80

    Use in Previous Research   80

    Operational Criteria   81

    Psychometric Criteria   81

General Procedures for Constructing Scales   81

General Procedures for Constructing Other Measures   84

    Open-Ended Measures   84

    Measuring Use of Medications and of Other
    Psychoactive Substances   86

        Measures as they appeared in the
        interview   87

        Derived measures of Valium use   88

Derived measures of use of other prescribed drugs   89

Use of street drugs, alcohol, caffeine, and tobacco   90

Measuring Stress   92

Measurement Quality of the Scales   93

Overview   93

Quality of the Raw Data   94

Retrospective data   95

Quality of the Data Processing   97

Quality of the Scales   97

Internal homogeneity   97

Estimates of construct validity   98

Agreement between focal respondent and significant others 100

Chapter 5 RESULTS 101

How Good Are the Data? 101

Indicator's of the Data's Quality 101

Internal reliability 101

Distribution 101

Coding reliability 102

Objective sources of validity 102

Retrospections 102

Convergent validity 103

Other evidence of validity 103

Summary 106

Portrait of Valium Users in the Study 106

Who Prescribed Valium? 107

How Supportive was the Prescriber? 107

How Was Valium Prescribed Versus Taken? . . . 108

How Did Patients Divide the Milligrams
They Took Over the Course of a Day?   109

Pattern of Use in the Last Six Weeks   110

Recency of Last Taking Valium   112

Across-Wave Variation in Valium Use   112

Respondents' Reasons for Taking Valium . . .   112

Decision Rules for Taking Valium   115

Respondents' Reasons for Not Continuing to
Take Valium   121

Health Status of Respondents   132

Comparison of the Health of Valium Users
and Nonusers   139

Use of Valium with Other Prescribed Drugs . .   145

Use of Valium with Alcohol, Cigarettes,
Caffeine, and Street Drugs   150

Professional Counseling and Valium Use . . .   157

Attitudes Regarding the Use of Valium and
Minor Tranquilizers   159

Summary of Portrait of Valium Users   160

Bivariate Analyses   161

Overview   161

Which Measures of Valium Should Be Used? . .   162

Milligram-weighted versus unweighted
measures   162

Pattern of use   163

Any use versus nonuse   163

Therapeutic dose   165

Check for Curvilinear Relationships   165

Stabilities in Means, Standard Deviations and
Relationships Over Time   166

Means   166

Standard Deviations   168

Relationships   168

xiii

Bivariate Relationships at Various Lags . . . 168

    Purpose and nature of the analyses . . . 168

    Results for Quality of life-as-a-whole and anxiety 171

    Results for Valium-taking and anxiety . 172

    Results for Valium-taking and quality of life-as-a-whole 173

    Results for Valium-taking and many major variables 173

    Conclusions 175

Searching for Spurious Effects 175

Potential Moderators of the Relationship Between Valium Use and Outcome Measures . . . 177

    How should potential moderators be selected? 178

    What methods and criteria should be used to detect moderator effects? . . . 178

Valium Use as a Moderator of the Stress-Strain Relationship 183

    Analysis I 183

    Analysis II 184

    Analysis III 184

    Analysis IV 185

    Conclusions 185

Summary of Bivariate Analyses 186

Multivariate Analyses 187

Overview 187

Multivariate Modeling: Theory and Method . . 187

    Results--Model A 191

    Results--Model B 197

    Conclusions 201

Correlations among Changes in Valium, Anxiety, and Life Quality 201

Purpose and nature of the analysis . . .   201

Results   203

Changes in Stress, Strain, and Performance
among the Highly Anxious: A Comparison
of Valium Users and Nonusers   207

Anxiety and other emotions   209

Caffeine, cigarettes, and alcohol . . .   210

Stress   211

Quality of performance   212

Quality of life   212

Mental health of the personal other . .   215

Summary   216

Summary of Multivariate Analyses   232

Within-person Analyses of Valium-taking,
Anxiety,and Quality of Life   232

Research Questions   232

Nature of the Analysis   233

Within-person Relationships for the
"Typical" Individual   234

Are There Some Individuals for Whom
Valium Shows "Beneficial" or
"Detrimental" Results?   236

Searching for Systematic Differences
Between People Who Showed "Beneficial"
and "Detrimental" Effects.   236

Summary   238

A Case Study Approach to Changes in Anxiety
and Quality of Life   239

Analysis I   240

Analysis II   240

Analysis III   242

Summary and Conclusions   243

Alternative Ways of Dealing with Anxiety   243

Effects of Valium Use on Significant Others in
Personal Life and Work Life   251

   Personal Other Results   251

      Who were they?   251

      Was the focal respondent's formal
      relationship to the personal other
      associated with characteristics of
      the personal other or
      of the focal respondent?   251

      Relationships between Valium use
      by the focal respondent and the
      well-being of the personal other. . . .   255

      Validity of the personal other data . .   257

   Work Other Results   258

      Who were they?   258

      Was the relationship of the work other
      to the focal respondent associated
      with any characteristics of the
      focal respondent or of the work other?   258

      Relationships of Valium use by the
      focal respondent to the
      well-being of the work other.   260

      Validity of work other measures   260

      Summary   262

   Chapter Summary   262

Chapter 6 SUMMARY AND DISCUSSION   263

   Summary of Purposes   263

      Social Effects   263

      Relationship of Valium Use to Use of Other
      Psychotropic Substances   264

      Anxiety   264

      Other Affective Strains   264

   Summary of Methods   265

      Recruitment   265

      Characteristics of the Respondents   266

Initial contact with respondents   267

Refusal and Continuance Rates   267

Quality of the Raw Data   268

Construction of Indices   268

Summary of Results: Portrait of the Valium User .   269

Summary of Results: Social Effects of Valium . .   270

Main Effects: Quality of Life   270

Analysis of Covariance: Social Effects . . .   272

Interaction Effects: Quality of Life and
Other Outcomes   273

Case Study Analyses: Quality of Life   274

Within-Person analyses: Quality of Life . . .   275

Effects of Use of Valium on Other Variables .   276

Interpretations: Social Effects   278

Interpretation 1   279

Interpretation 2   279

Interpretation 3   279

Interpretation 4   279

Interpretation 5   280

Summary of Results: Effects of Valium on Anxiety   281

Main Effects: Anxiety   281

Analysis of Covariance: Anxiety   283

Search for Interactions: Anxiety   283

Case Study Analyses: Comparing Pre- and
Post-Valium Anxiety   284

Interpretations: Anxiety   285

Interpretation 1 . . . ., ... ,. .   286

Interpretation 2   287

Interpretation 3   287

Interpretation 4   287

Limitations in the Clinical Trials   290

    Summary   290

Other Findings of Interest   291

Relevance of the Findings for Social Issues and
Questions   292

    1. Does the use of Valium numb patients so
that they are unaware of feelings and
emotions and cannot report them to others? .   292

    2. Does Valium use dull one's perception of
external reality?   293

    3. Does use of Valium decrease one's self-
esteem?   294

    4. Does the use of Valium affect patients'
perceived ability to control their lives? . .   294

    5. Is it true that people come to view Valium
as essentially a social and recreational
drug, not unlike alcohol? Do those who use
Valium consume more alcohol?   295

    In Conclusion   295

Appendix A   DESIGN OF RESPONDENT SELECTION PROCEDURES .   297

Appendix B   INITIAL LETTER TO POTENTIAL RESPONDENTS . .   299

Appendix C   PERSUASION LETTER   299

Appendix D   CERTIFICATE OF AGREEMENT   300

Appendix E   INITIAL LETTER TO POTENTIAL PERSONAL OTHERS   300

Appendix F   INITIAL LETTER OF POTENTIAL WORK OTHERS . .   301

Appendix G   FIRST THANK-YOU LETTER   301

Appendix H   SECOND THANK-YOU LETTER 302

Appendix I   TIME 4 QUESTIONNAIRES   302

Appendix J   DEFINITIONS OF INDICES, DERIVED
              MEASURES, AND SELECTED ITEMS   350

Appendix K   MEANS AND STANDARD DEVIATIONS OF INDICES
              AND SELECTED ITEMS   356

Appendix L   CRONBACH's ALPHAS FOR INDICES   361

Appendix M   EXACT PHRASING OF ITEMS IN INDICES AND
             SELECTED OTHER ITEMS   364

Appendix N   CODES FOR OPEN-ENDED MEASURES   377

Appendix O   COMMON THERAPEUTIC USES AND DRUG EFFECTS
             FOR DRUGS ON INTERVIEW FOLLOW-UP LIST AT WAVE 1   388

Appendix P   ESTIMATING THE NUMBER OF PILLS OF VALIUM
             TAKEN DURING "THE LAST 7 DAYS" PRIOR TO EACH
             INTERVIEW   388

Appendix Q   AN EXPLANATION OF THE CODING SCHEMES OF
             COMMON THERAPEUTIC CATEGORIES AND EFFECT
             CODES OF MEDICATIONS   392

Appendix R   NUMBER OF RESPONDENTS AT EACH TIMEPOINT
             TAKING MEDICATIONS CLASSIFIED BY COMMON
             THERAPEUTIC USE   394

Appendix S   CODING SCHEME FOR "MULTIPLE STRESS"
             MEASURE   397

Appendix T   DETAILED DESCRIPTION OF MODERATOR
             ANALYSES   398

References   405

OVERVIEW

This study examined the effects of Valium®[1] use on quality of life, affect, perceived performance, stress, social support, perceived control, coping and defense, and a number of other social-psychological variables related to mental health. A longitudinal survey was conducted in which a heterogenous group of 675 persons were interviewed four times, six weeks apart. In addition, questionnaire data were obtained from a significant other in the respondent's personal life and, if the respondent was employed, from a significant other at work. "Personal others" were interviewed for approximately 92% of the focal respondents at each timepoint. "Work others" were interviewed for approximately 70% of the focal respondents who were working at each timepoint. There were 367 respondents who used Valium at some time during the study and 308 who did not.

Although the pool of respondents was not intended to be a random sample of the population, it was selected to represent a broad array of social and demographic characteristics. Nearly all of the respondents were selected from pharmacy records in the Detroit Metropolitan Area and had filled a prescription approximately six weeks prior to the first interview.[2]

Participation was voluntary, by informed consent, and all information gathered was rendered anonymous. Approximately 48% of the people contacted agreed to participate, and 85% of those remained in the study through all four interviews.

---

[1]Valium is a registered trademark of Hoffmann-LaRoche, Inc. The generic name is diazepam.

[2]A few people were randomly selected from other lists so that interviewers would not know of the respondent's use of a pharmacy until the interviewer elicited that information.

At each interview, data were gathered assessing quality of life, anxiety, and use of Valium during each of the previous six weeks, including the current week. As a result there were 24 weekly data points on these variables covering the entire study. Other data, collected at each interview (such as stress, performance, subjective health, social support), focused on the current week.

Interview items intended to measure most of the various concepts were formed into indices. In general, these indices had acceptable internal reliabilities, good distributions, and good evidence of validity.

The most common dosage of Valium taken by respondents was 5 to 10 mg consumed once or twice per day, an amount within prescription limits indicated in the package insert. The most common prescribers were physicians in general practice, internal medicine, osteopathy, and psychiatry, in that order. This pattern of prescribers is similar to that found in the National Center for Health Statistics 1980 national survey of physicians and of their drug prescriptions for ambulatory care.

Users of Valium tended to take less Valium than prescribed. Reported use in excess of maximum recommended levels for the medication was extremely rare. Reported use of street drugs was also extremely rare.

Users of Valium tended to report that their physicians were supportive, taking time to listen to their concerns and answer their questions. Users also generally rated Valium as helpful in controlling their emotions.

The large majority of Valium users reported taking the medication for reasons related to anxiety disorders. Nevertheless, analyses were performed to determine if the effects might be different for persons taking it for anxiety compared to those taking it for other reasons. No such differences were found.

Many different analyses were performed to examine the relationship of Valium use to potential social effects and to anxiety. It was found that use of Valium was weakly associated cross-sectionally with low quality of life, high anxiety and other indicators of distress. This type of association has been found in national sample surveys; that is, users of minor tranquilizers report more distress in their lives.

When several different multivariate, longitudinal analysis techniques were used (structural equation modeling, analysis of covariance), this positive relationship between distress and use of Valium dropped virtually to zero. Longitudinal analyses generally showed no effect of Valium use, either harmful or beneficial, on a large number of outcomes. These outcomes included global quality of life; quality of performance in personal life; perceived control by others and by oneself over one's personal life and over one's emotions; perceived health; anger, anxiety, and depression; and the well-being of a significant other in personal life and in work life.

Analyses were also performed on subgroups to determine whether or not these effects might differ for selected groups of respondents. For example, daily Valium users were compared with nonusers, males with females, blacks with whites, and so on. There were a very small number of statistically significant findings that may be of value for future basic research. There was no notable evidence, however, of any harm or benefit of Valium use within any of these subgroups.

Analyses were also performed to determine whether or not the use of Valium might either decrease (buffer) or increase (exacerbate) the effects of various life stresses on emotional strain and on performance. These analyses tended to yield more evidence of buffering (that is, Valium use reduced the effects of stresses on anxiety and on other strains) than of exacerbating effects, except in the area of performance, where exacerbating effects were more common. The interpretation of these findings, however, is difficult. Their primary value may be to suggest further directions for research rather than to provide conclusions about the actions of Valium.

Use of Valium was unrelated to use of caffeine or of tobacco. Users of Valium did, however, tend to consume less alcohol in the weeks when they used Valium compared to the weeks when they did not. The findings may reflect a tendency to avoid simultaneous use of alcohol per the recommendations

3

for use. The findings may also reflect a tendency to substitute the medication for alcohol as an alternative psychoactive substance. Data from this study cannot serve to evaluate specifically the validity of each of these explanations.

Each respondent had 24 points of data regarding weekly use of Valium and weekly global quality of life and anxiety. These data were used to further determine if certain <u>individuals</u> might show a positive relationship between Valium use and these outcome measures whereas others might show a negative relationship. Correlations of use of Valium with quality of life and with anxiety were computed for each user over the 24 weekly data points using various time lags between Valium use and quality of life or anxiety. Only a small number of persons showed a negative relationship between Valium use and anxiety or a positive relationship between Valium use and quality of life. Comparisons of these individuals with the other respondents on over 80 variables showed no significant differences of note. Thus the few persons that did show notable relationships among these variables were considered to represent chance occurrences.

A number of explanations were considered for the general absence of effects of Valium use on the variables examined in this study. Since many of the Valium users who were studied had been using Valium for some time before the study began, it was suggested that perhaps this study examined people after they had already experienced the potential harms or potential benefits of the medication. If so, the study would detect no changes because they had already occurred. Analyses of respondents who were new users, and of users who were off Valium at least six weeks and then started taking it, again did not support this explanation.

It was also suggested that persons might not have had high enough levels of anxiety to show benefits or harmful effects. Analyses were therefore conducted specifically considering persons with the relatively high entry levels of anxiety found in clinical drug trials. These analyses did not change the basic findings.

4

It was also suggested that some people may take the medication prophylactically, in anticipation of a stressful event. In such cases differences in anxiety from pre- to post-Valium use would not necessarily appear. The study was not designed to evaluate the effect of such use.

With regard to the social effects of Valium use, then, this study generally found no evidence of beneficial or harmful effects with durations as short as one week or as long as 24 weeks. The absence of effects of Valium on anxiety suggests either that Valium has no anxiolytic effects, or that if it has effects, they stabilized for most respondents prior to the study or were too short-lived to be detected. Short-lived effects could occur if persons took the medication for the temporary relief of short-lived symptoms (much as aspirin is taken for relief of a headache). Clinical trials have consistently demonstrated the anxiolytic effect of Valium and other benzodiazepines. It may be of interest in future clinical trials to evaluate the relationship of prophylactic and temporary, short-term use of anxiolytics on short-term and weekly levels of anxiety in order to further evaluate these topics. It may also be useful to include some of the social-psychological variables from this study in clinical trials in order to investigate their effects in controlled experimental settings.

In summary, this study found no evidence that Valium had adverse or beneficial effects on a wide variety of social and psychological variables including anxiety. Further research is necessary to determine the generalizability of these findings.

CHAPTER 1

SOCIAL EFFECTS OF MINOR TRANQUILIZERS: OVERVIEW

This report describes a longitudinal panel study of the social and anxiolytic effects of one of the most widely-used medications in North America (Koch, 1982a): the minor tranquilizer, Valium (diazepam).[3] This investigation attempts a comprehensive examination of a wide array of social effects by gathering 24 weeks of longitudinal interview data from a panel of outpatient users and nonusers of Valium (total n=675 across four major interview waves) and from a panel of significant others in their lives.

Valium is one of a class of compounds known as benzodiazepines. A large body of clinical trial literature reflects the effectiveness of these compounds as anxiolytic medications (see Greenblatt & Shader, 1974). Valium is one of those benzodiazepines. Unlike a clinical trial, this is a study of Valium under conditions of actual use in society. The effectiveness demonstrated in the clinical trials is relevant to the extent that it can be regarded as predictive of effectiveness under conditions of actual use.

Social and Anxiolytic Effects

Social effects as considered here include possible effects of tranquilizer use on the nature and quality of people's lives and on the well-being of those close to them. A detailed

---

[3]Throughout this report the name "Valium" rather than "diazepam" will be used because this is the name by which the medication was mentioned, almost without exception, by the respondents. For purposes of documentation, it seemed important to refer to the proprietary name in order to avoid any ambiguity that might arise later on, should there be other proprietary forms of diazepam.

description of some of these possible social effects is presented in the next chapter.

Anxiolytic effects refer to a subset of indications for a benzodiazepine medication such as Valium. Valium in particular is:

> ...indicated for the management of anxiety disorders or for the short-term relief of the symptoms of anxiety. Anxiety or the tension of everyday life usually does not require treatment with an anxiolytic (Hoffman-LaRoche, Inc., 1982).

It is likely that most physicians rely on such guidelines when prescribing, rather than reviewing the detailed medical literature on the topic (see, for example, Avorn, Chen, & Hartley, 1982). Both our review of the literature on benzodiazepine efficacy and our discussions with people at Hoffmann-La Roche indicate that it is difficult to formulate more specific guidelines for prescription because the indicated applications of these medications are diverse, and evidence about efficacy under different conditions is complex (for example, see Rickels, 1981).

Social Significance of This Study

Prevalence. The use of minor tranquilizers is a matter of public interest because of the social issues that surround their use (e.g., Waldron, 1977; United States Senate, Committee on Labor and Human Resources, 1980; Koumjian, 1981) and because of the prevalence of their use. With regard to prevalence, according to 1980 nation-wide surveys by the National Center for Health Statistics, minor tranquilizers were prescribed, depending on the demographic group, in 11 to 20 out of every 1,000 medical visits (Koch, 1982a). The majority of prescriptions were written by internists and by general family practitioners (Cypress, 1982). These physicians comprise the most common categories of medical practice. Drugs used more frequently than Valium (the 11th most frequently prescribed drug in 1981; Koch, 1983) include antibiotics, medication for high blood pressure, and polio vaccine. By one conservative estimate, 10 million Americans used benzodiazepines in 1978 (National Disease and Therapeutic Index, 1979).

7

Public attitudes. Part of the potential social interest in tranquilizers is indicated by national survey findings about public attitudes toward tranquilizers. Ninety percent of those interviewed in the 1970s believed that it was morally better to use one's will-power than to use tranquilizers (Manheimer, Davidson, Balter, Mellinger, Cisin, & Parry, 1973). This attitude has been called "pharmacologic Calvinism" (Klerman, 1972). The relatively prevalent use of minor tranquilizers coupled with widespread pharmacologic Calvinism suggests that society has some ambivalence regarding the use of this class of medications.

Part of the ambivalence toward the use of tranquilizers may stem from the social stigma which surrounds mental, as compared to physical, illness (e.g., Gurin, Veroff, & Feld, 1960). Negative attitudes toward tranquilizers may derive in part from the association of tranquilizers with the treatment of a stigmatized illness.

This study, of course, does not address the morality of drug use. Nevertheless, it can provide some information regarding the effects of anxiolytic medication beyond the reduction of anxiety.

Effects and use. In the past few years, other social and psychological issues have been raised regarding the prescribing of minor tranquilizers. There is both scientific and social interest in whether or not certain uses of minor tranquilizers may lead to physiological and psychological dependence (e.g., Falk, Schuster, Bigelow, & Woods, 1982; Owen & Tyrer, 1983; Pevnick, Jasinski, & Jaertzen, 1978; Winokur, Rickels, Greenblatt, Snyder, & Schatz, 1980; Woods, Katz, & Winger, 1982). A careful review of the research on dependence (Woods, Katz, & Winger, 1982) shows that a small number of patients have developed physiological but not psychological dependence. The review found "...no compelling evidence that this dependence liability is associated with significant individual or social detriment, i.e., abuse liability" (p. 62).

Another social issue has arisen based on the observation that minor tranquilizers are prescribed more often for females than for males (see the review of this literature by

8

Cooperstock & Parnell, 1982). These findings have led to the following debates:

1. To what extent do physicians tend to prescribe anxiolytic medication on the basis of sex role stereotypes (e.g., Mcree, Corder & Haizlip, 1974; Prather & Fidell, 1975)?

2. To what extent are such demographically-linked differences in prescribing habits grounded in sound medical knowledge (Armitage, Schneiderman & Bass, 1980; Verbrugge, 1979)? Despite evidence of sex differences in anxiety (e.g., Dohrenwend & Dohrenwend, 1976; Gove, 1978), no research has yet been done which would determine systematically whether physician behavior is indeed driven by sound medical evidence, by sex differences in the willingness to present symptoms (Kessler, Brown, & Broman, 1981), or by stereotypes.

From a scientific point of view, these debates have not been settled.

Perhaps the most significant issue is whether or not the use of minor tranquilizers is a form of social control (Cooperstock & Parnell, 1982; Koumjian, 1981; Lennard, Epstein, Berstein, & Ransom, 1971). The argument has been made that these drugs allow medical personnel and allied professions to carry out their own work more easily, and in the process remove the patient's control over their own behavior and activities.

These and related issues have received national recognition both by the media and by the government. The congressional hearings on the "Use and Misuse of Benzodiazepines" (United States Senate, Committee on Labor and Human Resources, 1980) and reviews of these social issues and the scientific literature bearing on them (e.g., Cooperstock & Parnell, 1982; Koumjian, 1981) lead to the following conclusion: It is generally acknowledged that there is inadequate scientific information about the presence or absence of potential social effects of minor tranquilizers. As noted below, this ignorance may be due, in part, to the lack of studies of the effectiveness of minor tranquilizers as they are used in the general population.

Population Studies of Benzodiazepine Effectiveness

The most commonly cited studies of population symptomatology and tranquilizer use are the national random sample surveys of psychotherapeutic drug use in the United States (e.g., Mellinger, Balter, Manheimer, et al., 1978; Uhlenhuth, Rickels, Fisher, Park, Lipman, & Mock, 1966). Notwithstanding the cross-sectional designs of these studies, even experimentalists have been generous in applying causal explanations to the results. For example, the common interpretation of a positive correlation between psychic distress and use of psychotherapeutic drugs is viewed as evidence of appropriate drug use (e.g., Rickels, 1981). The conclusion is that if those taking the medication are more distressed, it is being used appropriately.

Appropriateness, however, refers to a process of medication use that involves both the presence and the absence or reduction of those conditions for which the medication is indicated. These cross-sectional studies do not deal with the disappearance of indications. Consequently, conclusions about appropriate use are speculative rather than scientific.

Indeed, there are several other competing interpretations of the positive relationship between psychic distress and use of psychotherapeutic drugs which cannot be ruled out by these cross-sectional studies. They include:

1. Tranquilizers increase psychic distress.

2. Psychic distress leads to tranquilizer use, but such use is ineffective, hence the correlation remains positive.

3. Psychic distress leads to tranquilizer use and such use reduces psychic distress but only over an interval too short to detect in such a survey.

Such studies were never intended to judge appropriateness or efficacy (Mellinger, personal communication, December, 1982). Consequently, the appropriate use of such research is to view it as purely descriptive and not indicative of causal relationships.

Clinical Studies of Benzodiazepine Effectiveness

There are numerous clinical trials demonstrating the anxiolytic properties of benzodiazepines (see reviews by Greenblatt & Shader, 1974; Hollister, 1974). It is important to note these clinical data because it is of practical consequence for interpreting the findings on social effects in this study. Many of our hypotheses about possible social effects (described in a following section) assume that those effects occur because of changes in anxiety. For example, consider the hypothesis that Valium can improve (or worsen) social role performance. One could base this hypothesis on the assumption that any improvement (or worsening) in the performance of social roles occurs via reductions in anxiety and its attendant discomforts as produced by the drug. Hypotheses of this sort, however, need not make such assumptions. For example, one can hypothesize that the mere act of taking an anxiolytic medication may have a placebo effect which would improve or worsen a person's sense of control over emotions, above and beyond the actual effect of the medication.

In theory, any assumed effects of diazepam via an intervening change in anxiety can be tested in this study. This testing is possible because the study includes measures of anxiety as well as of quality of life, sense of control, and other variables that can be examined as social effects.

What this Study Can and Cannot Examine

Different types of questions may require different designs (double-blind placebo-group trials versus longitudinal surveys, for example) and different types of samples (for example, long-term versus short-term users of a medication). This study was designed to examine a particular subset of questions regarding potential social effects of the use of a minor tranquilizer. Although a large number of concepts were examined, some social issues regarding Valium use were intentionally omitted because they can be better studied using a different design. Some of these issues are briefly described in the following paragraphs.

To begin with, this study was not designed to examine drug dependence or the effects of the illicit use of minor tranquilizers as street drugs. These questions require special procedures and samples.

Nor was this study designed to determine whether or not physicians are following sex-role stereotypes when prescribing minor tranquilizers such as Valium. A study of potential stereotyping would need to gather data on physicians as well as on their patients. This study did not gather such data.

This study also does not address questions about the effects of minor tranquilizers on objective performance measures such as eye-hand coordination, memory, and other basic aspects of human cognitive and psychomotor performance. Such behavioral outcomes have been examined primarily in the experimental laboratory (for reviews, see Johnson & Chernik, 1982; Kleinkecht & Donaldson, 1975; Wittenborn, 1979) and occasionally by experiments in the field (e.g., O'Hanlon, 1981; O'Hanlon, Haak, Blaauw & Riemersma, 1982).

This study has examined whether and how the use of Valium affects people's perceived quality of life, feelings of control, social support, perceived health, coping, and the performance of work and personal life roles as these people go about the business of their daily lives. The study has also examined the effects of using Valium on the well-being of significant others in these individuals' lives. These significant others include someone from the respondent's personal life (such as a spouse, relative or a close friend), and someone at work.

Finally, although the set of respondents is not intended to be representative of a particular population, steps were taken to ensure that a variety of demographic groups were included. The study includes males and females, blacks and whites, and persons spanning a wide range of ages, levels of education, occupations, and income.

12

CHAPTER 2

BASIC THEORETICAL MODEL

This section presents a model, Figure 2.1, representing some of the most basic hypotheses about the social effects of minor tranquilizers. Table 2.1 provides some examples of the variables assessed for each major construct in Figure 2.1. A number of alternative models are discussed in more detail in the Results.

The model in Figure 2.1 serves a number of purposes. It introduces key concepts. It also leads to a review of some of the literature regarding processes by which stress affects well-being, and by which Valium might have social effects beyond the reduction of anxiety.

The following is a brief summary of the major paths in Figure 1, after which follow definitions of the concepts and a more detailed discussion of the hypotheses. The model in Figure 1 depicts stressors as demands on the person or threats to need-fulfillment. Stressors can be internal problems (such as a chronic illness) or can originate from work or other environments. These stressors may lead to affective responses such as anxiety and to somatic responses such as the heart beating hard (Figure 2.1, arrow 1). These responses are called strains.

Both stressors and strains may stimulate coping and defense (arrows 2 and 3), including the use of minor tranquilizers. Defense may involve reducing the perception that stressors or strains are present without a corresponding change in the objective nature of stress or strain. Coping may involve direct attempts to reduce objective stressors, such as by working harder or by asking for a reduction in work load, or may involve direct management of strains such as when anxiolytic drugs are used to control anxiety.

13

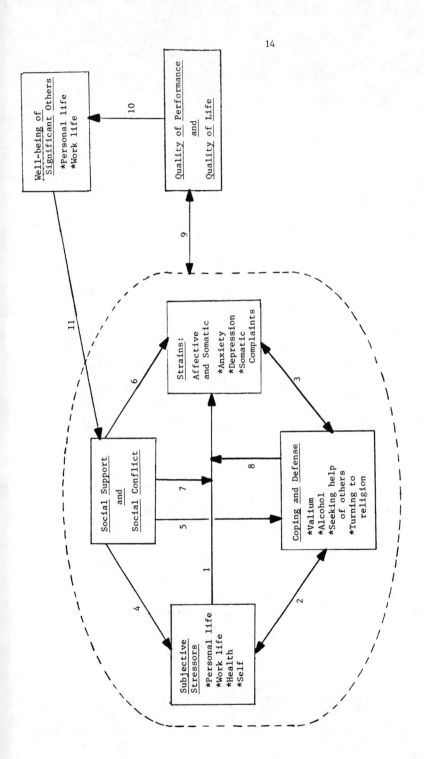

Figure 2.1 Schematic of major hypothesized links in the study of social effects of Valium. For ease of presentation, not all hypothesized paths are shown. The arrow originating from the dashed circle indicates that all variables within the circle may contribute to the hypothesized relationship. Arrows that intersect other arrows represent moderators of relationships. Social support and social conflict are represented separately from the other stressors in order to call attention to their role as moderators. See the text for additional explanation.

Table 2.1

Some of the Variables Assessing Each Construct

Stressors

Role ambiguity in personal life and in work life
Role conflict in work life
Negative life events and conditions
Misfit on internal control, control by others, control by
chance
      *over personal life
      *over emotions

Social Support and Social Conflict

Social Support
      *emotional support
      *informational support
Social conflict
Significant other's ratings of social support and conflict

Coping and Defense

Getting help from others
Reinterpretation of events
Taking a positive approach
Religion
Use of Valium
Use of alcohol, tobacco, and other psychotropic substances

General Affects and Somatic States

Anxiety
Depression
Anger
General positive affect
General negative affect
Somatic complaints
Perceived quality of health
Quality of sleep
Cardiovascular symptoms

Quality of Performance

In work life: social and technical
In personal life: social and technical
Work performance as assessed by work other
Personal life performance as assessed by personal
      others

Quality of Life (regarding:)

Personal life
Work life
People
Material well-being
Life as a whole
Work other's ratings of focal respondent's quality of work
        life and life as a whole
Personal other's ratings of the focal respondent's
        quality of personal life and life as a whole

Well-Being of Significant Other (rated by significant other)

Work other
Personal other

Note: Details regarding these and other related measures appear
in Chapter 4, "Measures."

Social   support   and   social   conflict,   described in more
detail shortly, are hypothesized to directly influence the intensity of stressors by providing aid or hindrances (arrow
4).[4] Social support and conflict may directly reduce or increase acts of coping and defense by encouraging or discourag-
ing such acts (arrow 5), and may directly increase or decrease
the   level   of various affects such as anxiety and depression
(arrow 6). Social support is also hypothesized to buffer the
effects of stressors on strain whereas social conflict is
hypothesized to enhance or exacerbate the effects of stressors
on strain (arrow 7). Coping and defense may also have buffering   (and   perhaps   enhancing) effects on relationships of
stressors to general affects (arrow 8).

These four sets of variables--stressors, strains, coping
and   defense,   and   social support and social conflict--are

----

[4]Too little social support and too much social conflict
can also be conceptualized as stressors. They have been kept
separate in order to depict their role as moderators of the
relationship between other stressors and strain.

16

hypothesized to influence quality of performance and quality of life (arrow 9). Quality of performance refers to how well, in the person's perception, he or she meets certain obligations associated with the roles occupied in work and in personal life. Quality of life refers to the person's evaluation of how good (or bad) life is. Quality of life should depend in part on the person's quality of performance because quality of life includes the perception of how well one performs one's roles. Arrow 9 is double-headed because the quality of performance is expected, ultimately, to reduce stressors and, under some circumstances, to reduce strains.

Quality of performance has direct consequences for the well-being of others because it involves performance in social roles (arrow 10). The person's quality of life also influences the well-being of others to the extent that others worry and feel bad when those close to them are having difficulties.

The remaining sections of this chapter provide more detailed definitions of these concepts and a fuller discussion of the hypotheses. Both general hypotheses about stress and strain and specific hypotheses regarding how Valium use is related to them are described.

Stressors

The term "stressor" is a broad term that refers to perceived circumstances which make demands on a person's abilities or threaten attainment of needs. Stressors may represent demands on the person (e.g., to produce work, to deal with interpersonal conflict) or they may represent deficits of supplies needed by the person (such as supplies of caring and esteem, of money, or of opportunity to control one's personal life). Poor health can be a stressor to the extent that it decreases the person's abilities and thereby increases the difficulty of fulfilling certain needs or places demands on the person.

Stressors are hypothesized to provoke emotional, somatic, and physiological responses. These hypothesized responses to stressors will be referred to as "strains," another broad term. Responses, such as elevated levels of anxiety, use of alcoholic

17

beverages, and disturbances in sleep patterns, can be viewed as strains to the extent that they deviate from levels that would be considered normal baseline states. Strains, in a cyclical process, can themselves become stressors.

Objective vs. Subjective Stressors

An important distinction is made between objective stressors (or stress) and subjective stressors (e.g., Levi, 1972; McGrath, 1976: French & Kahn, 1962). Objective stressors are those which can be assessed independently of the person's perceptual processing and potential distortion of them. Subjective stressors are those which are <u>perceived</u> by the person. A subjective perception that a stressor is present will accurately reflect the existence of an objective stressor to the extent that the person has access to and attends to accurate information (Ericcson & Simon, 1980) and to the extent that the person is not motivated to distort or repress that information (French, Caplan & Harrison, 1982).

In this study the measures of stressors are subjective. That is, they are based on respondents' perceptions. The choice of subjective stressors was guided by two considerations. First, although there has been progress in measuring physical stressors, such as decibels of noise and degrees of temperature, it is very costly to develop methods for assessing objectively the complex social-psychological stressors found in day-to-day settings. Second, those studies which have compared the predictive effects of objective and subjective measures of the same stressor on well-being have generally found that subjective measures were better predictors (French & Caplan, 1973; Kraut, 1965; French, et al., 1982). Other research has shown that people's emotional and physiological responses to objective stressors is influenced by the way they perceive those stressors (Lundberg & Frankenhaeuser, 1978).

The general superiority of subjective over objective measures of stress as predictors of well-being may be due to two reasons. One of these is the already acknowledged difficulty of measuring objective stressors. Second, most theories of psychological stress and well-being hypothesize that objective stress leads to subjective stress which in turn

18

leads to emotional and physiological strain. According to these theories, subjective stressors should be stronger predictors of strain and well-being because they are closer than objective stressors in the causal chain leading to strain. Furthermore, if individuals perceive stress, they are likely to exhibit strain regardless of whether the stress is objectively present or not.

The problem of developing measures of objective stressors still remains. To partly address this need for objective measures, this study obtained ratings of the person's well-being and performance from two significant other persons. These ratings, of course, are still based on opinion, and measure subjective outcomes rather than stress.

Five major subjective stressors were examined in this study--role ambiguity, role conflict, misfit on control, poor subjective health, and negative conditions and events. They are described in the following sections.

Role Ambiguity

Role ambiguity refers to the extent to which a person is uncertain about how to carry out a particular role in life. This study examines the ambiguity people experience as they attempt to fulfill their social roles in their work and personal lives. Personal life refers to all nonwork settings including leisure, friendship, and family relationships.

Role ambiguity was selected for study because of its potential association with anxiety. Ambiguity or uncertainty has been suggested as a central precursor of anxiety (Archer, 1979; Arieti, 1970). In a study of 22 different white and blue collar occupations, role ambiguity was found to be one of the most important work conditions predicting anxiety (Caplan, Cobb, French, Harrison & Pinneau, 1980). National sample research found that role ambiguity was related to low self-confidence and a sense of futility (Kahn, Wolfe, Quinn, Snoek, & Rosenthal, 1964).

Role Conflict

Role conflict refers to the "simultaneous occurrence of two or more role expectations such that compliance with one

19

would make compliance with the other more difficult" (Katz & Kahn, 1978). These conflicting demands can come from the same person or from more than one person. Conflict is most strain-producing when it comes from persons of great importance to the individual (e.g., one's immediate supervisor; Kahn & Quinn, 1970).

Role conflict was examined as a stressor in work life partly because previous research had shown that it was related to low job satisfaction and high job-related tension (Kahn, et al., 1964). This research found that nearly half the respond-ents reported working under conditions of conflict. In a more recent national survey, 31% of the sample reported role con-flict (Quinn & Shepard, 1974).

Role conflict was also selected for study because of its potential links to anger (Maier, 1949) and to anxiety. A study of stress in 22 different occupations had found that role con-flict was positively correlated with anger-irritation, anxiety, and depression (Caplan, et al., 1980).

Misfit on Control

The third major stress we have selected is person-environment misfit with regard to control over one's personal life and emotions. The term "control" refers to people's beliefs about who or what determines outcomes in their lives. For example, people who believe they determine what happens in their lives are said to have "internal" perceptions of control (Rotter, 1966). On the other hand, people who believe that what happens to them is a matter of luck or chance or is highly influenced by other people are said to have "external" beliefs about control (Levenson, 1973, 1974; Lefcourt, 1982). The dis-tinction between control by others versus by chance may be use-ful on the grounds that control by others may be perceived by the person as more or less predictable than control by chance or luck (Levenson, 1973; Sherman & Rykman, 1980). Research in-dicates that many of the beneficial effects of control can be explained by predictability alone (Schulz, 1978).

There is evidence that repeated lack of control over situations the person expects to control is likely to lead to

20

giving up, or "learned helplessness" (Seligman, 1975). This helplessness response is particularly likely when the person attributes lack of control to himself or herself (i.e., self-blame) and perceives that this lack of control is unlikely to change (Abramson, Seligman, & Teasdale, 1978). Learned helplessness has been associated with impaired cognitive, affective, and behavioral functioning (Seligman, 1975; Abramson, Seligman, & Teasdale, 1978).

Whereas lack of control appears to increase adrenal-medullary response (increased adrenaline and increased cortisol), presence of control can suppress this response (see review by Frankenhaeuser, 1980). The importance of control in people's lives is demonstrated by a national sample survey of the work force which studied the relative importance of 33 facets of work (Quinn & Cobb, 1977). Multivariate analyses indicated that control over conditions of work was one of the most important predictors of job satisfaction and a significantly more important predictor than other key facets of work such as pay. It should be noted that studies of work participation also involve the concept of control and have found similar effects on well-being.

Person-environment (PE) fit theory (French, Rodgers & Cobb, 1974) provides a useful conceptual framework for taking into account situations in which people have too little, too much, or the right amount of control. PE fit theory considers the effects on well-being of a mismatch between one's needs and abilities (P) and the commensurate environmental (E) supplies (for those needs) and demands (for those abilities).

The concept of PE fit regarding control is useful because more control is not always preferable to less. People differ in how much control they prefer (e.g., Burger & Cooper, 1979). In some situations people may have too much control over outcomes (Rodin, Rennert, & Solomon, 1980; Bazerman, 1982). They may like someone else to handle particular matters. For example, most of us would feel overwhelmed by being given the opportunity to decide just which procedure should be used at each step of having a tooth extracted. Both too little and too much control may be expected to increase strain. From

21

the literature on learned helplessness (e.g., Seligman, 1975) and locus of control (e.g., Lefcourt, 1982), it is known that perceptions of low personal control appear to increase symptoms of depression and anxiety. It is not known whether excessive subjective control increases anxiety or depression or both. This seems a reasonable hypothesis, however, considering that under certain conditions (such as being held responsible for poor decisions), personal control is associated with lower self-esteem (Rodin, et al., 1980) and poorer performance (Bazerman, 1982).

One can measure PE fit on control by examining the amount of control the person needs (P) and has (E). For a detailed discussion of evidence regarding PE fit theory, the reader is referred elsewhere (Harrison, 1978; French, et al., 1982; Kulka, 1979; Caplan, 1983). No previous research has applied the theory of PE fit to the study of control.

Poor Health as a Stressor

Poor physical health is a stressor which differs from the others that have been discussed in that its locus is always the person. In this study ratings of physical health were obtained from the person but actual diagnoses from a physician were not available. Accordingly, the measure of physical health primarily indicates subjective perceptions.

Life Events

There has been a great deal of interest and research regarding acute life events (Holmes & Rahe, 1967; Dohrenwend & Dohrenwend, 1974) as predictors of psychiatric and physical illness. Nevertheless, the magnitude of relationships has generally been weak (correlations rarely exceeded the upper .20s; see review by Rabkin & Streuning, 1976). Furthermore, research has suggested that life events are a relatively weak predictor of psychological affects measured by the Hopkins Symptom Checklist (Derogatis, et al., 1974) when compared with the predictive power of measures of daily "hassles" and "uplifts" (Kanner, et al., 1981). Whatever variance in emotional strain was due to life events could be explained, in multivariate analyses, by daily hassles and uplifts.

As a result of these findings, a life events scale was excluded from the interview schedule (a number of such choices had to be made to keep the interview within reasonable limits). Nevertheless, certain open-ended questions on the degree to which the person mentioned positive and negative events and conditions were coded. The use of these coded measures will be described in more detail later.

Strains

This study's measures of affect reflect changes in symptomatology rather than in a specific diagnosis. There has been a considerable amount of research validating the self-report measures of anxiety and depression symptomatology. Research shows good, but not perfect, agreement between psychiatric diagnoses and self-report measures of related symptoms (e.g., Derogatis, et al., 1974). Consequently, although affect-related findings from this study might differ depending on whether one used psychiatrist or self-ratings, evidence would suggest that the conclusions drawn would be similar regardless of the form of assessment. We expect any differences to be ones dealing with the magnitude rather than the direction of relationships.

Anxiety, Anger and Depression

The most obvious strain for study is anxiety because it is the primary affect treated by minor tranquilizers. Depression was also included for a number of reasons. Physicians and psychiatrists have a very difficult time separating anxiety from depression when making diagnoses. Furthermore, the two affects tend to be correlated (e.g., Caplan et al., 1980). There is also evidence that anxiolytic drugs are not effective when depressive symptomatology is equal to or greater than anxiety symptomatology (Rickels, 1981; Prusoff & Klerman, 1974). Consequently, it may be useful to examine the relative amounts of anxiety and depression as potential predictors of the social effects of minor tranquilizers.

A measure of anger was included because role conflict tends to relate specifically to anger (Caplan, et al., 1980). Also, because of anger's potentially harmful social consequen-

23

ces, it was measured as a potential social effect of the use of Valium.

Somatic Complaints

Measures of a number of somatic complaints (e.g., heart beating hard, shortness of breath, and sweaty palms) were also included in the study. These symptoms are often found to be associated with the experience of negative affective responses such as anxiety and other emotions that might be influenced by the use of a minor tranquilizer.

Coping, Defense, and Affect Management

Coping and Defense

Following definitions derived from PE fit theory (French, et al., 1974), coping is behavior aimed at producing a change in the objective self (abilities, needs) or the objective environment (demands, supplies). For example, obtaining help from another person can be coping if the aim is to produce better objective fit with regard to some demand (such as asking coworkers to help complete a task, or having a supervisor reduce the work load).

Defense is defined as a response aimed at changing subjective perceptions of the stressor without producing a change in the objective stressor. Denial that a serious objective threat exists is an example of a defense. This defense is common among persons who fall victim to disasters in which there are adequate advance warnings (e.g., Janis, 1974). The use of defenses such as denial and repression may be useful in some circumstances and harmful in others (Lazarus, in press). Over the short run, defense mechanisms may, as part of a cycle, enable people to gain respite from a persistent stressor. Defenses may also allow people to approach stressors in a detached manner which will not interfere with their performance in attempting to overcome them. On the other hand, over the long run, distortion of reality may interfere with performance or disrupt social relationships. When distortion is used to deny the existence of a serious, treatable illness, it may even prove fatal.

24

Little is known, however, about the conditions under which coping and defense and their subcategories are helpful or harmful in promoting long- versus short-term well-being. Nevertheless, there is evidence that the more coping of all types people use, the weaker the effects of controllable stressors on strain (Pearlin & Schooler, 1978). Thus, coping may buffer the effects of stress on strain (Figure 2.1, arrow 8). There is also evidence that affects such as depression may trigger the seeking of information and emotional support (Coyne, Aldwin & Lazarus, 1981).

Taking steps to manage affect (such as taking a tranquilizer, attempting to relax, and so on) can be categorized as coping to the extent that they are intended to change the objective emotional state of the person.[5] This study assesses the use of Valium as well as other psychotropic substances to determine whether such affect-managing behaviors are beneficial for the person. The other substances whose use was studied include caffeine, alcohol, tobacco, and other stimulants and depressants.

Each act of coping or defense may occur independently or may be related to other coping and defense behaviors. For example, studies of arousal-seeking suggest that people who use one type of psychotropic substance (e.g., tobacco) are also more likely to use other substances (e.g., alcohol; for example, Schubert, 1964; 1965). All of the substances examined in this study (tranquilizers, alcohol, tobacco, and so on) tend to be of social interest because they are used frequently in our society.

As noted earlier, the study does not include measures of objective stressors. Accordingly, this study cannot formally investigate the effects of coping and defense because their assessment, by definition, requires measures of the objective and subjective stressor. Therefore, although the actual hypotheses apply to coping and defense, tests of these hypotheses are limited to predictions that involve coping-like and defense-

---

[5]The use of a tranquilizer may also change the person's other coping behaviors, thereby indirectly influencing the objective nature of stressors.

like measures. Coping-like responses are judged on theoretical grounds to be aimed largely at changing the objective nature of the person or the environment. Defense-like items are judged to be directed primarily towards distorting perceptions of the objective self and objective environment or of repressing such perceptions altogether. The nature of those measures is discussed in Chapter 4, "Measures."

Main Effects of Coping, Defense, and Affect Management

It has been noted that affect management (such as "keeping one's cool" or taking a tranquilizer) may occur in response to emotional strains and somatic complaints. Similarly, affective and somatic strains may also be influenced by coping and defense (Figure 2.1, arrow 3).

Anxiety may signal the person (Freud, 1959) to focus on affect management. Anxiety may also signal the person to engage in coping and/or defense in an attempt to alter objective and subjective stressors (Figure 2.1, arrow 2).

When a stressor is only a threatened or anticipated one-- for example, an upcoming speech for someone who is deathly afraid of facing large audiences--the effect of the stressor may be to trigger anticipatory or preventive affect management. Under such conditions, high levels of anxiety and other unpleasant affects may not necessarily precede the use of a minor tranquilizer. The only clue that anticipatory affect management is taking place may be the presence of high levels of anticipated stressors in combination with moderate to low levels of strain.

Moderator Effects

Coping and defense, including various forms of affect management, may also moderate (or condition) the relationship between stressors and strains. For example, a positive correlation is predicted between the amount of role ambiguity and anxiety a person experiences. This relationship may be weaker or nonexistent, however, for a person who has taken a minor tranquilizer. This will be the case if the anxiolytic medication has attenuated the reactivity of the person to the stressor above and beyond directly reducing the level of anxiety. The presence of coping may reduce the effect of stressors on strains through problem-solving or emotion-focused action.

What evidence is there of such moderator effects? Some studies suggest that coping can buffer or reduce the effects of stressors on strain (Pearlin and Schooler, 1978 ; Caplan, Naidu & Tripathi, 1982); other studies do not find such evidence (Felton, Revson & Hinrichsen, 1981). A comparison of these studies suggests that coping is more likely to have a buffering effect when the stressor is something over which the person can exert a reasonable amount of control (Caplan, et al., 1982).

Outcomes of Stressors, Coping and Defense, and Strains: Quality of Performance and Quality of Life

Quality of Performance

Performance can be conceptualized as the responses people make in attempting to fulfill role demands. Quality of performance is defined as how well people execute these responses with regard to some standard of excellence. The study of performance in natural social settings has received the greatest attention by psychologists studying employees in work organizations and students in school.

There have been numerous attempts to determine the dimensions of performance in social settings. The two most common elements of performance in these studies are (1) meeting the demands of the task, which is an instrumental type of performance, and (2) social-emotional performance, or how well the person gets along with others (for example, Blake & Mouton, 1964; Bales, 1950; Bowers & Seashore, 1966).

Use of a minor tranquilizer and of other modes of coping and defense may influence task and social-emotional performance. The hypothesized effects of these variables on such performance are left unspecified and will be explored as a research question. If tranquilizer use helps individuals manage their affect, they may perform more effectively. This may not be the case, however, if there are motor and cognitive effects of the tranquilizer that interfere with performance (e.g., Wittenborn, 1979; Gottschalk, 1977; Kleinknecht & Donaldson, 1975).

Emotions and related symptoms may also influence performance. Some symptoms may linearly decrease performance such that high strain produces poor performance. For example, somatic symptoms may distract the person and increase irritability to the point where it is difficult for the person to pay attention to all the internal and external cues that are required for excellent performance. On the other hand, an early experiment on anxiety found that anxiety had a curvilinear effect on test performance (Yerkes & Dodson, 1908). Very high and very low levels of anxiety both resulted in lower performance than did intermediate levels of anxiety. To illustrate, a physician preparing for grand rounds may fail to make a good presentation if he is not sufficiently anxious to be motivated to prepare. Similarly, a physician suffering excessive anxiety of stage fright would also perform inadequately during grand rounds.

Stressors also can interfere with performance. For example, a certain amount of role ambiguity may inspire some useful discretion about how to best achieve a work goal. An excessive amount of such ambiguity on the other hand may make it impossible to decide what that goal is. As another example, conflicting demands from others (role conflict) may lead to failure to satisfy these demands, particularly if the person cannot resolve the conflict such as by prioritizing or by having one demand eliminated (Kahn, et al., 1964).

Performance should reduce stressors to the extent that it handles demands of the situation and satisfies the needs of the person. One should not expect, however, that the relationship will be perfect. Some aspects of life, for example, are inherently unalterable (such as certain health problems). Some conflicts are inherently, or at least basically, unresolvable (for example, some disagreements represent basic differences in values). Furthermore, many problems are misdefined, and such mislabelling makes them nonresponsive to performance. For example, a person may mistakenly believe that improving social relationships is merely a matter of getting a new set of

28

clothes and a better stereo system, when the problem is actually more related to the person's tendency to dominate social interaction.

In all of these instances, the quality of performance may be judged by how hard the person tried rather than by actual performance. This especially may be the case for tasks which have insurmountable demands. Those who try and fail may be judged better than those who failed to try. Such considerations suggest that if irrelevant standards of performance are assessed, the effect of performance on stressors (and strain) will be weak.

Quality of Life

The subjective quality of life is an important aspect of people's emotional experience (Campbell, Converse, & Rodgers, 1976). Studies of the quality of life demonstrate that, although subjective experiences of material wealth and security do covary with socioeconomic classes in meaningful ways, feelings of deprivation and satisfaction with social-psychological aspects of life vary within rich and poor alike (Brickman & Campbell, 1971). Consequently, subjective quality of life was selected as a potentially important social effect in this study. Quality of life (QOL) was hypothesized to be influenced by stressors, by coping and defense, and by emotional and somatic states.

The study examined quality of life within a number of domains, such as work, personal life, and emotions. According to theories of quality of life, people assess overall life quality or "life as a whole" as a function of the quality of life in specific domains. These domains include (among others) work, personal life, and self (for a national sample study of the content of these domains, their importance to people, and their interrelationships, see Andrews & Withey, 1976). As is shown in Figure 2.2, these domains combine to produce the overall assessment of subjective well-being, global quality of life. McKennell and Andrews (1980) suggest that subjective quality of life is a function of emotional feelings one has and of an evaluation (a cognition) of how well one is doing with regard to some standard (Figure 2.3). Positive and negative

29

affect combine to produce an overall feeling of hedonic tone (positive to negative, pleasant to unpleasant) which Bradburn (1969) refers to as the "affect balance." It was expected that anxiety should influence quality of life primarily via negative rather than positive affective components of life quality. It was hypothesized that minor tranquilizers should have a stronger effect on the negative rather than on the positive affective components because such tranquilizers are expected to reduce anxiety rather than to increase positive affect.

Figure 2.4 shows that each domain of quality of life, as with life as a whole, is affected by components of positive and negative affect and by cognition. The model represents the hypothesis that each domain's affective and cognitive components influence the affective and cognitive components of life as a whole. Figure 2.4, thus, represents one logical integration of Figures 2.2 and 2.3.

The theory that life quality is the result of joint effects of the balance of positive affect, negative affect, and cognitive evaluations has received only preliminary exploration (McKennell & Andrews, 1980). This study is one of the first in which the models shown in Figures 2.3 and 2.4 are tested by attempting to develop separate measures of affect and cognition.

Based on results of multivariate analyses of national sample data by Andrews and Withey (1976), five domains of quality of life were selected for study because of their importance as predictors of overall life quality: personal life, self, work, health, and life as a whole. The domains that were omitted play a more minor role in overall life quality (for example, satisfaction with government and with the nation as a whole).

Social Support and Social Conflict

Social Support

There are a variety of definitions of social support (e.g., Caplan, 1979; Wortman, 1983). Nevertheless, they basically emphasize the following qualities: affirmation of thoughts, beliefs, and feelings, encouragement, expression of

30

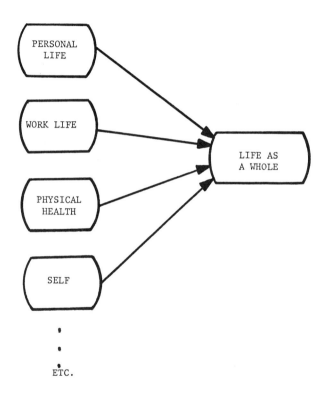

Figure 2.2   Overall quality of life (life as a whole)
             is hypothesized to be the result of the perceived
             quality of life in specific domains.

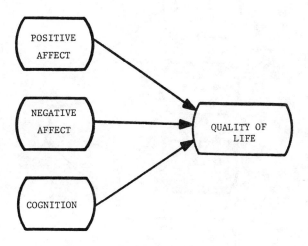

Figure 2.3 Quality of life shown as a hypothesized function of
positive affect, negative affect, and cognition.

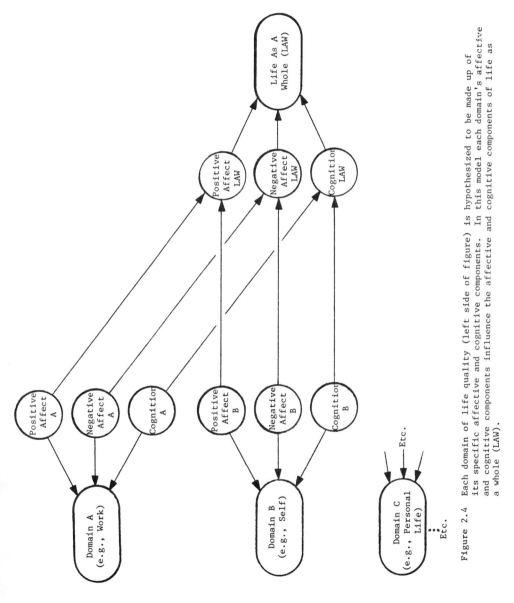

Figure 2.4 Each domain of life quality (left side of figure) is hypothesized to be made up of its specific affective and cognitive components. In this model each domain's affective and cognitive components influence the affective and cognitive components of life as a whole (LAW).

33

positive regard and affection, and certain kinds of direct aid (Katz & Kahn, 1978).

Social Conflict

Social conflict is defined as the disaffirmation of a person's thoughts, beliefs, and feelings, the expression of negative regard and disaffection, and certain kinds of direct withholding of aid or erection of barriers. Such behavior may occur by intention, but it can also result during well-intentioned interaction. For example, advice may be provided that is unwanted or manipulative. The social support literature has focused largely on the expectation that support is beneficial to well-being (reviews by Cobb, 1976; House, 1981; Kaplan, et al., 1977). More recently, the literature has been tempered by findings suggesting that well-being may be undermined by excessively dense, homogeneous social networks (Hirsch, 1980), highly emotional family environments (Leff & Tarrier, 1981), and aid which threatens the recipient's self-esteem (Abbey, Holland, & Wortman, 1980; Fisher, et al., 1982).

Although social support and social conflict may be inversely correlated when coming from the same person (the more social support, the less conflict), there is little or no relationship between the overall amount of support and the overall amount of conflict that people experience in their lives (Abbey, Abramis & Caplan, 1981). This finding seems reasonable in that, both within and across domains of life, people may encounter others who vary in the degree to which they are supportive, apathetic, or contentious.

Main and Conditioning Effects

Social support is expected to directly reduce stressors (e.g., Caplan, et al., 1980) as well as directly reduce strain (see reviews by House, 1981, and by Kaplan, et al., 1977). Social undermining or conflict is hypothesized to increase stressors and strains.

As with stressors, a distinction is made between objective and subjective support and conflict. This study does not include measures of objective social support and conflict. The study assesses the focal respondent's perceptions of received

34

social support and conflict. Also, significant others in personal life and work report on the social support and conflict they receive from and provide to the focal respondent. As a result, the two sources of measurement of social support and of social conflict can be compared.

Social support and social conflict are hypothesized to affect coping and defense. Social support may promote strategies of coping and defense which help the person and discourage strategies that harm; social conflict may do just the opposite. At this time, there is no published research regarding these effects.

Social support is hypothesized to have buffering effects on the relationship between stressors and strains. Buffering means that social support reduces the positive relationships between stressors and strains from what they might be without support.

By contrast, social conflict is hypothesized to have exacerbating effects on stress-strain relationships. Exacerbating effects refer to the potential ability of social conflict to increase the effects of stressors on strains, perhaps by reducing the person's emotional resistance to stressors.

There is research supporting the buffering effect (see reviews by Cobb, 1976, and by House, 1981, and research by Abbey, Abramis, & Caplan, 1981; LaRocco, House, & French, 1980; Caplan, 1971; French, 1974; Kadushin, 1981; and Vanfossen, 1981). There is also research finding no evidence for buffering (Pinneau, 1975; Frydman, 1981). Consequently, the conditions under which one does and does not find buffering remains a topic of exploration (e.g., Thoits, 1982).

Much of the discussion of when buffering occurs centers on methodological issues regarding how to search statistically for interaction effects. It is also important to consider just how buffering works substantively. If the effects of stress on strain operate largely via coping and defense, then social support may buffer the effects of stress on strain by altering the quality of coping and defense (Caplan, 1979). This study contains the basic elements for evaluating this hypothesis.

35

Social Support and Anxiolytic Therapy

Research suggests that anxiolytic drugs are more likely to be effective when the physician's attitude toward the patient is supportive (e.g., Rickels, 1978). If the anxiolytic effectiveness of a minor tranquilizer depends on the level of social support, there will be an interaction or conditioning effect of social support on the effect of tranquilizer use on anxiety and other potential outcomes.

There are at least two rationales for the importance of professional support in conditioning the effects of a minor tranquilizer on anxiety. One rationale is that the physician needs to communicate confidence in the medication to promote patient compliance. Inadequate compliance may reduce the efficacy of the medication. Second, the physician or therapist may need to be on hand when anxiety is reduced to a manageable level, in order to help the patient cope with those facets of illness or of other life stresses which generated the anxiety in the first place.

The physician and therapist, of course, are not the only sources of social support or conflict for the patient. Persons in the larger social network including family, friends, and those at work, also play a role in this relationship. For example, in a study of schizophrenic outpatients, the supportiveness of the home environment enhanced the effectiveness of medication prescribed to these patients. Lack of home supportiveness reduced medication effectiveness to the point where reinstitutionalization was required (Goldberg, et al., 1976). Consequently, both the physician and others in the person's life may be important as parts of the adjunctive milieu in which anxiolytic therapy takes place. As a result, the study examined the perceived social support from physicians and therapists as well as from others.

The Well-being of Others

As members of society, people are accountable to others as well as to themselves. Therefore, the broad definition of the social effects of a minor tranquilizer may reasonably include

36

the well-being of others who interact with the user of Valium
as well as of users themselves.

This research examines the well-being of two key persons
in the patient's life--a significant other in the domain of
personal life and, if the focal person is employed, a significant other in work life. The quality of life of these
others and their emotional well-being may be affected by the
well-being and performance of the Valium user.

The performance of the focal person should have a direct
effect on the significant other to the extent that the significant other depends on the focal person to satisfy various
needs. Some of these needs may be social-emotional (for example, needs for affiliation, for expressions of care and concern, and for maintenance of affects promotive of well-being).
Some of these needs may be for tangible support (for example,
the focal person's ability to share in household, family, and
work role responsibilities). The focal person's social-
emotional performance should have a stronger effect on well-
being of a significant other in personal life (e.g., a spouse)
than in work life. This prediction is made because motives for
affiliation are theoretically a stronger basis for personal
life than for work life relationships.

The links between the well-being of the focal person and
of significant others form a potential feedback loop. It is
likely that the well-being of significant others influences
their ability to provide social support and to avoid social
conflict (Figure 2.1, arrow 11). That support, in turn, may
have consequences for whether the patient responds favorably or
unfavorably to anxiolytic treatment. (For a discussion of how
the health care provider's own support-giving behavior is
dependent on the social support of the patient and others, see
Caplan, 1979; Harrison, Caplan, French, & Wellons, 1982; and
Caplan, Harrison, Wellons, & French, 1980b.)

Summary

There are several major hypothesized determinants of the
effectiveness with which people deal with their lives. These
determinants include the stressors that come from the environ-

ment and from illness conditions, emotional and somatic strains, and coping and defense responses aimed at dealing with these stressors and strains. Among these responses to stressors and strains is the use of minor tranquilizers, the effects of which form the major focus of this study.

Stressors, strains, and coping and defense may influence one another and may influence the performance of social-emotional and task-oriented behavior. Social support and social conflict generated in interaction with others may influence the intensity of stressors and strains and influence the use of coping and defense responses. The amount of social support may determine the extent to which anxiolytic therapy reduces anxiety and consequently influences the person's ability to master potentially anxiety-provoking situations.

A broad definition of the social effects of any medical intervention, including the use of a minor tranquilizer, includes the effects of the patient's well-being on the well-being of others. Those significant others may themselves be important sources of social support to the person taking the tranquilizer.

CHAPTER 3

METHOD

Rationale

As described in detail in the previous two chapters, the purpose of this study was to examine the social effects of Valium use and of untreated anxiety. To achieve this purpose, it was not necessary, or even desirable, to obtain a random sample of the population. Although Valium is one of the country's most commonly prescribed medications, the frequency of use is low,[*] so obtaining an equal-probability sample with a sufficient number of Valium users for detailed analysis would have been costly and inefficient. Other researchers have collected descriptive data about Valium users (Mellinger, et al., 1978; Parry et al., 1973; Uhlenhuth, et al., 1978), and description was not the primary goal of this study. Instead, the study was designed to oversample some groups, such as males and senior citizens, to ensure an adequate number of respondents in these categories for detailed subgroup analyses.

The strength of this study is in its capacity to examine relationships among variables both cross-sectionally and longitudinally. The use of a heterogenous set of respondents, selected to show variation on variables of key importance to the study, permits the use of the types of multivariate analyses required to test the major hypotheses. Although there is no reason to believe that these findings will not generalize to all Valium users, this assumption should be tested in future research.

---

[*]According to random sample national survey results, only two percent of Americans report taking Valium on any particular day (Opinion Research Corporation, 1983).

Procedures Considered but Rejected

The original goal of this study was to compare persons who were about to start a course of anxiolytic drug therapy with persons who did not receive a prescription for any anxiolytic but had similar high levels of anxiety. Both groups would be followed over time. Their use of any other psychotropic medications or substances would be measured during that period and taken into account in subsequent analyses.

Two strategies were considered and explored for meeting this goal: recruitment via clinics and private practice, and recruitment on-site at pharmacies. Each of these strategies proved to have serious disadvantages, and each strategy involved compromises in the original goal mentioned above. These disadvantages and compromises are described below so that the reader will understand the ultimate choice of the method of respondent selection described in the Procedures Section of this chapter.

Recruitment Via Clinics and Private Practice

Recruitment from clinics and private practices had the advantage of allowing selection of respondents at locations where the likelihood of receiving a prescription for Valium was higher than in the general population. Recruitment in these health care settings would have reduced the costs of screening dramatically. Using this technique, it would be possible to contact patients with a prescription for Valium just before they began taking their medication. By contacting patients before they took their medication, baseline measures of anxiety and other variables of interest in the study could be obtained.

To explore the feasibility of this approach, a series of surveys was conducted. In the first survey, almost every Health Maintenance Organization (HMO) and large multi-practice clinic in the Detroit Metropolitan Area and in a second nearby metropolitan area, Toledo, Ohio, were contacted.

Three types of evidence from these contacts suggested that prescribing of minor tranquilizers at these sites had declined from earlier levels. One source of information was the physicians' comments. Physicians talked about a shift towards

40

reduced prescribing of anxiolytic medication. They mentioned seminars and staff meetings in which physicians were urged to use alternatives to anxiolytic medication, such as the increased use of counseling.

Another source of information was tallies of outpatient intake and prescriptions at some large clinic sites. These tallies indicated that very small numbers of patients were prescribed Valium and other minor tranquilizers. As a third source of information, pilot tests were conducted in a large HMO in which patients were recruited as they left the physician's office. This too indicated that it would be extremely difficult and time-consuming to obtain a sufficient number of patients for the study using HMOs and large clinics as sites.

Was this also the case for smaller practices? To answer this question, a survey of physicians in private practice was conducted. In the physician survey, the names of 85 physicians were randomly drawn from the Detroit Yellow Pages (psychiatrists, oncologists, internists, gynecologists, cardiologists, general practitioners and surgeons). The doctors were sent a letter describing the proposed survey of their prescribing of Valium. One week later they were contacted by phone by an interviewer.

Interviewers were able to contact 55 of these physicians (18% being lost to refusal to participate and the balance being unavailable by phone or having moved). From this survey it was concluded that there was wide variation in the number of prescriptions for Valium written per patient and per practice in small, private practices. The range of prescriptions was from zero to eight per day per practice with estimates of zero to 20% of the patients per practice taking Valium.

It was evident that the logistics of having an interviewer contact patients prior to their filling a prescription would be formidable because of the small numbers of Valium patients available in each practice. One could, of course, seek cooperation from a minority of physicians who wrote an unusually large number of prescriptions for Valium. That approach, however, would fail to provide the broad range of patients and of patterns of usage desired for the study.

Recruitment at Pharmacies

The third strategy that was examined involved recruitment from pharmacies. An advantage of recruiting at pharmacies is that each pharmacy serves as a catchment for patients from a large number of practices. Furthermore, it might be possible to obtain baseline data by interviewing patients at the pharmacies before they took any medication. Even if it was not possible to interview all such persons before they had taken their medication, a history of recent usage could be obtained and this information could be taken into account in the analyses. The nonValium group could be drawn from the same pharmacies, as a comparison group. They would be similar in the sense that they, like the Valium patients, would have recently visited a physician.

As the first step in exploring the feasibility of this strategy, a random survey of 50 outpatient, noninstitutional pharmacies was conducted to determine how frequently they filled prescriptions for Valium. The pharmacies were sampled from the directory of the Detroit Pharmaceutical Association.

By telephone survey, trained interviewers were able to contact 38 pharmacies (response rate = 76%) in Detroit and its suburbs regarding a one-day (a Friday) activity of filling prescriptions for Valium.

Two key things were learned from the survey. One was that pharmacists were relatively cooperative, even when being contacted by phone. Second, in one day, 38 pharmacies (about 4% of the total directory) filled 110 outpatient, noninstitutional prescriptions for Valium of which more than two-thirds were classified as new prescriptions rather than refills. (Federal regulation limits refills on each Valium prescription to a six-month period).

These results were encouraging. Consequently, a pilot test of patient recruitment procedures at pharmacies was conducted. A number of pharmacy chains volunteered to allow interviewers access to their drug stores. The procedure for selecting patients was as follows: If the client presented a prescription for Valium to the pharmacist, the pharmacist or clerk asked the client if he or she would like to meet with an interviewer from The University of Michigan who could describe more about the study. The pharmacist mentioned that the University would pay $10 for the first interview.

This procedure had a number of difficulties. Pharmacy clients generally did not have an hour to spare for an interview on the spot. They were often in the middle of errands or other commitments. So even if they wished to cooperate, it was difficult. A large recreational vehicle was used as a mobile interviewing station, and it too created problems. The vehicle proved difficult for the interviewers to move and use. Heating it in the upcoming winter would be complicated. Third, a walkie-talkie beeper was used to help pharmacists summon the interviewer. That too, without a cumbersome external antenna, was unreliable. Thus ended the "mobile home" phase of the pilot testing.

If clients could not spend time being interviewed at the pharmacy, could they call the University to schedule an interview at a later time? To test this strategy, pharmacists explained to any qualified client that The University of Michigan was conducting a study on stress and daily life and was paying for interviews. The pharmacist was to tell clients that, if they wanted more information, they could phone a number on an information sheet that was given to each client. Some sheets even had coins attached to pay for the phone call.

The outcome of this strategy was unsatisfactory. Those who were motivated enough to phone were frequently desperate for the interview money. They included the impoverished, drug addicts, and prostitutes, all of whom were challenging to interview and unrepresentative of the majority of Valium users. This attempt concluded the last of the unsuccessful methods for recruiting patients for the study.

At that stage, the interviewers pointed out that the Survey Research Center had over 20 years of outstanding success in eliciting respondent cooperation, when the interviewer was the first person to make contact with the potential respondent:

"Give us a chance to talk to respondents and we'll be successful. Pharmacists aren't trained in this type of recruiting."
This led to the procedure that was finally adopted, as
described below.

Respondent Recruitment Procedures

The following procedures were used to obtain respondents
for the study. First, approval for the study was obtained from
two sources. In November, 1981 the final study protocol was
approved by the University of Michigan Human Subjects Review
Committee, which agreed that the proposed research would
protect the rights and welfare of human subjects (approval of
an earlier version of the protocol was obtained in 1980). The
investigators also submitted the study protocol to the Michigan
State Board of Pharmacy. The Board, under Michigan law, can
approve direct access to pharmacy records for certain research
purposes. The Board evaluated the procedures and the expected
outcomes of the study, using the following criteria: a) protec-
tion of respondents' confidentiality and safety, and b)
benefits of the study for the people of Michigan. The Board
approved the study in December, 1980.

In the second stage of respondent recruitment, a sample of
pharmacies was drawn from a pool of large-volume pharmacies in
the greater Detroit area. Large-volume pharmacies were used to
increase the efficiency of case-findings. Although it was not
the researchers' intent to obtain a representative sample of
the population, or even a representative sample of Valium
users, it was desirable to obtain respondents who were
heterogeneous with respect to standard demographics. Thus,
using ZIP codes of 137 pharmacies, the Sampling Section of the
Institute for Social Research drew a systematic sample of 50
pharmacies stratified by county (urban and suburban areas),
neighborhood income, and racial composition. In addition, 50
more pharmacies were sampled to match the first 50 (on county,
income, and race) in anticipation of a low pharmacy recruitment
rate; when a given pharmacy declined to participate in the
study, its matched replicate was substituted. When the
research staff contacted the sampled pharmacies to obtain permission to examine their records, the actual pharmacy recruit-

ment rate was low enough that 97 pharmacies were ultimately contacted and 39 (40%) consented to allow their client records to be sampled. These 39 pharmacies did provide a distribution which represented the geography, income, and racial composition of the greater Detroit area reasonably well.

The Sampling Section then sampled 2131 client names from the combined lists of all the pharmacies that consented to participate. Pharmacy records were sampled to include a) 50% males and 50% females, and b) 66% people who had filled a prescription for Valium within the prior six weeks and 33% who had filled a prescription for a medication other than Valium, other antianxiety agents, antidepressants, antipsychotics, or antihistamines in the prior six weeks. This was done to ensure that control group members would not be taking medications which could conceivably have been prescribed for a psychological problem. Individuals taking these medications were omitted because this would provide the clearest comparison of the effects of taking versus not taking a medication prescribed for an emotional disorder—the disorder in this case being anxiety. The 2131 names drawn from pharmacy records were combined with a small number of names from business mailing lists to provide additional confidentiality for respondents. In this way, an interviewer contacting a particular respondent did not know in advance if that respondent was taking any medication. Furthermore, only the interviewing staff had access to the names of the respondents. The project staff had access only to the anonymous questionnaires and could not tell the source from which a person's name was drawn. Both pharmacies and respondents were viewed as participants in the study; therefore, to ensure confidentiality, neither interviewers nor respondents were told the specific sampling methods of the study. (See Appendix A for a precise description of the Sampling Procedures.) Instead, both interviewers and respondents were told that names came from an assortment of legally obtained lists.

Pilot Testing of Procedures Used in the Study

Procedures Used

In March of 1981, the specific procedures used in this study were pilot-tested. (Numerous other pilot tests which were conducted to test other procedures and the questionnaire are described in other sections of this chapter.) The source of pharmacy records was asked to provide records from the previous six weeks from three different pharmacies in different parts of the Detroit Metropolitan area. Two lists were provided. The first included all individuals who had filled a prescription for Valium during the previous six weeks. The second included all individuals who had filled a prescription for a nonpsychoactive medication during the previous six weeks.

The purpose of this pilot test was to ensure that (1) the source of respondents could provide their records within the specified time period, (2) the interviewers' supervisor could promptly distribute names of potential respondents to interviewers, (3) the pharmacy information was accurate (i.e., with respect to phone numbers, identification of clients' sex and age, and prescription information), and (4) a reasonable number of pharmacy clients would be willing to be interviewed. All of these checks of the procedures were accomplished successfully. Pharmacy lists were provided promptly, and, although they were not error-free, the number of errors was fairly small. Fifty-four percent of the interviews attempted with Valium users (25 out of 46) and 48% of the interviews attempted with nonusers (20 out of 42) were successfully completed. This was considered to be an adequate acceptance rate for a pilot test (interviewers did not try hard to persuade reluctant individuals or to contact hard-to-reach individuals because the pilot test was to be completed within one week).

Implications of These Procedures

These same selection procedures, that is, contacting individuals who had filled a prescription during the prior six weeks, were used in the main study. This provided a heterogeneous set of respondents who were well suited for the relational analyses described later in this report. These analyses included a variety of statistical controls for differences between respondents in levels of stress, health, and anxiety. Of course, it was not possible to assess most respondents' anxiety or quality of life prior to their Valium-taking using this procedure. However, some respondents had

46

stopped taking Valium at a later interview and some of these had resumed Valium use at a still later interview. And a few other respondents, who were not taking Valium at Time 1, began taking it at some later point. Special analyses of these individuals who provide both pre and post measures of Valium use, anxiety, and quality of life are described in the Results Chapter.

Procedures of Data Collection

Interviewer Training

General training. Survey Research Center interviewers collected the data for this study. These interviewers are carefully trained professionals. Interviewers are typically well-educated individuals willing to work part-time with flexible hours. All of the 37 interviewers who worked on this study were females between the ages of 25 and 65.

All interviewers had been taught about (1) the objectives of social research, (2) interviewing techniques, (3) sampling techniques, and (4) administrative procedures. Interviewers were trained to use structured questionnaires, to record respondents' answers verbatim, to use non-directive probing techniques, and to provide respondents with appropriate feedback to encourage precise answers (Survey Research Center, 1976). Interviewers were also trained how to contact potential respondents and how to encourage participation without being too pushy. Interviewers were told that they should never attempt to counsel a respondent or to request counseling from a respondent. If specifically asked by respondents for help, interviewers provided them with the names of regular, recognized public agencies. All interviewers signed a pledge in which they promised to keep all respondent information completely confidential.

Interviewers were carefully monitored. Each interviewer had a supervisor who trained her and monitored her performance. Also, a member of the field office in Ann Arbor (the study manager) coordinated communication between the interviewers and the study staff. This standard training was supplemented with

specialized training by the project staff for this specific
interview and procedures.

Pilot tests. The entire project staff met with pilot test
interviewers before and after each pilot test. Pilot tests
were conducted by a small number (5-7) of interviewers with experience in many previous studies. They had permission to
deviate from the standard respondent contact procedures or the
precise phrasing of a question in the interview if either did
not appear to be working successfully. Their impressions of
the pilot test were thoroughly described to the project staff.
Their comments were useful and contributed to the quality of
the questionnaire.

Prestudy briefing. Once the procedures and questionnaire
were finalized and the study was ready to enter the field, the
project staff met with the entire interviewing staff for a full
day to describe the study. First, the purpose of the study and
the potential value of its findings were explained. Then some
of the major variables were described and their locations in
the questionnaire were pointed out. Actual hypotheses were not
mentioned so interviewers would not be biased while administer-
ing the questionnaire. Based on previous experiences of the
project staff and the field office, we felt it was important
to convey to the interviewers the value of the study. Interviewers who felt that they were working on something important
were expected to try harder than interviewers who were less
convinced of the value of their work.

The exact procedures for obtaining and contacting respondents were also described at the meeting. Then the format of
the questionnaire was explained. A few potentially difficult
sections of the questionnaire were discussed in detail. Interviewers were given plenty of time to ask questions about any
aspect of the study.

Prior to the meeting each interviewer had been given a
copy of a 197-page instruction book which was designed specifically for this study. This book contained (1) a review of the
purposes of the study and its procedures, (2) a sample questionnaire completed for a fictional respondent, and (3)
detailed question-by-question instructions which described the

purpose of each question and special instructions about skip patterns and probing techniques. Interviewers were asked to read the book and conduct one practice interview before the meeting. Interviewers were also given a worksheet in which several situations were presented for which they were to determine the appropriate action. This training gave interviewers enough experience with the materials so that they came to the meeting prepared to discuss any procedures which were still unclear to them.

Quality Control

The field supervisor reviewed the practice interview conducted by each interviewer to ensure that it was completed properly. Any problems were discussed with the interviewer before she conducted her first interview with a respondent. In addition, the field supervisor met with all new interviewers after they completed their first five interviews to assess their performance. Interviewers could call their supervisor, the study manager, or the project staff at any time with questions, and many did, especially at the beginning of data collection.

Interviews were carefully examined when they arrived in the field office by the study manager and a member of the project staff. They checked the portions of the interview which were known to be somewhat complicated (e.g., the medication section, the work status section). Interviewers were notified of any errors they had made so they could avoid making the same error in the future. The interviewer was asked to call the respondent if possible to collect any missing information. If several interviewers made the same error, a memo was mailed to all interviewers which described the proper procedures. Although these procedures were time-consuming, they seemed warranted, to ensure the quality of the data, in view of the length and complexity of the interview.

Interviewer Morale

Interviewers were required to conduct a large number of interviews within a relatively short time. The interview was fairly personal and many respondents shared intimate information with interviewers. In view of the fact that virtually every respondent had filled a prescription for a medication recently, and that two-thirds of these were for Valium, it was not surprising that the respondents were on the average more physically ill and anxious than respondents in most surveys. Interviewers were trained to keep respondents from digressing and to avoid giving advice, but many respondents insisted on telling sad stories about their lives. For these reasons, although interviewers enjoyed conducting interviews, they found it to be a somewhat stressful experience. The supervisor was available to discuss these issues with interviewers. Also, the project staff held two meetings with the interviewers during the course of the study: the first was held after two months of data collection, the second was held after four months of data collection. During these sessions, interviewers were allowed to discuss any problems they had with respondents or procedures. In many cases other interviewers had encountered similar problems so there was a group discussion of how best to handle these situations.

During these sessions materials for the later waves of data collection were also distributed. Again instructions and work sheets were provided and difficult questions were reviewed. Our many sessions with interviewers were time-consuming; however, we feel that they contributed to the quality of the study.

Contact with Potential Respondents

A letter was mailed to potential respondents approximately 1-2 weeks before they were to be contacted by an interviewer. The letter stated that The University of Michigan's Survey Research Center was conducting a study on the effects of stress on health, work, and everyday life, and was interested in interviewing a wide range of people, including them. The letter assured them that their answers would remain confidential. It also gave them the name of their interviewer and indicated that she would be calling soon to set up an appointment (see Appendix B).

When possible, potential respondents were assigned to interviewers who lived near their homes. This minimized travel

50

costs because most interviews were conducted in respondents' homes. A few days after respondents should have received the letter, interviewers called them to set up an appointment for an interview. The instruction book contained a sample script which interviewers were allowed to modify. Respondents who were reluctant to be interviewed were sent a persuasion letter (see Appendix C) and were called back by another interviewer. Potential respondents were not told exactly how their names were sampled (nor were interviewers). If they asked, interviewers told them that names were obtained from a number of lists that were legally obtained and were chosen to achieve a heterogenous group of respondents.

Some of the potential respondents were eliminated for various reasons. All respondents were to be at least 18 years of age (one 17-year-old was mistakenly interviewed). Individuals living in nursing homes or who were currently hospitalized were not eligible for participation. Also, individuals who were clearly too senile or emotionally disturbed to provide valid data were excluded from participation. Interviewers were told to make this last judgment cautiously. If in doubt they were told to begin an interview and then end it if it became obvious that the individual could not understand the questions. (This procedure was never necessary.)

Interview Setting and Procedures

After an individual agreed to be interviewed, an appointment was made for the earliest possible date. Interviews were usually held in a respondent's home. If the neighborhood was a known high-crime neighborhood, interviewers were allowed to schedule the interview at the local library or a quiet coffee shop. If the interview was conducted in the respondent's home and other people were there, the interviewer asked if there was a room in which they could meet privately. Most respondents were interviewed alone; for 71% of the respondents no one else was present at any point during the interview.

Before beginning the interview, the interviewer carefully described the study to respondents. They were given a booklet which explained the purpose of the study, how they were selected, what types of questions they would be asked, an assurance of confidentiality, a description of the benefits of the study, and information about how to contact the study staff if they had additional questions. They were also asked to sign a Certificate of Agreement. This specialized consent form stated that (1) they were voluntarily agreeing to be interviewed four times, (2) they understood that accurate, carefully considered responses and participation in all four waves were vital, and (3) they should not participate if they were unwilling to make this commitment. Previous research indicates that respondents asked to sign such a consent form appear to provide more accurate responses (Oksenberg, Vinokur, & Cannell, 1979). Another paragraph guaranteed that the University would (1) pay them $5.00 for each of the first three interviews and $10.00 for the final interview, and (2) keep their responses totally confidential. The interviewer, as a representative of the University, signed this portion of the form while respondents signed the portion referring to their obligations. Respondents were allowed to keep this certificate (see Appendix D).

After the respondent signed the Certificate of Agreement the interview began. Respondents were given booklets which contained the various scale options used throughout the questionnaire. This made it easier for respondents to consider each option carefully before making a choice. At the point in the interview where respondents were asked about events in their lives for the previous six weeks (see Chapter 4 for a description), they were given a small appointment book which they were encouraged to use in the future to improve their recall at later interviews.

At the end of the interview, arrangements were made for interviewing one person in the respondent's personal life and another in his/her work life if the respondent was employed. If the personal other lived with the focal respondent and was home at that time, the interviewer conducted the interview at that point. Otherwise, a letter introducing the study and a response booklet was left with the focal respondent for both the personal and work others (see Appendices E & F). The respondent was asked to meet the personal and work others within 24 hours to give them the letters and booklets and to inform them that an interviewer would be calling.

Interviews with personal and work others were conducted as soon as possible after the focal respondent's interview, usually within one week. If the focal respondent had not given the other individuals the materials, the interview was conducted anyway. If the potential personal or work other refused to be interviewed, the interviewer called the focal respondent and asked for a second candidate.

Approximately two weeks before focal respondents' second interviews were scheduled to take place, they were sent a letter from the project staff thanking them for their participation and reminding them that they would be called by their interviewer again soon (see Appendix G). Focal respondents, personal others, and work others were sent a similar letter prior to the fourth interview (see Appendix H). Many respondents spontaneously mentioned to their interviewers that they appreciated receiving this letter. Respondents were also encouraged to complete a post card which would allow us to send them a copy of the findings when the study was completed. We think that such signs of appreciation improved response rates and general attitudes about the study.

Acceptance and Refusal Rates

Acceptance Rate at Time 1[7]

The Sampling Section of the Survey Research Center selected 2,131 names from the available lists (see section on Respondent Recruitment Procedures). Sixty-one of these names included errors (e.g., address not in tri-county area, duplicate names) which reduced the number of names to 2,070. Of these, 62 individuals were on extended vacations and therefore could not be interviewed; 77 individuals were judged by the interviewer to speak English too inadequately or be too ill or senile to be interviewed, 305 individuals could not be located, usually because the addresses provided were incomplete or incorrect, 534 individuals refused to be interviewed, and an additional 44

---

[7]The terms "Time" and "Wave" are used interchangeably throughout the text to refer to the interview timepoint.

53

Table 3.1

ACCEPTANCE RATES AT TIME 1

Outcome:	N	%
Interviewed	784	37.9
Foreign speaking, too ill, too senile	77	3.7
On vacation	62	3.0
Never located	305	14.7
Evasive; never interviewed	264	12.8
Someone else refused interview for the individual	44	2.1
Refused an interview	534	25.8
	2,070	100.0

refused through another individual; and 264 individuals neither refused nor accepted an interview (labeled "evasive"). Seven hundred and eighty-four individuals were successfully interviewed (see Table 3.1). This was satisfactorily close to our original goal of 773 initial interviews. While this was not intended to be a representative sample of Valium users or nonusers, the refusal and evasion rates were comparable for individuals prescribed Valium and other individuals (refusal rate: Valium: 28.7%; Other: 25.6%, evasion rate: Valium: 13%; Other: 12%). Approximately 48% of the people contacted agreed to be interviewed.

For 92% of the focal respondents a personal other was interviewed. Focal respondents who were employed 15 or more hours a week were asked to identify a significant other from their work life. Of the 385 focal respondents who met this criterion, 270 (71%) identified work others who were successfully interviewed (see Table 3.2).

Continuation Rate at Follow-up Interviews

The continuation rate from Time 1 to Time 2 was 91% (Table 3.2). Table 3.3 indicates the reasons for the dropouts. Ninety percent of the individuals selected as Valium users were reinterviewed at Time 2, while 94% of the individuals selected as nonusers were reinterviewed. For 91% of the Time 2 focal respondents a personal other was interviewed at Time 2. For 70% of the Time 2 focal respondents employed at least 15 hours a week, a work other was interviewed at Time 2. (See Table 3.2.)

The continuation rate from Time 2 to Time 3 was 96%. Once a respondent had missed a wave of data collection, no attempts were made to reinterview him or her at later waves. Table 3.4 indicates the reasons for the dropouts. Ninety-five percent of the individuals selected as Valium users who were interviewed at Time 2 were reinterviewed at Time 3, while 96% of the individuals selected as nonusers were reinterviewed at Time 3. For 91% of the Time 3 focal respondents a personal other was interviewed. For 70% of the Time 3 focal respondents employed at least 15 hours a week, a work other was interviewed (See Table 3.2).

The continuance rate from Time 3 to Time 4 was 98%. Table 3.5 indicates the reasons for the dropouts. Ninety-eight percent of the Time 3 respondents who had been selected as Valium users were reinterviewed, while 99% of the individuals selected as nonusers were reinterviewed. For 92% of the Time 4 focal respondents, a personal other was interviewed. For 67% of the Time 4 focal respondents employed at least 15 hours a week, a work other was interviewed (see Table 3.2).

This high continuance rate can be attributed to several factors. Respondents seemed to find the questionnaire interesting and enjoyed being interviewed. This appears to be due to their intrinsic interest in the content of the questionnaire and the interviewers' ability to make respondents feel comfortable. Interviewers were very skillful at encouraging reluctant respondents to continue participating in the study. Also, many respondents spontaneously mentioned appreciating the thank-you letters they were sent. The high continuance rates suggest

Table 3.2

CONTINUATION RATES FOR FOCAL RESPONDENT,
PERSONAL OTHER, AND WORK OTHER

	Focal Respondent	Personal Other	Work Other
Time 1	784	719 (92% of FR)	270 (71% of FR's working $\geq$ 15 hours)
Time 2	716 (91% of T1)	655 (91% of FR T2)	251(70% of FR's working $\geq$ 15 hours)
Time 3	686 (96% of T2; 88% of T1)	625 (91% of FR T3)	238 (70% of FR's working $\geq$ 15 hours)
Time 4	675 (98% of T3; 86% of T1)	624(92% of FR T4)	228(67% of FR's working $\geq$ 15 hours)

that the time spent training and monitoring interviewers, attempting to keep the questionnaire clear and interesting, and
providing respondents with positive feedback for participation
was well spent.

Continuation Rates for Subgroups of Respondents

As indicated in Table 3.2, 784 respondents were initially
interviewed. Of these, 675 respondents participated throughout
the entire study, while 109 discontinued prior to participating
in all four interviews.[8] To determine whether certain types
of individuals were more likely to drop out of the study than
others, continuation rates for various subgroups were examined.

---

[8]Most of the analyses discussed in this report were conducted on the 675 respondents who completed all four interviews.

Table 3.3

CONTINUATION RATE AT TIME 2

Outcome:	N	%
Reinterviewed	716	91.3
FR refused	39	5.0
Other refused for FR	2	.3
FR could not be contacted	1	.1
FR too ill	2	.3
FR on vacation	2	.3
FR deceased	2	.3
FR evasive	17	2.2
FR could not be located	3	.4
	784	100.0

Table 3.4

CONTINUATION RATE AT TIME 3

Outcome:	N	%
Reinterviewed	686	95.8
FR refused	13	1.8
FR could not be contacted	2	.3
FR too ill	1	.1
FR deceased	1	.1
FR evasive	12	1.7
FR could not be located	1	.1
	716	100.0

Table 3.5

CONTINUATION RATE AT TIME 4

Outcome:	N	%
Reinterviewed	675	98.4
FR refused	3	.4
FR too ill	4	.6
FR evasive	3	.4
FR could not be located	1	.1
	686	100.0

Table 3.6 provides descriptive characteristics for focal respondents who participated in all four interviews versus those with less than four interviews. The characteristic showing the largest difference in continuation rates was race: blacks were more likely to drop out of the study than whites. Study dropouts also were somewhat more likely to be taking Valium or some other psychotropic drugs' and to be male, less educated, and have lower income. Continuation rates were independent of age, reported anxiety, depression, and subjective quality of health.

Although dropouts had a somewhat different profile than those who participated throughout the study, this was not considered a serious problem given the goals of the study. As stated earlier, respondents were not intended to represent a random sample, which would be biased by selective dropout. Furthermore, despite higher discontinuation rates among certain types of respondents (e.g., blacks and males), there were still sufficient numbers in these various groups to permit examination of moderator effects (which are described in Chapter 5).

'This includes prescribed anti-depressants, anti-psychotics, stimulants, and sedative hypnotics other than Valium.

Table 3.6

CHARACTERISTICS OF FOCAL RESPONDENTS' WHO PARTICIPATED IN
4 INTERVIEWS VS. <4 INTERVIEWS (PERCENTAGES)

CHARACTERISTIC	4 WAVES	<4 WAVES
During Previous 6 Weeks at Wave 1		
Took Valium but no other psychotropic	46	50
Took other psychotropic but not Valium	8	10
Did not take Valium or other psychotropic	41	34
Took both Valium and some other psychotropic	5	6
	100%	100%
Sex		
Male	42	59
Female	58	41
	100%	100%
Race		
Black	18	33
White	81	66
Other	1	1
	100%	100%
Age		
MEAN CODE VALUE	4.3	4.5
1=17-24	8	6
2=25-29	9	11
3=30-34	12	6
4=35-44	19	17
5=45-54	21	25
6=55-95	31	35
	100%	100%

Table 3.6

CHARACTERISTICS OF FOCAL RESPONDENTS' WHO PAR-
TICIPATED IN 4 INTERVIEWS VS. <4 INTERVIEWS
(continued)

CHARACTERISTIC	4 WAVES	<4 WAVES
Years of Education		
MEAN CODE VALUE	5.1	4.8
1=0-4	1	2
2=5-7	2	3
3=8	4	11
4=9-11	20	23
5=12	35	33
6=13-15	23	17
7=16+	15	11
	100%	100%
Annual Family Income (in thousands of dollars)		
MEAN	4.8	4.2
1=Under 5	9	11
2=5-9.9	11	16
3=10-14.9	13	18
4=15-19.9	10	8
5=20-24.9	14	15
6=25-34.9	17	10
7=35-49.9	18	17
8=30+	8	5
	100%	100%
Perceived Health		
MEAN	3.4	3.3
1.0-1.4	7	11
1.5-2.4	16	20
2.5-3.4	24	19
3.5-4.4	33	32
4.5-5.0	20	18
	100%	100%

Table 3.6

CHARACTERISTICS OF FOCAL RESPONDENTS' WHO PAR-
TICIPATED IN 4 INTERVIEWS VS. <4 INTERVIEWS
(continued)

CHARACTERISTIC	4 WAVES	<4 WAVES
Anxiety (Hopkins Scale)		
MEAN	1.6	1.6
1.0-1.4	49	48
1.5-2.4	41	43
2.5-3.4	9	9
3.5-4.0	1	0
	100%	100%
Depression (Hopkins Scale)		
MEAN	1.8	1.8
1.0-1.4	37	33
1.5-2.4	51	54
2.5-3.4	11	12
3.5-4.0	1	1
	100%	100%

'Respondents with 4 interviews, N=675
Respondents with <4 interviews, N=109

Interview Design

A major task during the early part of the project was to design the interview schedules. These schedules would be used to collect data from the focal respondents and from the two other people who were significant in the focal respondent's life, the personal other and work other respondents. As with any major study, it was necessary to design a set of questionnaires and related materials that would yield useful measures of the desired concepts within the time and economic constraints of the study. We also wanted these materials and interviews to be interesting and attractive to the respondents and the interviewers.

Great effort was devoted to this task over a period of about one year. There was a rich array of concepts that seemed potentially relevant to the study and, for many of them, a variety of promising ways they might be measured. Results from previous research, relevant social and psychological theory, and a series of six pilot tests, most with multiple waves of data collection, were used to develop a set of final question- naires and related materials.

The developmental sequence began with the project staff drafting a series of interview questions. Then the team worked with personnel in the Survey Research Center's Field Office to assemble the questions in an appropriate format as an interview schedule for a pilot interview. This pilot interview was then tested by about a half dozen of the Center's most experienced interviewers in the Detroit region. The interviewers ad- ministered the interview to 30-50 respondents specially selected for this purpose.

After the pilot test data had been collected, the inter- viewers, Field Office personnel, and project staff met together to discuss all aspects of the interviewing procedures. Taking account of the problems that had been identified and the sug- gestions for solving them, the project staff then revised the interview schedule, and the process was repeated. Since the study was to involve repeated interviews with the same focal respondents, and interviews with two other people significant in the life of each respondent, these aspects of the data col- lection had to be considered and tested as part of the general developmental sequence.

During the period from June 1980 to May 1981 a series of six pilot tests was conducted. The first pilot test involved three waves of data collection (spaced about six weeks apart), and the third and sixth pilot tests each involved two waves of data collection. In each of these three pilot tests, inter- views were conducted with personal other and work other respondents as well as with focal respondents. The fifth pilot test was a less inclusive effort intended to test the useful- ness of certain procedures for presenting some of the materials. The second and fourth pilot tests were specifically designed to carefully determine how to measure two specific concepts: (1) perceived social support and interpersonal conflict and (2) perceptions of internal control, control by others, and control by chance. Detailed descriptions of these two pilot studies have been reported elsewhere (Abbey, Abramis, & Caplan, 1981; Conway, Abbey, & French, 1983). Altogether, these six pilot tests involved ten distinct data collections.

The final products of this interview schedule development were the questionnaires used to collect data from the focal respondents at the four waves of the main study, the questionnaires to collect data from the personal other and work other respondents at each of the four waves, and a large number of other supporting materials. These supporting materials included a booklet for the interviewers describing the study, a set of detailed instructions for the interviewers, various address and accounting forms for the interviewers, an initial contact letter that was sent to potential focal respondents, various follow-up letters, a booklet for respondents describing the study, a booklet for respondents that presented various answer scales for questions in the interview, a respondent agreement form, and materials to assist the focal respondent in soliciting participation of the personal and work other respondents.

Copies of the questionnaires used at Wave 4 of the study for the focal respondent, personal other respondent, and work other respondent are included as Appendix I. The Wave 4 questionnaires are virtually identical to the questionnaires used at the preceding waves but include at the end a few additional items for the focal respondent.[10]

As can be seen by inspecting the questionnaires, the data collected from the focal respondent were much more extensive than those obtained from the personal and work other respondents. In actual operation, the median length of a focal respondent interview was about 90 minutes, the median length of

---

[10]Copies of the other questionnaires and of the various forms and booklets can be obtained for a modest fee (to cover duplication, postage, and handling) by writing to the authors at the Survey Research Center.

a personal other interview was about 17 minutes, and the median length of a work other interview was about 14 minutes.''

Most questions are of the closed variety (i.e., have specific response choices from which the respondent chooses) and employ 4- to 7-category ordered scales. These have been found in previous survey work to produce useful information along dimensions preselected by the investigators and to do so in an efficient manner. In addition, there are, scattered throughout the interviews, a number of open questions to which respondents were invited to respond in their own words (which were recorded verbatim by the interviewers and coded for content by the study staff). As can also be seen, questions are grouped according to topical content and ordered in what the pilot tests showed to produce an easy-to-manage and interesting flow. One of the design considerations that is not obvious from a simple inspection of the questionnaires is the inclusion of multiple indicators (i.e., questionnaire items which measure the same concept but are phrased differently) for all of the important concepts being assessed. Such multiple indicators permit the formation of scales (indices) to measure the concepts (assuming certain conditions are met, as more fully described in the next chapter), which can be expected to result in higher measurement quality.

Procedures of Coding

Interviews were coded by professional coders at the Survey Research Center at the Institute for Social Research. The questionnaires were coded in two stages. First, the closed-ended responses (e.g., Likert-type scales, yes/no questions) were coded. The code values for most responses were included in the questionnaire so coders only needed to transfer these values to codesheets. During the coding operation, 9% of all interviews were selected at random to be check-coded. The coding supervisor recoded these interviews and compared her responses with those of the coders. All errors were then noted

---

''The precise median was slightly different at each timepoint.

64

and corrected. Table 3.7 shows the error rate for each wave of the study.

Table 3.7

ERROR RATE IN CLOSED-ENDED QUESTIONS

Wave	Error Rate[*]	Percent Error
1	0.56	0.06%
2	1.08	0.11%
3	0.81	0.09%
4	0.85	0.09%

[*]Average number of errors per interview. There were approximately 950 variables coded for each interview.

The second stage of coding involved coding the open-ended responses. Eleven different open-ended codes were developed (see Chapter 4 for a description of these variables). Due to the complexity of some of these codes, coders were extensively trained by a member of the project staff. The purpose of each variable and detailed coding criteria were presented to coders in the first training session. Then they were all asked to code the same ten interviews. At the next session, their choices were compared and disagreements were discussed to help clarify code boundaries. This cycle of coding and comparing answers was repeated several times until nearly perfect agreement was achieved. After training, each coder's first thirty interviews were checked by a member of the study staff for accuracy. A random 5% of the remaining interviews were check-coded. Two coders coded the same questionnaire; all disagreements were decided by a member of the study staff. Table 3.8 shows the percent of perfect agreement for each open-ended question.

Table 3.8

AGREEMENT RATE BETWEEN CODERS FOR OPEN-ENDED QUESTIONS

Variable coded	Percent Agreement
Positive events	92
Positive salience	96
Negative events	84
Negative salience	94
WHO health codes	83
Why stop taking Valium	78
Reasons for taking Valium	94
When FR takes Valium	77
Why stop taking other medication	81
Why not fill a prescription	81
Why FR thinks tranquilizers are used too much	79

Procedures of Data Management

A methodical series of procedures was followed to trans-
form coded questionnaire information into a "clean," computer-
analyzable set of data. Figure 3.1 provides an overview of
this process. These procedures were designed to maximize the
likelihood of finding coding, keypunching, and file-building
errors so they could be corrected prior to substantive data
analysis. Initially, each of the four waves of data was
treated separately. Coded questionnaire information was
keypunched onto computer cards, and all cards were verified for
accuracy. Information from these cards was then transferred to
computer files in the University of Michigan computing system.
The OSIRIS.IV (1982) software system was used for all subsequent data management.

After creating a dictionary of variables to describe the
coded questionnaire information, univariate frequency distribu-
66

FLOWCHART OF DATA-CLEANING AND ASSOCIATED PROCESSES

Figure 3.1

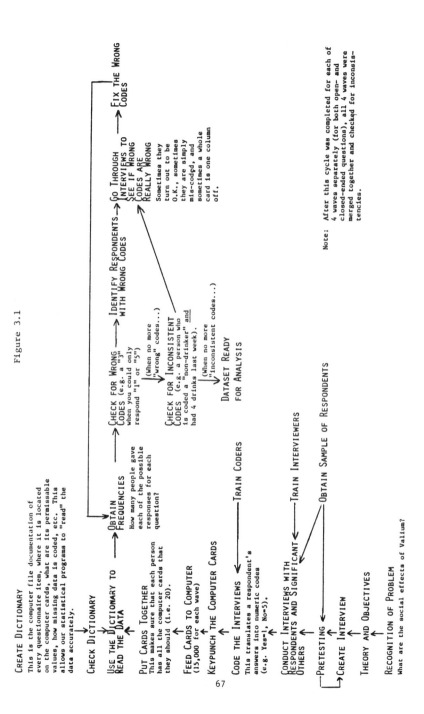

tions were obtained for all variables. Each of these distributions was checked for "wild" codes which could not possibly be valid, and steps were taken to correct these invalid values. Additionally, numerous consistency checks were made by looking for incompatible responses to related questions. For example, people who were coded as having taken no medications in the last seven days should not also have had codes specifying names of medications taken during that same period. Similarly, people coded as unemployed during the last six weeks should not have had an estimate of the number of times arriving late to work during the last two weeks. Any such inconsistencies were checked against original questionnaire responses and appropriate corrections were made.

These procedures for file-building and data cleaning were done separately for each wave of data. Then the files containing separate waves of data were merged into a single file containing information on all individuals included in the study at each of the waves. Frequency distributions were rerun for all variables and again checked for wild codes. Additional consistency checks were made comparing codes for related variables across different waves. For example, sex and race of a respondent were expected to be coded the same at each wave. Again, wild codes and any apparent inconsistencies were checked against the original questionnaire responses and appropriate corrections were made on computer files.

These steps assured the absence of invalid codes and indicated the data had been merged correctly. Overall, more than 55,000 merge checks, 450,000 consistency checks, and 2,500,000 wild code checks were made on the data. Fewer than 2,000 keypunching and coding errors were found with all these checks, indicating an error rate of less than .07% prior to data cleaning. Following data cleaning procedures, the error rate in the data set finally used for analysis must be extremely small.

Descriptive Characteristics of Respondents

Focal respondents

Comparisons with 1979 U.S. Census data. Respondents in this study were not intended to be representative of Americans as a whole. However, a few demographic comparisons were made with 1979 U.S. Census data to see how closely the respondents matched the American adult population on selected characteristics (Statistical Abstract of the United States, 1980). Respondents in this study were very similar to the American population with respect to distributions of sex, age, and education. There were only four differences greater than 3.6%. Respondents in this study were slightly less likely than Americans as a whole to be 25-29 years of age (10.2% compared to 14.3%) and slightly more likely to be 45-54 years of age (23.8% compared to 18.2%). Also, respondents were slightly more likely to have completed 9-11 years of education (20.3% compared to 14.0%) and 13-15 years of education (21.0% compared to 14.7%). No obvious interactions existed between age and education or between sex and education.

With respect to race, differences were more pronounced. Respondents in this study were more likely than Americans as a whole to be black (20.5% compared to 9.8%), and less likely to be white (78.6% compared to 88.4%). There was a moderate interaction of race and education; black respondents in this study were substantially more educated than the American black population. These differences are likely to be explainable by the geographic region from which respondents were drawn; the percentage of blacks in the Detroit area is greater than for the country as a whole.

Descriptive characteristics of Valium users and nonusers. Because of the study's central interest in Valium use, descriptive characteristics of respondents were examined separately for those who reported Valium use during the six weeks prior to the first interview versus those who did not. Table 3.9 indicates percentages of initial Valium users versus non-users for selected descriptive characteristics. The final group of respondents included somewhat more female than male users. There was also a somewhat higher proportion of whites reporting Valium use than blacks. On the average, Valium users also tended to be slightly older, less educated, and have lower income compared to non-users. At the first interview, Valium

69

users also reported lower subjective quality of health, higher anxiety, and higher depression.

Quality of life evaluations compared to national samples. Some of the items included in this study to assess quality of life were similar to items which have been used previously in national surveys conducted during 1972-1976 (Andrews & Withey, 1976). Although the respondents in this study were selected to represent a heterogeneous group of Valium users in the Detroit Metropolitan area, it is of interest to compare their life quality evaluations with representative samples of American adults.

These comparisons are not exact, however, for the following reasons: (a) the time span for assessment differed--i.e., "the last seven days" for the present study rather than "the last year and what you expect in the near future" for the national surveys; (b) a few slight wording changes--e.g., "work" in the present study and "job" in the national surveys; also, "wife/husband" and "marriage" were combined into a single item in this study, but kept separate in the national studies; (c) "life-as-a-whole" was a single item in this study, whereas it was an average of two items in the national data; and (d) possible historical context differences related to date of data collection--1972 to 1976 for the national surveys and 1981 for the current data. Although these factors could have produced some differences in the evaluations given in this study compared to the national surveys, it is unlikely that such effects would be very large.

Table 3.10 compares mean levels for responses to life quality items by Valium users and nonusers at Wave 1 with mean data from the representative national samples.[12] The means are along a 7 point scale coded as follows: 7=delighted, 6=pleased, 5=mostly satisfied, 4=mixed, 3=mostly dissatisfied, 2=unhappy, 1=terrible. Nonusers of Valium tended to give average life

---

[12]For descriptive purposes, only Wave 1 life quality responses of Valium users and nonusers in this study were compared with those from representative national samples. A more detailed analysis of changes in perceived life quality over the course of the study is reported in Chapter 5.

Table 3.9

PERCENTAGES OF VALIUM USERS AND NON-USERS
FOR SELECTED CHARACTERISTIC[1],[2]

CHARACTERISTIC	VALIUM	NO VALIUM
Sex		
Male	39	46
Female	61	54
	100%	100%
Race		
Black	15	22
White	84	78
Other	1	0
	100%	100%
Age		
MEAN CODE VALUE	4.5	4.0
1=17-24	5	11
2=25-29	10	9
3=30-34	8	16
4=35-44	17	21
5=45-54	25	17
6=55-95	35	26
	100%	100%

(Table continues)

Table 3.9

PERCENTAGES OF VALIUM USERS AND NON-USERS
FOR SELECTED CHARACTERISTIC[1],[2]
(continued)

CHARACTERISTIC	VALIUM	NO VALIUM
Years of Education		
MEAN CODE VALUE	5.0	5.3
1=0-4	1	0
2=5-7	3	2
3=8	4	4
4=9-11	22	18
5=12	38	32
6=13-15	21	26
7=16+	11	18
	100%	100%
Annual Family Income **(in thousands of dollars)**		
MEAN	4.5	5.0
1=Under 5	9	8
2=5-9.9	14	8
3=10-14.9	14	12
4=15-19.9	9	10
5=20-24.9	15	14
6=25-34.9	17	17
7=35-49.9	16	21
8=50+	6	10
	100%	100%
Perceived Health		
MEAN	3.0	3.9
1.0-1.4	12	2
1.5-2.4	23	8
2.5-3.4	30	17
3.5-4.4	27	40
4.5-5.0	8	33
	100%	100%

(Table continues)

Table 3.9

PERCENTAGES OF VALIUM USERS AND NON-USERS
FOR SELECTED CHARACTERISTIC[1],[2]
(continued)

CHARACTERISTIC	VALIUM	NO VALIUM
Anxiety (Hopkins Scale)		
MEAN	1.8	1.4
1.0-1.4	32	67
1.5-2.4	53	29
2.5-3.4	14	4
3.5-4.0	1	0
	100%	100%
Depression (Hopkins Scale)		
MEAN	1.9	1.6
1.0-1.4	25	50
1.5-2.4	57	45
2.5-3.4	17	4
3.5-4.0	1	1
	100%	100%

[1]Valium use category based on use at any time during the six weeks prior to the Wave 1 interview; N=345 reported using Valium during that period, N=330 did not report Valium use.

[2]Percentages based on the 675 respondents who participated in all four interviews.

quality responses which were similar to those given by respondents in national surveys. Valium users, however, tended to rate their life quality lower than nonusers on all items, but especially for health. Average responses for these two groups differed by .2 or less on all life quality items except that nonusers of Valium in this study felt somewhat more positive about their children but less positive about their spouses/ marriages and coworkers than did the national survey respondents (see Table 3.10).

Table 3.10

MEAN EVALUATIONS OF LIFE QUALITY ITEMS BY VALIUM
USERS AND NONUSERS AT WAVE 1 COMPARED TO RESPONDENTS
IN NATIONAL SURVEYS OF AMERICAN ADULTS

Life Quality Items	Valium Users	Nonusers	National Data' (1972-1976)
Handle Problems	4.8	5.1	5.2
Work	4.7	5.2	5.3 to 5.5
Children	5.6	5.9	5.6
Spouse/Marriage	5.4	5.8	6.2 to 6.3
Friends	5.3	5.5	5.6
Coworkers	5.1	5.3	5.6
Accomplishments	4.4	4.9	5.0 to 5.2
Health	3.8	4.9	5.1 to 5.3
Income	4.2	4.6	4.2 to 4.8
Self	4.6	5.2	5.2
Sleep	4.4	4.9	5.0
Financial Security	4.0	4.5	4.5
Adjust to Change	4.6	5.0	5.2
Work Itself	5.0	5.4	5.6
Life as a Whole	4.7	5.3	5.3 to 5.5
How Happy	1.8	2.0	2.1 to 2.2
How much worry	3.5	3.0	2.8 to 2.9

'See Andrews and Withey, 1976

Significant others

Percentages indicating the characteristics of personal
(PO) and work others (WO) interviewed at Wave 1 are presented
in Table 3.11. While the sex of WO's was evenly split between
females and males, a much higher percentage of PO's were
females (70%). The highest percentage of PO's were spouses

(45%) of the focal respondents, followed by friends (23%). Most WO's were coworkers (56%), followed by bosses/supervisors (27%). On the average, focal respondents had known PO's many more years than they had known WO's (22 versus 7 years, respectively). PO's also tended to be slightly older and less educated than WO's.

Descriptive statistics on significant others are presented only at Wave 1 for two reasons. First, a majority of both PO's and WO's did not change for focal respondents who participated throughout the entire study. Of 632 focal respondents with PO's at all four waves, 482 provided the same PO at each interview; 137 of 247 WO's were the same at each interview. Second, the statistics describing all significant others at Waves 2-4 are very similar to those for Wave 1. The only differences worth noting were that the average age of the significant others and the number of years focal respondents had known them decreased slightly after Wave 1.

Table 3.11

DESCRIPTIVE STATISTICS (PERCENTAGES) FOR
SIGNIFICANT OTHERS' AT WAVE 1

CHARACTERISTIC	Personal Other	Work Other
Sex		
Male	31	48
Female	69	52
	100%	100%
Age (years)		
MEAN	42.4	38.8
16-24	11	12
25-29	11	14
30-34	16	14
35-44	20	28
45-54	20	21
55-95	22	11
	100%	100%
Years of Education		
MEAN CODE VALUE	12.5	13.4
1=0-4	1	0
2=5-7	1	1
3=8	3	0
4=9-11	16	8
5=12	42	41
6=13-15	24	25
7=16+	13	25
	100%	100%

(Table continues)

Table 3.11

DESCRIPTIVE STATISTICS (PERCENTAGES) FOR
SIGNIFICANT OTHERS' AT WAVE 1
(continued)

CHARACTERISTIC	Personal Other	Work Other
Relationship to FR		
Spouse	46	
Parent	5	
Child	13	
Brother/Sister	7	
Other Relative	3	
Romantic Friend	2	
Friend	23	
Other	1	
	100%	
Boss/Supervisor		26
Coworker		56
Subordinate		4
Relative		6
Friend		7
Colleague		1
		100%
Length (years) of Relationship with FR		
MEAN	21.6	7.2
1 yr. or less	2	22
2-5	12	38
6-10	13	21
11-15	10	6
16-20	12	6
21-30	26	4
31+	25	3
	100%	100%

'Note: At the 1st interview: N=633 Personal Life Significant Others; N=247 Work Life Significant Others. Only
significant others of focal respondents who participated in
all four interviews were included in this table.

CHAPTER 4

THE MEASURES

This chapter describes the measures used in the study. The chapter begins with a brief methodological discussion about the nature of scales and indices, how they are used in analysis, and why they are preferred over single-item measures. Section 2 of the chapter describes criteria that governed the selection and design of the scales that were constructed for this study. Section 3 presents the data analysis procedures that were followed in implementing the above criteria for all of the scales. Section 4 provides details on procedures used in the construction of other measures. Section 5 discusses the quality of the measurements and some quantitative evidence about their validity and reliability. The questionnaires used to obtain information from the focal respondents, personal others, and work others can be seen in Appendix I; the questionnaires are those used at Wave 4, but are identical in all but a few ways to those used at the other Waves.

On the Nature of Scales and Indices

The data for this study come from the answers people gave to the series of questions asked by the interviewers. Each question, whether a "closed" question, in which respondents chose from among set answers, or an "open" question, which respondents answered in their own words, constitutes a questionnaire item. Answers to individual items were coded and form the basic raw variables (i.e., measures) for analysis.

Although substantive survey analyses can be carried out using single questionnaire items, more dependable results are usually obtained by using scales or indices. (In this report the terms are used synonymously.) A scale or index is a set of items, all of which tap the same construct (e.g., level of anxiety, or quality of life-as-a-whole), that have been combined to form a new variable on which each respondent has a score. In this study, the combining was usually a simple averaging process and is more fully described below.

A scale usually provides a better measure of an underlying construct than does information from just a single questionnaire item because some of the measurement errors and other idiosyncrasies that affect answers to single items are cancelled out when the items are combined. Social scientists' use of multiple items to form scales is based on the same logic as obtaining multiple measurements to assess physical-science constructs. For example, one would generally expect to get a more precise indication of the efficiency of an automobile (miles-per-gallon) by taking several measurements and averaging them.

Well-designed surveys usually include the components of many scales among the items included in the interview. Typically, a survey designer identifies a concept as important for the study and then includes in the questionnaire several items intended to tap that concept. Sometimes the survey designer may be able to draw directly on previous research in which a scale tapping a needed construct has been developed and validated. In this case, it is a straightforward matter to include those items in the new questionnaire. An example of this in the present study is the measurement of anxiety: one of the measures of anxiety is a scale based on items from the Hopkins Symptom Checklist. In other cases, however, a survey researcher may not know of any previous attempt to measure a desired concept using items that would be appropriate for the new study, and it is necessary to write new items which--the researcher hopes--will be combinable into a scale for measuring the desired concept. In this case the researcher must do an analysis to show that the items all reflect the desired construct. One piece of evidence is that the items covary--i.e., that respondents who give a certain kind of answer to one item also tend to give similar answers to other items in the set. Other evidence includes the appearance of similar content among the items, the stability of inter-item relationships across different subgroups of the respondents, and the demonstration that the scale scores relate in theoretically reasonable ways to measures of other constructs.

Because of the improved validity of scales as compared to measures based on single questionnaire items, most of the measures employed in the main substantive analyses for this study are scales. In the design of the study, a significant effort was made to include multiple items to tap the important constructs of the study. After the data were collected, considerable attention was devoted to checking the appropriateness of the items intended to tap each construct and to combining selected items to form each scale.

Criteria for Selection and Design of Scales Used in this Study

The scales used in this study were selected or designed to meet a number of distinct criteria. These include the following:

Conceptual Relevance

The concepts (or "constructs") considered relevant for the goals of the study, described in Chapter 1, were derived from theory and previous research. An attempt was made to construct a multi-item scale as the empirical measure for each important theoretical concept. Appendix J presents brief conceptual definitions for each scale and some selected items.

Use in Previous Research

Most of the concepts investigated in the present study had been used in previous research. In some cases questionnaire items for assessing these concepts could be taken directly from earlier work conducted by ourselves or others, and in some other cases this could be done if minor adaptations were made in the items (e.g., changing the time span of an item to match "the last seven days" that was adopted as the standard reporting period for the present study). Where relevant scales were available from previous research, we attempted to use them because this reduced the work needed to develop new scales and

80

allowed the results from the present study to be placed in the wider scientific context of previous research.

Operational Criteria

Attention was given to the ease and efficiency with which the data for a scale could be collected. Attempts were made to keep the number of items needed for each scale rather small (3-5 items, in most cases), to use one of a limited set of standard response formats, and to use items whose wordings were as simple and straightforward as possible. Also, questionnaire items referred to a standard reporting period, the "last seven days," whenever possible (sometimes referred to in this text as "the prior week"). A select few items referred to "the last six weeks," "since you were last interviewed," or "the last year."

Psychometric Criteria

All scales, whether or not used in previous research, were evaluated with respect to their variance, skew, and internal homogeneity. Each scale should be able to distinguish differences among respondents, i.e., show some variance; no scale should clump most respondents together at one end while spreading the rest toward the other end--i.e., be extremely skewed; and within every scale the items (if intended to tap the same construct) should show substantial covariation--i.e., be internally homogeneous. Quantitative reports of variance (squared standard deviations) and internal homogeneity (Cronbach's alphas) of each scale are presented in Appendices K and L. While skews are not reported for each scale, all were reasonably low, as detailed below.

General Procedures for Constructing Scales

A six-step procedure was used to develop most of the indices used in data analyses. Indices measuring various aspects of affective states, quality of life, coping and defense, social support, social conflict, perceptions of control, performance, role ambiguity, role conflict, attitudes about Valium, attitudes about tranquilizers in general, and interviewers' ratings of respondents were created using this technique.

For each of the above families of concepts, items measuring each specific concept were enumerated. For example, quality of life can be broken down into concepts concerning the respondent's personal life, work life, health, and several other domains (e.g., Andrews & Withey, 1976). Questions about quality of life were also asked of three different types of respondent: the focal respondent, personal other, and work other. Items designed to measure each concept were identified for each respondent source. Furthermore, other items which were designed to measure different concepts but were quite similar to the target concept were also identified. For example, items measuring depression were expected to form a distinct concept, but, because of their similarity to some items measuring quality of life, they were included in the exploratory analyses of the life quality items.

Once this list was developed, frequency distributions were computed for all items relating to a particular concept. Items that were moderately skewed (skewness > 2.00) were bracketed such that categories with few cases were combined. Items that were extremely skewed (skewness > 3.50) were omitted from further analyses since their useful variance was so slight.

Then, correlation matrices of these items were created using the data from all respondents at Time 1. These matrices were examined carefully and correlograms were drawn to clarify the relationships observed in the matrices. In addition, orthogonal factor analyses were conducted to examine the relationships in the matrices. For most concepts, oblique factor analyses were also conducted. (In all cases, results from the orthogonal and oblique factor analyses were quite similar.) None of the conceptually distinct items (e.g., depression and quality of life) loaded together highly on the same factor, so separate indices could be formed for each concept.

At this point, potential indices for each concept were proposed. We were concerned, however, that the factor structure for items tapping some of these concepts might differ for some groups of respondents. For example, the factor structure of the anxiety items might differ between Valium users and individuals not taking a psychoactive drug. Because of this concern, seven different groups were identified: females, males, Valium users, nonusers who also were not taking a psychoactive drug on the medication list,[13] high education respondents (at least some college), low education respondents (did not graduate from high school), and all respondents at Time 3. This final group was included in case time or familiarity with the questionnaire altered the factor structure of the items.

Correlation matrices were created for each of these groups to confirm that interitem relationships found for all respondents at Time 1 were similar to those relationships found for each group. Cronbach's alpha, a measure of reliability that assesses internal homogeneity, was computed for each proposed index across people in each group. As can be seen in Appendix L, which indicates the reliabilities of the indices for each group, and for all respondents at each timepoint, alphas were quite similar across groups. Consequently the factor structure of the indices appeared to be stable for different groups of respondents and across time. In many cases, alphas were somewhat higher at later timepoints; this may have been due to greater familiarity with the questionnaire.

When possible, comparable indices were computed for different domains (such as work and personal life) and for different respondents. A slight drop in internal consistency was accepted if it allowed us to include the exact same items in the set for each subgroup of respondents or relevant domain.

The Hopkins Symptom Checklist Anxiety Subscale has frequently been used in research on psychological states in general, as well as on Valium's effects on anxiety (e.g., Rickels, 1981). Consequently all the Hopkins items from the subscales on anxiety and depression and the majority of items from

---

[13]As described in the section below on measuring the use of medications, a list of the most commonly prescribed psychoactive medications was included in the questionnaire. Respondents who reported taking any of these medications were asked specific questions about their pattern of use. Because this list was not exhaustive, this "no medication on list" group may contain individuals taking a psychoactive drug not on the list. This occurred infrequently, however, so this group can be thought of as being nonusers of psychoactive medications.

the Somatic Complaints Subscale were included in the questionnaire.[14] The procedures described above confirmed that these scales had adequate reliabilities, so they were used as our principal measures of anxiety, depression, and somatic complaints.

In most cases, the items being combined into an index used the same response scale and had similar variances. For a few indices, items were from different response scales or had quite different variances. In these cases, items were either standardized or weighted to equate variances. Items were then summed and divided by the number of items in the index to create indices whose scores reflected the mean of the responses to the index's components. When data for some items in an index were missing for a given respondent, the index score was developed based on the other items of that index; when data on more than half the items in an index were missing, no index score was included for that respondent. The amount of missing data was quite small; most respondents had complete data for each index.

Frequency distributions were computed for all indices. Variances and skews were examined to ensure that there was adequate variability for analysis. Appendix J presents the name of each index and a brief description of what it is meant to measure. Appendix M presents the exact items on which each index is based. Cronbach's alphas for each index are presented in Appendix L. Appendix K presents the mean and standard deviation for each index at each timepoint.

General Procedures for Constructing Other Measures

Open-Ended Measures

Numerous open-ended questions were included throughout the interview. Many of these were necessary to provide information which could not be assessed as completely using a closed-ended response format. For example, respondents were asked when they

---

[14]Those items measuring somatic complaints which had the lowest factor loadings in previous research were omitted.

took Valium, why they took it, and, if appliable, why they stopped taking it. Codes were created for any responses mentioned more than 3 times so that a thorough depiction of responses was preserved. Appendix N includes the coding scheme used for each open-ended variable which was coded.

Several other open-ended questions were asked primarily to break up the monotony of closed-ended responses and to provide the respondent with a chance to talk. Most of these questions were not coded because responses were quite varied and did not appear to tap an underlying construct.

Each respondent's health status was derived from several open-ended questions to which health-related answers were frequently given. These responses were coded using the International Classification of Diseases (World Health Organization, 1977). After extensive training (see the Procedures of Coding Section of the Method chapter for a description of the training), coders translated respondents' answers into the broad categories of this classification scheme (see Appendix N for the actual coding scheme used). These codes must be viewed with two issues in mind. First, they are based on self-reports by patients and are therefore subject to the usual biases of such reports. However, self-reports have been the basis for many important health surveys (for examples, see Ware, et al., 1978). Second, even though interrater reliability was high (83% agreement), interviewers did not probe ambiguous responses because the decision to use this coding scheme was made after the data were collected. These health codes are used in the report primarily for descriptive purposes to provide the reader with a general appreciation of the health status of the respondents.

While reading through transcripts of open-ended responses, several members of the project staff were struck by two common themes: (1) positive and negative life events or conditions in respondent's lives, and (2) the importance of other people in respondents' lives. There are a variety of scales which measure life events (e.g., Holmes & Rahe, 1967); however, a decision was made not to use any of them in this study since these scales present a number of methodological problems

85

(Thoits, 1981; Vinokur & Selzer, 1975). Respondents did, however, clearly vary in the overall positiveness or negativeness of their lives. Consequently, detailed coding schemes were developed to measure the amount of positive life events or conditions and negative life events or conditions a respondent reported (see Appendix N for the actual coding scheme). Further information on these measures is also presented in Appendices J and K.

Respondents also clearly differed in the extent to which they mentioned other people in response to open-ended questions. For example, when asked about the positive occurrences in their lives in the last six weeks, some respondents mentioned people-oriented events such as their child's graduation or spouse's birthday, while others mentioned self-oriented events such as doing well at work or buying some new possession. It was hypothesized that this "salience of others" measure might relate to social support and social conflict, and so two variables that attempted to reflect these differences among respondents were coded (see Appendix N for the actual coding scheme). Further information on these measures is also presented in Appendices J and K.

Measuring Use of Medications and of Other Psychoactive Substances

Reviews of the literature on assessment of medication use (e.g., Dunbar, 1979) show that there is no one ideal method. Self-report measures were selected in this study because of their ease and economy of collection. It should be noted that physicians' and patients' ratings are not highly convergent. Roth & Caron (1978), for example, reported a correlation of .48 between patient and physician estimates of use of antacids among ulcer patients; pill counts and patient ratings correlated .42. Pill counts and biochemical assays each have their own documented weaknesses (Dunbar, 1979). Evidence also suggests that there are systematic biases which go beyond forgetting. Patients tend to underreport what they perceive as socially undesirable use of medication. Thus, patients are more likely to underreport than overreport noncompliance with a medical regimen (Haynes, Sackett, Gibson, et al., 1976; Park &

Lipman, 1964). Nevertheless, self-reports of medication use do tend to be related to treatment outcomes for which they are indicated (e.g., Caplan, et al., 1976). In this study, the amount of Valium which respondents reported taking was related to the amount of emotional strain with which they had to deal (see Chapter 5).

Measures as they appeared in the interview. Section F of the interview was devoted almost entirely to the assessment of medication use (see Appendix I, p. 32-41). Information was obtained not only about Valium use, but also about the use of all other prescribed medications which had been taken in the 6-week period prior to each interview.

For each medication mentioned, the interviewer asked to see the container in which it came, and from the prescription label obtained the following information: name of the drug, when it was filled, the strength and units prescribed (e.g., 5 mg. or 100 cc), the number of times per day it was prescribed (including "take as needed"), the number of pills to be taken each time (when applicable), and the number in the container when it was full. When prescription labels could not be obtained, respondents were asked to report the above information from memory; for each drug mentioned, interviewers recorded whether the information was obtained from the label or from the respondent's memory.

Detailed information about actual drug use was obtained only for a selected group of 79 drugs. This limitation was imposed because: a) to follow up in detail on every drug mentioned would have lengthened the interview, making it too burdensome to respondents and too economically costly to administer, b) many drugs mentioned were not expected to change the impact of diazepam use, and were thus judged not worth following up, and c) it was unlikely that any one drug besides Valium would be mentioned often enough to make it possible to analyze a subgroup of respondents taking it. The 79 drugs on which detailed use information was obtained were selected by a pharmaceutical expert at Hoffmann-La Roche, Inc., Donald Green, M.D., based on two criteria: 1) having psychoactive properties and 2) being among the most commonly used drugs in the United

States. These 79 drugs are listed in Appendix I, Section F, p. 33.[15]

Whenever one of these 79 drugs was mentioned as having been taken in the last six weeks, interviewers asked respondents for the following information about how they used the drug: "are you still taking it?" ("if not, why not?"), "for what reason(s) are you taking it?", date of first use, the date of last use, number of times per day usually taken, number of units (e.g., pills, capsules) usually taken, pattern of use over the last year (e.g., see item F13 in Appendix I), and pattern of use over the last 6 weeks (e.g., see F14).

Whenever respondents mentioned Valium, they were asked some additional questions about their physician (see F14-F17 and F28B), how they decided when to take it (F22), and the degree to which they found it beneficial (F23-F27). Also, they were asked to fill out the retrospective calendar for each of the last 6 weeks (or the number of weeks since they were last interviewed) with respect to: a) their pattern of use of Valium during each week (F18), and b) the number of Valium pills they took during each week (F20).

Derived measures of Valium use. Most of the measures of drug use described above were not used by themselves in analyses. Rather, they were frequently combined with one another or recoded in some way to produce more reliable and conceptually meaningful measures. An example of a combined or "derived" measure is one measure of the amount of Valium prescribed per day (VY618)[16]; this measure is a multiplicative

---

[15]At Wave 1, respondents reported having been prescribed 1,593 drugs in the last 6 weeks which were judged by pharmacy experts to have effects similar or opposed to that of diazepam (this figure is the total number of drug mentions--not the total number of different drugs). (See "Derived Measures of Use of Other Drugs.") Of these, 67% (59% excluding Valium) were among the list of drugs about which more detailed information was obtained. (See Appendix O).

[16]The notation VY_ _ or VX_ _ refers to a variable or index which appears in more than one Wave. The letter "V" abbreviates the word "variable" and "X" or "Y" represent the Wave number. Wave numbers range from 1-8, with 1 and 5 representing Wave 1, with 2 and 6 representing Wave 2, with 3 and 7 representing Wave 3, and with 4 and 8 representing Wave 4.

combination of the number of times usually taken per day (F11), the number of pills taken per time (F12), and the number of milligrams in each pill (F3B). These derived measures are described here briefly; for more detailed explanations, see Appendix J.

Besides this measure of the amount of Valium prescribed per day, numerous other measures were formed and tested to see which would be the most useful in analyses. (The results of these tests are presented in Chapter 5 in the section on bivariate analyses.) Estimates were derived for the amount of Valium taken in "the last 7 days" and over the last 6 weeks prior to the interview, based on respondents' reports of when they last took Valium (F10), how many times per day they usually took it (F11), how many pills they usually took each time (F12), and the number of milligrams in each pill (F3B). In addition, measures were created which did not take the number of milligrams per pill into account, so that, by comparison, it could be determined if the number of milligrams per pill made any difference in the analyses.

A second estimate was also derived for the amount of Valium taken in "the last 7 days," based on the retrospective calendar report of number of pills taken during the week of the interview and the number of milligrams per pill.[17]

Finally, a measure of compliance with the prescribed regimen was derived by simply subtracting the estimate of the amount of Valium usually taken per day from the amount of Valium prescribed per day (VY620). Further information on these measures is presented in Appendices J and K.

Derived measures of use of other prescribed drugs. Because no one drug other than Valium was mentioned often enough to permit analyses on such a subgroup, two methods were used to combine other medications in ways which would allow at least a

Thus, V2618 is variable 618 at Wave 2, or the amount of Valium prescribed per day at Wave 2.

[17]The procedures for deriving this estimate of Valium consumed in "the last 7 days" is rather complex, and is thus reported in greater detail in Appendix P.

superficial examination of their effects. Both methods required "recoding" of each drug. The recoding was done by a
consultant team of doctors of pharmacy at the University of
Michigan School of Pharmacy: Drs. Eddie L. Boyd, Duane M. Kirking, and Leslie A. Shimp. They used two methods of recoding:
1) assigning each drug up to three codes for its common
therapeutic use(s) (e.g., a drug might be used as both an an-
tihistamine and an antitussive and would receive a code for
each of these uses--see Appendix Q), and 2) placing each drug
into one of five effect categories. These effect categories
were: 1) containing active ingredient(s) that could be expected
primarily or secondarily to produce an effect similar to that
of diazepam, 2) opposite to that of diazepam, 3) both similar
and opposite to that of diazepam (e.g., combination products),
4) neither similar nor opposite to that of diazepam, or 5)
unknown effect. (See Appendix Q for a more detailed description of these procedures).

Appendix R shows the number of respondents at each
timepoint taking medications as they were classified by common
therapeutic effect. Of the 1,227 mentions of drugs having effects similar to those of diazepam at Wave 1, 82% were on the
questionnaire follow-up list (72% excluding Valium); for the
170 mentions of drugs with opposite effects, 9% were on the
follow-up list; and, of the 196 mentions of drugs judged to
have both similar and opposite effects to those of diazepam,
30% were on the follow-up list (see Appendix O).

These drug effect codes were used to derive two measures
for each respondent. One measure was the number of drugs used
in the prior six weeks which were expected to have an effect
similar to that of Valium (VY610). The other measure was comparable, but for drugs expected to have an effect opposite to
that of Valium (VY611). Further information on these measures
is also presented in Appendices J and K.

Use of street drugs, alcohol, caffeine, and tobacco. Use
of street drugs, alcohol, caffeine and tobacco was assessed in
Section G of the interview. Additional information regarding
several of these measures is presented in Appendices J and K.

Use of street drugs was assessed with respect to the use of each drug both in the 6 weeks and in the 7 days prior to each interview. Street drug use was assessed with questions G11-G14 in the interview (Appendix I), which asked about "...street drugs such as PCP, Uppers, Downers, Speed, Quaaludes, Mescaline, Marijuana, Heroin, or Methadone." The number of street drugs mentioned was fairly low (only 64 respondents at Wave 1 mentioned having used one or more street drugs in the prior 6 weeks). Consequently, only an overall measure of street drug use was created for each respondent—number of times all street drugs were used in the prior 6 weeks (VY617).

Alcohol use was measured with questions G8-G10 (following Cahalan, et al., 1969). From responses to these questions, two measures were derived for each respondent: 1) the number of alcoholic drinks consumed in the prior 7 days (VY412), and 2) the number of alcoholic drinks consumed in the prior month (VY413).

The approximate number of milligrams of caffeine consumed by each respondent in the prior 7 days (VY411) was derived from questions G16-G18, which assessed consumption of coffee, tea, and cola drinks. The number of drinks of each type was multiplied by an estimated number of milligrams of caffeine in a commonly consumed quantity of each drink. One "average" cup of coffee (8 oz.) was estimated to contain 171 mg of caffeine, 1 cup of tea (8 oz.) was estimated to contain 64 mg., and one cola drink (12 ozs.) was estimated to contain 47 mg. of caffeine. These estimates were derived from the Journal of the American Dietetic Association (Bunker & Williams, 1979). Such estimates are obvious compromises, given the variety in sizes of cups people use, in how full they fill them, and in how people prepare them.

Tobacco use was measured using questions G15-G15a, which asked about use of cigarettes, cigars, and pipes in the prior 7 days. Three hundred eighty-two of the respondents reported smoking (Wave 1), and 95% of these smoked only cigarettes. Only the usual number of cigarettes smoked in the prior 7 days was examined in detail (VX641) because the number of respondents smoking cigars and/or pipes was so small, and because the

91

comparability of cigarettes, cigars, and pipe tobaccos with respect to their physiological effects is questionable.

Measuring Stress

Stresses or demands of daily life which may threaten individuals were measured in two domains: in work life and in personal life. As described in Chapter 2, in the work domain role ambiguity or feelings of uncertainty about what is required on the job (VY242), role conflict or receiving conflicting demands on the job (VY241), and uncertainty about continued future employment (VY583) were measured. Role ambiguity was also measured separately for the personal life domain (VY243).

In addition to these life demands, several other stressors, which are discussed in more detail elsewhere in this report, were measured: social conflict (Y352), person-environment (PE) fit on control, and open-ended assessments of negative life events and conditions (VY007).

Finally, two additional measures of stress were derived from those noted above in order to increase both the reliability and validity of our measures. There is no theoretical reason to assume that all of the various different kinds of stress should be intercorrelated. For example, just because one's role seems very ambiguous doesn't necessarily mean it will also involve many conflicting demands; the two types of demands are potentially independent. Consequently, averaging these stresses together to form an overall index as described in Section 3 of this chapter did not seem appropriate; averaging procedures would require the assumption that each type of stress was essentially the same. It did seem appropriate, however, to use two other methods to combine these various aspects of stress into an overall measure of stress in order to achieve more sensitive and valid measures.

The first measure, which is referred to as "Multiple Stress" (VY262), uses role ambiguity in personal life, social conflict, and negative life events and conditions. Respondents who had high scores on all 3 were coded high on Multiple Stress; those with low scores on all 3 were given a low score on Multiple Stress; and those with medium scores on all three received medium scores on Multiple Stress. (The specific form of the coding scheme is presented in Appendix S.) The logic of this stress measure is based on the assumption that individuals experiencing high levels of several types of stress simultaneously will experience the most stress.

The second measure, which is called "Highest Stress" (VY261), assigns each respondent his or her single highest score from among 11 stress measures.[18] These 11 measures are: negative events, role conflict at work, role ambiguity at work, role ambiguity in the personal life, social conflict, and person-environment fit on internal control, control by others and control by chance in the domains of personal life and emotions. With this type of index, respondents' scores on Highest Stress could be high if they were high on only one of the 11 stresses, but could be low only if they were low on all 11 stresses. This logic is based on the assumption that respondents need to experience high levels of only one type of stress to perceive their overall level of stress as being high. Information about the means and standard deviations of these measures is presented in Appendix K.

Measurement Quality of the Scales

Overview

Evaluating the measurement quality of a scale can be a complex matter. The ideal scale would be perfectly valid, i.e., accurately reflect the respondent's true position on the construct being assessed. However, it is often difficult and sometimes impossible to know what the true position is. What is important, however, is to estimate and report _how_ accurate a measure is because no science expects its measures to be perfectly accurate. As indicated below, there are numerous indicators of the quality of a scale.

---

[18]In order to avoid the problem of some measures affecting Highest Stress more than others simply because of their arbitrary scales, this procedure was performed after standardizing each measure.

All of the indicators of measurement quality examined in this study lead us to believe the scales are of good quality. We believe they compare well with survey-based scales typically used in studies of this kind and that they are more than sufficiently precise to reflect the relationships the study set out to explore.''

Quality of the Raw Data

In considering the quality of measurement it is helpful to recall the process by which a measure was generated and to seek indicators of how well each step in the process went. For this study the data depend, initially, on the respondents' interest in and understanding of the interview and willingness to respond frankly. These were rated by the interviewers at the conclusion of each session with every respondent, and the results are good. Across the four waves of data collection the ratings tended to be very similar. The majority of focal respondents were rated "very" (the highest possible score) on the dimensions of interestedness, understanding the interview content, and frankness. (The percentages of such ratings of focal respondents at Wave 1 were 77%, 64%, and 74%, respectively.) Very few (less than 1%) were rated "not at all" by the interviewer on any of these dimensions.

Another indicator of how respondents reacted to the interview is provided by the proportion who did not answer a question that applied to them. High rates of missing data could be expected if a question were poorly phrased, conceptually difficult, embarrassing, asked for information respondents did not have, or was otherwise problematical. Missing data rates in this study, however, were satisfactorily low. Typical values are in the range 0% to 2%.

''Formal discussions of measurement error often distinguish between bias (an error, up or down, that is the same for all individuals) and dispersion (errors that vary from individual to individual). Although we have no reason to suspect any large biases, most of our measurement quality evaluations have focussed on dispersion. These are the kinds of errors that affect relationships (constant biases do not), and relationships provide the basis for the study's conclusions about the consequences of Valium-taking.

94

Information about how medicines were prescribed was obtained directly from the prescription label on the bottle whenever possible. The label was the source of information in about three-quarters of the reports on prescription medication, including Valium. (This proportion varies from 65% to 86% across the various medicines and waves of the study.) For the other one quarter of the medications, information was based on respondents' memories.

Retrospective data. One aspect of the raw data to which we gave particular attention was the quality of the retrospective data. In the "calendar" portion of the interview, respondents were asked to report, for each of the six weeks preceding the interview, their levels of anxiety and quality of life-as-a-whole, and the amount of Valium they had taken. Although various things were done to help respondents remember accurately (e.g., providing calendars on which respondents were encouraged to record significant events in their lives; having respondents review events which had happened each week before they made their ratings), there remained a concern about how accurate their retrospective reports would be. Anticipating this concern, several extra items were included in the interview to permit quality checks of these data.

One set of items asked respondents on what basis they had answered the retrospective questions. Respondents chose from a set of categories ranging from "remembered exactly" to "guessed almost all." For the questions about Valium-taking (both pills-per-week and the pattern of Valium-taking), about 55% of respondents said they "remembered exactly" and another 29% said they "remembered mostly"; only 4% said all or most of their answers were based on guesses. For the retrospective data about anxiety and life quality, answers based primarily on guessing were also rare (4% and 2%, respectively), but respondents were more likely to report that this information was "remembered mostly" than "remembered exactly." (About 56% of respondents answered "mostly" and 20% "exactly.") The substantial proportions of respondents who claimed to answer the retrospective items from memory rather than guessing are an encouraging indication about the quality of these data.

Another indication of the quality of the retrospective data comes from another set of special items, included at Waves 2, 3, and 4, that asked respondents to recall their anxiety, life quality, and Valium-taking during the week of the _preceding_ interview--6-7 weeks earlier for most respondents. From these items it is possible to see how closely respondents' retrospective reports agreed with what they had previously reported for that same week.

For each of the three concepts addressed here (anxiety, life quality, and Valium-taking) there were three independent checks of the quality of the retrospective reports (Wave 2 retrospective reports matched to Wave 1 concurrent reports, Wave 3 similarly matched to Wave 2, and Wave 4 matched to Wave 3). The differences among the three checks were small, so they are summarized by averaging. The mean correlations were: .81 for Valium-taking,[20] .48 for anxiety, and .56 for life quality.

From this check of the quality of retrospective data we conclude that the reports about Valium-taking 6-7 weeks ago were good, and that the 6-7 week retrospective reports about anxiety and life quality were fair. This difference probably reflects the fact that Valium-taking tended to be a more stable phenomenon than people's experience of anxiety or assessment of the quality of life-as-a-whole. It may also be easier to recall something concrete like a number of pills rather than a level of anxiety. When one recalls that these checks examine the longest memory span and that the other retrospective data involve shorter spans, it seems safe to conclude that the quality of· the retrospective data is more than sufficient to permit its productive use.

---

[20]This figure applies to the pills-per-week measure, after adjusting to compensate for short weeks as described earlier in this chapter and in Appendix P. The "calendar" section of the interview also included another item that asked about the _pattern_ of Valium-taking. These retrospective data were even more reliable than the pills-per-week measure: the mean correlation between retrospective reports and the previously obtained current reports on pattern of Valium-taking was .85.

Quality of the Data Processing

After the data were collected, they were coded for computer entry. Any errors introduced during the coding would detract from the quality of the final measures. In this study 9% of all answers (selected on an approximately random basis) to closed questions were recoded by a particularly experienced coder and compared with the original coding. For 99% of the codings, the match was perfect. The comparable figure for codings of open questions, where one expects substantially lower agreement rates, averaged 85%. (Further details appear in Chapter 3.) These figures suggest that coding errors will not significantly intrude on the final measures.

After coding, the data were punched onto machine-readable cards. This process was verified at a 100% rate by a different machine, run by a different operator, checking to see that the coders' work was accurately represented by the data on the cards. Any errors found were corrected, and hence the transfer of the data to the cards did not introduce new errors that could degrade the final measures.

Once the original data were in a computer file, they were checked for wild codes and inconsistencies. Every variable was checked for values outside the permissible range, and 324 combinations of variables were checked for logical inconsistencies. (Chapter 3 provides details.) This process removed most of the (relatively few) recording and coding errors not detected previously.

Quality of the Scales

Internal homogeneity. Once the raw data had been "cleaned" by the above process, the scales described in this chapter were formed. As noted previously, an important indicator of the quality of a scale is the extent to which its component items tap the same underlying construct. This is known as the scale's internal homogeneity, which can be quantified by Cronbach's alpha coefficient of reliability.[21] Alpha

---

[21]Two different types of reliability should not be confused. Internal homogeneity reliability, which is assessed and reported here, is distinct from stability reliability. Given

coefficients for each scale, computed for the total set of respondents at each of four waves and for several subsets, are presented in Appendix L. As can be seen there, nearly all measures have alphas in the range .60 to .90. (Alpha can range from .00 to 1.00.) The trend is toward the middle and upper part of this range for most measures having to do with quality of life, affect (anxiety, depression, anger), social support, and work life; and the trend is toward the middle and lower part of the range for most measures that tap coping and defense, role ambiguity in personal life, and social or technical performance in personal life. The measures reflecting amounts of control exercised by or desired from various sources vary across the whole range. The scales used most extensively in the analysis tended to have alphas in the upper part of the range. For only a few measures do we observe many instances of alphas lower than .60. These include: evaluations of relationships with other people as a component of life quality, social support from one's therapist, social support from the physician who prescribed Valium, and the extent of control that one desires other people to exercise over one's personal life. With the exception of these measures, for which internal homogeneity should be assessed as "mixed", all of the scales consistently show at least "adequate" internal homogeneity, and for many scales it can be assessed as good to excellent.

Estimates of construct validity. Another indicator of measurement quality is provided by some of the parameters in the causal models presented in the following chapter. As described there, these models allow us to take a set of measures (single questionnaire items and/or scales), link them to factors representing the constructs we hypothesize the measures reflect, and then examine the simultaneous and lagged linkages among these factors. It is the linkages between the measures and factors (and some of the associated error terms)

the longitudinal nature of the data, we have also examined the stability of measures over time. However, the six weeks between waves is long enough for substantial real changes to occur, so we do not regard these stability figures as indicators of the reliability of the measures.

that are of particular interest with respect to the quality of measurement.

These models assume that a measure is <u>caused</u> by the factor(s) to which it is linked. If one assumes a factor accurately represents the theoretical construct a measure was intended to reflect (which seems at least approximately true for anxiety, Valium-taking and quality of life-as-a-whole in these models), and if the model fits the data and meets various other criteria of acceptability reasonably well (which is also the case for these models), then one can interpret the strength of the factor-measure linkages as estimates of the construct validity of the measure.[22] Furthermore, the model also estimates the extent to which a measure reflects influences other than that of the main theoretical construct, and this information can be used to develop inferences about the amount of random and correlated measurement error included in the measure.[23]

Using estimates from the more complex of the two models presented in Chapter 5 (Model B), one finds the following estimates of construct validity (averaged across the four waves of the study): .91 for Valium-taking, .74 for the anxiety scale, and .84 for the quality of life scale.[24] The estimated construct validities of the single-item-based measures of anxiety and quality of life-as-a-whole are lower, as would be

---

[22]Construct validity is one of several kinds of validity and is often recognized as the most important kind. It refers to the extent a measure accurately reflects the theoretical construct it was intended to represent. Since theoretical constructs, the basic building blocks of science, are—by definition—different from measures, one can never directly observe or compute a measure's construct validity but can only develop estimates of that quantity.

[23]Correlated measurement error is a component of a measure's variance that does not reflect the intended theoretical construct but that differs between respondents and also occurs in one or more other measures included in the same analysis. Random measurement error is an unintended component that differs between respondents and occurs in only one measure.

[24]The measures for the other concepts in this model, health, stress, and performance, are not intended to be conceptually identical, and therefore it is not appropriate to interpret the strength of these factor-measure linkages as estimates of construct validity.

expected for such measures: .56 and .63, respectively. Estimates from the smaller of the two models in Chapter 5 (Model A) are close to these values or a bit higher. A check of the results reported for these two models shows that correlated errors, while clearly present (as expected), are not a major feature of these data.

Agreement between focal respondent and significant others. The use of a significant other in the focal respondent's personal life, and another in work life for employed respondents, provided the opportunity to examine the consensus between two observers. Such consensus can be examined for measures of performance, quality of life, social support and social conflict. As noted in the section on Measurement, significant others were asked to rate the focal respondent's quality of life, social support, social conflict, and performance with regard to the domain with which they were most familiar. For example, work others only rated performance with regard to work and not with regard to personal life.

Using data from Wave 1, which are typical, the personal others' and focal respondents' scores on technical and social performance in personal life were correlated .18 and .25 respectively. The respective correlations in the work life domain were .09 and .30. In both domains, consensus was higher regarding social-emotional than technical performance. Ratings of social support by the focal respondent related positively, but only in the low teens, with ratings by the significant others. On the other hand, the focal respondents' ratings of quality of life were moderately to strongly correlated with ratings by the personal and work others in the relevant domain (.61 and .44 respectively).

Given the generally good internal reliabilities of the measures from the focal respondent and significant others, the lack of high correlations between focal respondents and significant others is unlikely to be due to random measurement error (Quarm, 1981). It is probably best to consider the focal respondent and significant others as persons representing different perspectives (cf., Douglas & Wind, 1978), each perhaps having their own particular biases and access to information.

100

CHAPTER 5

RESULTS

This chapter begins by summarizing findings regarding the quality of the data. Then it presents the results of the analyses. The first part of the results describes how the Valium users take their Valium, who prescribes it, and some related aspects of Valium use. Then data are presented on the consequences of Valium use with regard to anxiety and social effects. Both bivariate (two variables) relationships and multivariate (three or more variables) relationships are described.

How Good Are the Data?

Indicators of the Data's Quality

Chapter 4, "The Measures," presented evidence that our measures have adequate reliability and validity. A brief summary of those findings follows.

Internal reliability. The indices in this study generally have alphas of .60 or higher, with most coefficients being in the .70s and .80s. These reliabilities held up even when examined within various subgroups such as males, females, Valium users, nonusers, and within different waves such as at Time 1 and Time 4.[25] The reliabilities are considered highly adequate for using these measures in research (Nunnally, 1967, p.226).

Distribution. All indices and single-item measures were carefully checked and found to be, with few exceptions, free from serious skew or restriction of range. Where skew was a problem, measures were rescaled to minimize skew. Consequent-

---

[25] The terms "Time" and "Wave" are used as synonyms throughout the text to refer to the interview timepoint.

ly, the measures have adequate distributions for examining their effects over a wide range of their values.

Coding reliability. For those few open-ended measures in the interview (for example, health, negative events), the judgment of the human coder is a source of potential unreliability. Checks of coding indicated high reliability among coders (ranging from 77% to 96% agreement). The reliability for closed-ended questions was much higher (percent error rate averaged .09) and all key punching was 100% verified.

Objective sources of validity. Up to nine medications were recorded by the interviewers at each of the four waves. These recordings involved the name of the medication, prescribed dosage, and prescribed schedule of use. Approximately 75% of such recordings came directly from the prescription label (for the other 25% it was based on recall of the prescription label). Information on actual use of medication was based on self-reports. Measures of use of street drugs, caffeine, and alcohol also relied entirely on the respondent's self-report, as did most measures of stress, coping, and strain.

As discussed in Chapter 4 on measures, there is no one best method of measuring medication use (Dunbar, 1979). In order to promote the objectivity of self-report data, the questionnaire was designed and pretested to minimize respondents' defensiveness. In addition, interviewers were trained to encourage complete, accurate answers by the respondents, and respondents signed a document at the start of the study agreeing to be accurate. Prior research suggests these procedures increase respondent accuracy (Cannell & Fowler, 1975).

Retrospections. At each interview respondents provided retrospective reports of the preceding six weeks for three variables: use of Valium, anxiety, and quality of life. Waves 2-4 also included retrospections about the week of the previous interview. These reports were compared with the report made at the previous interview. The correlations were moderately strong (r's ranged from .44 to .85). These coefficients might be considered the lower limit for the retrospective data in general, since they derive from the longest period that

102

respondents were asked to recall. These data suggest that the retrospective data from the calendar part of the interview were not subject to serious memory errors and appear to be reasonably accurate.

Convergent validity. This study includes multiple measures for anxiety, quality of life, and Valium (measures from the main body of the interview and measures from the retrospective calendar section). For example, anxiety is measured by the Hopkins Symptom Checklist and by the single-item scale in the calendar. As noted in the previous chapter, the agreement between different measures of the same construct was good.

Other evidence of validity. Another source of confidence in the measures stems from the extent to which measures of one construct, such as role ambiguity, predict to or correlate with measures of another construct, such as anxiety, in ways which make theoretical sense or replicate other findings. An extensive report could be written on this topic, given the large number of social-psychological concepts examined in this study. The following is just a sampling of such findings. They are all based on Time 1 cross-sectional analyses.

Examining quality of life, for example, Time 1 data showed that persons with high levels of anxiety and depression on the Hopkins Symptom Checklist had low evaluations of quality of life with regard to the self, personal life, life-as-a-whole, and the general negative affective component of quality of life (r's range from .6 to .7). There was also evidence of discriminant validity in that the Hopkins Somatic Complaint index was correlated -.71 with quality of life regarding health but correlated much lower (never higher than -.55) with quality of life in other domains.

One of the strongest links between specific stressors and the Hopkins measure of anxiety was the positive relationship between role ambiguity and anxiety. This replicates other research (e.g., Caplan, et al., 1980a; Archer, 1979; Caplan & Jones, 1975) which found that uncertainty per se tended to be associated with anxiety.

With regard to the work domain, measures of role conflict and role ambiguity were both associated with low quality of working life (r's in -.30s). Role ambiguity in particular was associated with poor social-emotional and technical performance. And poor performance was associated with poor perceived quality of life in the work domain. These findings paint a plausible picture of how ambiguity about what one is supposed to do undermines the quality of one's performance. The data suggest that both performance and role stress may be important determinants of a person's feelings of satisfaction and/or dismay about work. Other research has suggested that some individuals increase performance at a cost in social relations (generating conflicts) and that some individuals may sacrifice performance because of conflict (Miles & Perrault, 1980). The findings in this study relating role ambiguity to quality of life in the work domain agreed with other major studies of role ambiguity and of its undesirable effects on job-related tension (Kahn, et al., 1964).

One last set of findings illustrating construct validity deals with selected measures of social support, coping, and control. These measures showed plausible relationships to one another and to other variables. Figure 5.1 summarizes a pattern of findings which suggest that seeking the help of others has both benefits and costs for mental health. Help-seeking was positively correlated with both perceived social support from others and with control others have over one's personal life and emotions. Whereas social support had potential benefits, as it was negatively correlated with anxiety and depression, control by others had potential costs, being positively correlated with anxiety and depression. All such relationships were statistically significant, and the coefficients ranged from the .20s to the .40s. Lack of social support is a known correlate particularly of depression (e.g., Cobb, 1976). The literature on learned helplessness and depression suggests that the perception that one has low control over one's life is both a consequence and cause of depression (e.g., Depue & Monroe, 1978; Abramson, et al., 1978). Consequently, findings in this study are in line with other research in this area.

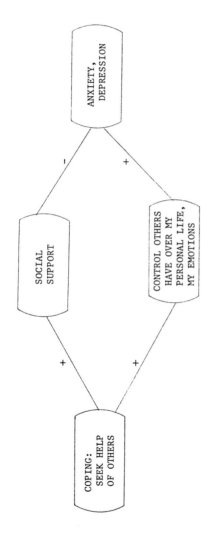

Figure 5.1.

Potential costs and benefits of seeking help from others. All correlations significant at p <.05 or higher (r's range from .20s to .40s).

Relationships between social support, social conflict, and other variables were strong and in the direction predicted by previous research (Abbey, Abramis, & Caplan, 1981; Cobb, 1979; Silver & Wortman, 1980). Social conflict strongly related to negative affect and quality of life (r's ranged from -.25 to .61 such that increased social conflict related to increased negative affect and decreased quality of life). Social support consistently buffered the relationship between stress (e.g., role ambiguity in the personal life and negative life events) and strain (e.g., negative affect and quality of life).

These results constitute a small sampling of the array of data and findings involving the measures of stress, coping, control, social support, affect, and other potential social effects of Valium. If we had not found such relationships among the measures in this study, we might have felt ill-prepared to proceed with a study of the social effects of Valium. These data, however, provide ample evidence of the construct validity of the measures.

Summary

Adequate reliabilities, good distributions, and a number of assessments of validity indicate that the measures used in this study were quite good on the whole. The quality of these data provides an important foundation for proceeding with an examination of the social effects of Valium.

Portrait of Valium Users in the Study

Before data are presented on the social effects of Valium, this section provides background on the use of Valium by the respondents: who prescribed Valium, how it was prescribed versus how it was taken, and why it was taken. This section also describes other types of drugs with which Valium was taken, general attitudes regarding the use of minor tranquilizers, and Valium users' feelings about the helpfulness of Valium.

To interpret the descriptive data which follow, it is important to recall that the respondents do not form a random sample. For example, respondents were selected so that half of the Valium users would be male and half female, even though in the general population more females than males use minor tranquilizers (e.g., Parry, et. al., 1973). Such deviations from representativeness of the population can produce results which are dissimilar to what might be found in a true sample of the population. If, for example, females in this study differ from males with respect to patterns of Valium use, then overall statistics on use in this set of respondents will overrepresent male patterns because males are intentionally overrepresented in the study where possible. Nevertheless, some indication will be given of the extent to which the descriptive statistics appear to be similar to published data available from random sample surveys of the population.

As already presented in Chapter 3, Valium users entered the study with somewhat higher levels of anxiety and depression and lower life quality than respondents who did not use Valium. The reader is referred to Chapter 3 for details on the demographic characteristics of Valium-using and non-using respondents.

Who Prescribed Valium?

Nearly all respondents (98.8%) who reported taking Valium at Time 1 had received a prescription for it. The most common source of prescriptions was general practitioners (just over 40%), followed by internists (almost 1/4 of all prescriptions). The next highest prescribing specialties were osteopaths and psychiatrists; each was responsible for five to six percent of all prescriptions. Data at Times 2 through 4 were similar to Time 1 data.

These data are similar in basic pattern to those reported by the National Disease and Therapeutic Index for 1978 (1978). In those data general practitioners accounted for 37% of the prescriptions, followed by internal medicine with 20% and psychiatry and surgery with 13% and 9% respectively. The 1980-1981 National Ambulatory Medical Care Survey (Koch & Campbell, 1983) showed similar results.

How Supportive was the Prescriber?

Previous research (Rickels, 1978; Uhlenhuth, et. al., 1966) suggests that the physician's own supportive attitude improves the effectiveness of Valium as an anxiolytic. In this study Valium respondents judged physicians as very supportive on the average. The mean rating at Time 1, which was almost identical to those at Times 2 through 4, was about four (where 1 = low support and 5 = high support). Consequently, most prescriptions were written by physicians who were perceived as reasonably warm by their patients and who were perceived as providing the time to discuss all the things the patient wanted to talk about.

How Was Valium Prescribed Versus Taken?

The data at Times 1 through 4 were very similar, so Time 1 data will be used here for illustration. The most frequent prescriptions for Valium called for 10 mg per day (17% of the Time 1 cases), 15 mg per day (25% of the cases), or 20 mg per day (18% of the cases). Less than 9% of the prescriptions were for 30 mg or more per day, and about 20% of the prescriptions were for 5 mg or less per day (the remaining 11% were prescribed "as needed"). Thus, there was a good range of dosages for examination in this study.

Patients tended to be conservative in their daily intake, underusing rather than complying exactly or overusing.[26] The most frequent ingestions per day were 2 mg (7.3% of all users at Time 1), 5 mg (36%), 10 mg (almost 25% of all users), 15 mg (7.3%), and 20 mg per day (7.3%).

An estimate of compliance in Valium use was obtained by computing the difference between the number of milligrams prescribed per day versus the estimated number the person actually took per day. Across all four waves the results were the same. Respondents took about 5 mg less than prescribed (the means for Waves 1 through 4 respectively were 4.6, 5.1, 5.8, and 5.0; the standard deviations were 8.4, 6.5, 6.7, and 6.9 respectively).

As for the distribution of compliance and noncompliance, the data from Time 1 were typical of those found at the other

---

[26] Nevertheless, there was a clear tendency for patients with higher dose prescriptions to report taking more than patients with lower dose prescriptions (Chi square = 1,109.3, $p < .0001$, df = 95; contingency coefficient = .89).

four waves. At Time 1 almost 40% of the Valium users who were prescribed a specific regimen (i.e., rather than "as needed") showed perfect compliance. Just under 3% (nine people) took more Valium than prescribed. Among those people, two-thirds (or six persons out of 286 users prescribed a specific regimen) took 1-12 mg more per day than prescribed and the other one-third (just three persons out of 286 users) took 30-60 mg more than prescribed. About 58% of all users took _less_ than prescribed, most commonly 5 or 10 mg less. Specifically, 25% of Valium users took 1-5 mg less than prescribed, 20% took 6-10 mg less, 6% took 11-15 mg less, and 7% took 16-30 mg less than prescribed. These findings agree with other research on patient compliance with tranquilizer regimens (Hulka, et. al., 1976), which found that the most common form of noncompliance is for patients to take less than the physician prescribes.

Although the actual distribution of milligram usage was quite similar across all four waves, there were slight shifts that may be of interest. These occurred with regard to the categories of 5- and 10-mg usage per day. The percentage of persons who reported using 5 mg per day increased slightly from Time 1 to Time 4 (from 36.4% to 44.3%) and the percentage of persons who reported using 10 mg per day decreased slightly from Time 1 to Time 4 (from 24.1% to 17.9%). All other categories had about the same percentage of users across waves. In the preceding paragraph we noted the overall tendency of patients to underuse Valium at any one timepoint. The data just presented suggest that a decrease in reported daily use over time from 10 to 5 mg might have occurred in this set of respondents without a comparable shift in prescriptions. An alternative interpretation is that persons taking 10 mg were more likely to stop taking Valium between Time 1 and Time 4. That too would have the effect of producing the above shift. Further analyses would be required to evaluate each of these interpretations.

How Did Patients Divide the Milligrams They
Took Over the Course of a Day?

The results here were very similar at all four waves. The most common patterns were 2 or 3 mg once per day (about 15% of

109

the Time 1 cases), 5 mg once per day (about 36% of the cases), 10 mg once per day (about 11% of the cases), 10 mg twice per day (about 12% of the cases), and 15 mg three times a day (about 7% of the cases). The remaining 35% were scattered across a range totalling 1-90 mg per day taken 1-5 times per day with no more than 5% in any one category. (The one person who reported "usually" taking 90 mg took Valium three times per day; this was verified by checking the original interview. This person represents far less than 1% of the total respondent pool at Time 1.) Overall, the large majority of patients took less than 15 mg per day and the most common number of times per day was once (almost 65% of the cases). The complete Time 1 data appear as Table 5.1.

Pattern of Use in the Last Six Weeks

The pattern of Valium taking over the six weeks preceding each interview showed some variety in use across individuals. The findings were virtually the same at Times 1 through 4, so Time 1 data are used for illustration.

During the six week period prior to the interview, 1/3 of the patients reported taking the medication "only once in a while," whereas almost half the respondents (47%) reported taking Valium "every day or every other day the whole time." The remainder took Valium periodically ("some weeks almost every day, other weeks not at all"; 11%) or at evenly spaced intervals but not as frequently ("at least once a week the whole time"; 9%). [27]

These patterns were associated with the number of milligrams taken per day (Time 1 Chi square = 73.51, p < .01, df = 45, C = .43). Persons taking higher dosages per day (10, 15 or more mg per day) tended to be "daily or every other day" users. Persons taking small dosages (2 and 3 mg per day) tended to take the medication "only once in a while." Persons taking 5 mg per day were about equally divided between daily or near daily use and use "only once in a while." The Time 1 data are presented in Table 5.2.

[27] Within this six week period, respondents took Valium for periods ranging anywhere from just one day to the entire six weeks. However, they were asked to describe their pattern of use over the entire six weeks (see Appendix I, question F13a).

Table 5.1

CROSSTABULATION OF TOTAL MILLIGRAMS OF VALIUM TAKEN PER
DAY BY NUMBER OF TIMES PER DAY VALIUM WAS TAKEN AT
TIME 1 (CELL ENTRIES ARE PERCENTAGES)[1]

Estimated Total mg Valium Taken Per Day (V5619)	Number of Times Per Day Valium Was Usually Taken (V1444)					Total Row%
	1	2	3	4	5	
1	1	0	0	0	0	1
2	8	0	0	0	0	8
3	7	0	0	0	0	7
4	1	2	0	0	0	3
5	36	1	0	0	0	37
6	0	0	1	0	0	1
8	0	0	1	1	0	2
10	11	12	0	0	<1	23
15	0	0	7	0	0	7
16	0	<1	0	0	0	<1
18	0	0	<1	0	0	<1
20	0	5	0	2	0	7
30	1	0	2	0	0	3
40	0	<1	0	1	0	1
60	0	0	<1	0	0	<1
90	0	0	<1	0	0	<1
Total Column %	65	20	11	4	<1	100%

[1]All cells indicated as <1% had only one person in that category.

111

Recency of Last Taking Valium

At Time 1 about 30% of the Valium users reported last taking Valium on the day of the interview, and another 30% reported last taking it the day before the interview. Another 18% last took Valium 2-6 days before the interview. Only 13% reported last taking Valium 7-20 days before the interview, and 9% reported last taking Valium more than 20 days before Time 1. Consequently, a large percentage of the respondents (83%) at Time 1 were interviewed within a week of last taking Valium. The distributions at Times 2 through 4 were essentially the same as at Time 1.

Across-Wave Variation in Valium Use

The preceding analyses, while indicating which patterns of use were most prevalent, also demonstrate that there was considerable variety in the use of Valium within each wave. Such variance is necessary for studying the social effects of different amounts and patterns of use of Valium.

It is also important to have some variation over the course of the study. As an initial check on the variation in Valium use over the course of the study, patterns of "on/off" use across the four waves were examined. As indicated by the categories listed in Table 5.3, there were 16 possible patterns of on/off use defined as whether a respondent took Valium during the six weeks prior to a given interview. Of the 675 respondents who participated in all four interviews, 367 (54.4%) used some Valium during the study while 308 (45.6%) did not report any Valium use. Category 1 shows that the majority (59%) of the Valium users took some Valium during each of the 6-week periods prior to the interviews. The other largest categories of use were those who took Valium only prior to the first interview (category 8, 15%) and those who took Valium prior to both the first and second interviews but not prior to the last two interviews (category 4; 10%).

Respondents' Reasons for Taking Valium

When respondents reported taking Valium, they were asked an open-ended question: "For what reasons are you taking

Table 5.2

CROSSTABULATION OF TOTAL MILLIGRAMS OF VALIUM TAKEN PER DAY BY PATTERN OF USE DURING 6 WEEKS PRIOR TO TIME 1
(Cell entries are percentages)[1]

Estimated Total mg Valium Taken Per Day	Pattern of Use				Row Total%
	1 Only once in a while	2 Some weeks almost every day;other weeks not at all	3 At least once a week the whole time	4 Every day or every other day the whole time	
1	2	0	0	0	2
2	4	1	2	2	9
3	4	<1	<1	2	6
4	<1	<1	0	2	2
5	13	4	5	15	37
6	0	<1	0	1	1
8	<1	0	0	1	1
10	6	3	2	13	24
15	1	1	<1	5	7
16	0	0	0	<1	<1
18	<1	0	0	0	<1
20	2	2	<1	3	7
30	1	<1	0	2	3
40	0	<1	0	1	1
60	0	0	0	<1	<1
90	0	<1	0	0	<1
Column Total%	33	11	9	47	100%

[1]All cells indicating <1% had only one person in that category.

113

Table 5.3

ACROSS-WAVE PATTERN OF VALIUM USE FOR RESPONDENTS
PARTICIPATING IN ALL FOUR INTERVIEWS

Category[*]	Wave 1	Wave 2	Wave 3	Wave 4	Frequency	% of Total	% of Valium Users
1	+	+	+	+	217	32.1	59.1
2	+	+	+	—	18	2.7	4.9
3	+	+	—	+	10	1.5	2.7
4	+	+	—	—	36	5.3	9.8
5	+	—	+	+	4	0.6	1.1
6	+	—	+	—	1	0.1	0.3
7	+	—	—	+	4	0.6	1.1
8	+	—	—	—	55	8.1	15.0
9	—	+	+	+	3	0.4	0.8
10	—	+	+	—	3	0.4	0.8
11	—	+	—	+	1	0.1	0.3
12	—	+	—	—	8	1.2	2.2
13	—	—	+	+	1	0.1	0.3
14	—	—	+	—	4	0.6	1.1
15	—	—	—	+	2	0.3	0.5
16	—	—	—	—	308	45.6	—
TOTAL					675	100%	100%

[*]Note: All possible patterns of Valium use during the 6-week period prior to each of the four interviews are represented.

+ = Some Valium use during 6-week period prior to interview.
- = Did not report Valium use during this period.

114

Valium?" This question was asked to provide information about individuals' explanations for their use of Valium.

Respondents' reasons for taking Valium are presented in Table 5.4 (see Chapters 3 and 4 and Appendix N for descriptions of the coding procedures). Column one presents the first reason respondents mentioned, while column two presents the number of respondents who mentioned each reason at any point during their response to the question (up to 5 reasons were coded for each respondent). This distinction was made because it was thought that respondents might first mention a socially acceptable reason, such as poor health, while admission of psychological reasons might be more prevalent for later mentions.

By far the most commonly mentioned reason for taking Valium was tension or anxiety (code 051); 45% of respondents' first reason was anxiety, while an additional 38 respondents (11% of Valium users at Time 1) later mentioned anxiety as a reason for taking Valium. Another 8% of respondents' first reason for taking Valium was to keep calm or relaxed (code 502), a reason quite similar to anxiety-reduction. An additional 10% of Time 1 Valium users' first reason for taking Valium was insomnia (code 059). Another 7% mentioned a pulled back or sore muscles for their first reason (code 131); this was the only commonly mentioned physical reason for taking Valium.

In sum, the majority of these respondents reported taking Valium for reasons related to anxiety. Only 5% reported taking it for hypertension (code 072), 1% for ulcers (code 092), and another 4% due to a stressful situation (code 602).

Decision Rules for Taking Valium

Respondents reporting Valium use were also asked in an open-ended question: "How do you decide when to take Valium?" Little is known about the decision process individuals go through prior to taking Valium, or indeed most medications, once they have a prescription. Consequently, responses to this question should provide insight into this decision-making process. Table 5.5 catalogues Valium users' answers to this

Table 5.4

RESPONDENTS' REASONS FOR TAKING VALIUM AT TIME 1[1]
(N=345)

Code	Reason	N(%)[2] First Mention	N(%)[3] Any Mention
C20	Neoplasms	0	1(0.2)
030	Endocrine, nutritional and metabolic diseases & immunity disorders	0	4(0.7)
040	Diseases of the blood & blood forming organs	0	1(0.2)
050	Mental disorders	2(0.6)	5(0.9)
051	Tension, anxiety, nerves, "keyed up"	156(45.2)	194(36.3)
052	Depression, blues, sadness	2(0.6)	2(0.4)
053	Fears, phobias, apprehension	0	2(0.4)
054	Upset or emotional	12(3.5)	21(3.9)
057	Withdrawal from other prescribed medication or dependence on other prescribed medication (e.g., Darvon, Tranxene).	0	1(0.2)
059	Sleep disorders, insomnia, any problems with falling to sleep	36(10.4)	57(10.7)
060	Diseases of the nervous system	3(0.9)	6(1.1)
061	Epilepsy	4(1.2)	5(0.9)

Table 5.4

RESPONDENT'S REASONS FOR TAKING VALIUM AT TIME 1 [1]
(continued)

Code	Reason	N(%) [2] First Mention	N(%) [3] Any Mention
063	Paraplegia and quadraplegia	0	1(0.2)
065	Diseases of the sense organs	2(0.6)	3(0.6)
070	Diseases of the circulatory system	4(1.2)	11(2.1)
072	Hypertension & high blood pressure	6(1.7)	16(3.0)
073	Ischaemic heart disease, angina pectoris, myocardial infarction & heart attack	0	2(0.4)
090	Diseases of the digestive system	1(0.3)	3(0.6)
092	Gastric, duodenal, & peptic ulcers & gastritis	2(0.6)	4(0.7)
093	Stomach disorders including indigestion, habitual vomiting (unless due to pregnancy), & acid stomach	1(0.3)	5(0.9)
100	Diseases of the genitourinary system	1(0.3)	1(0.2)
101	Diseases of the male or female genital organs	0	1(0.2)

Table 5.4

RESPONDENT'S REASONS FOR TAKING VALIUM AT TIME 1'
(continued)

Code	Reason	N(%)² First Mention	N(%)³ Any Mention
102	Menopausal or post menopausal disorders or symptoms (e.g., cramps, or flushing IF due to these conditions)	2(0.6)	4(0.7)
130	Diseases of the musculoskeletal system & connective tissue	4(1.2)	4(0.7)
131	Pulled back, sore muscles, stiff muscles, sore back, sprains & strains of muscles & joints, & muscle spasms	23(6.7)	30(5.6)
160	Symptoms, signs, & ill-defined conditions	6(1.7)	9(1.7)
165	Dizziness, giddiness, vertigo	1(0.3)	3(0.6)
167	Shaking	3(0.9)	7(1.3)
170	Symptoms involving nervous & musculoskeletal systems	1(0.3)	1(0.2)
171	Symptoms involving skin	0	1(0.2)
173	Symptoms involving head & neck	4(1.2)	6(1.1)
174	Symptoms involving cardiovascular system	2(0.6)	5(0.9)
175	Symptoms involving respiratory system	2(0.6)	5(0.9)

Table 5.4

RESPONDENT'S REASONS FOR TAKING VALIUM AT TIME 1'
(continued)

Code	Reason	N(%)² First Mention	N(%)³ Any Mention
176	Symptoms involving digestive system	0	1(0.2)
180	Injury & poisoning	1(0.3)	3(0.6)
190	Surgery, dialysis	2(0.6)	4(0.7)
501	Anger, temper, "pissed off"	0	1(0.2)
502	To keep calm, relax, "keep cool"	29(8.4)	49(9.2)
503	Cry, want to cry	0	1(0.2)
506	Unspecified discomfort; uneasy feeling	1(0.3)	1(0.2)
601	Tried other things that didn't work, so trying the medication	1(0.3)	6(1.1)
602	Stressful situation (e.g., tragedy in family, financial problems, job stress, etc.)	5(1.4)	12(2.2)
603	Stressed but not clear if it is due to a situation, "can't cope" but source of problem is not specified	4(1.2)	10(1.9)
604	Used to prevent an anticipated emotional state	1(0.3)	2(0.4)

Table 5.4

RESPONDENT'S REASONS FOR TAKING VALIUM AT TIME 1 [1]
(continued)

Code	Reason	N(%) [2] First Mention	N(%) [3] Any Mention
605	Used to prevent an anticipated situation	0	1(0.2)
606	To cope with anticipated situation	1(0.3)	3(0.6)
701	Requested by health care professional (e.g., M.D., nurse, psychiatrist, counselor, psychologist)	7(2.0)	10(1.9)
703	Requested by unspecified other	0	1(0.2)
801	As prescribed: either the box is checked or R says so	1(0.3)	1(0.2)
802	R follows regular rules (e.g., "every night before bed","three times a day")	2(0.6)	3(0.6)
803	R takes as needed including "how I think I should take it"	1(0.3)	2(0.4)
860	To get high	1(0.3)	1(0.2)
997	Other	2(0.6)	2(0.4)
998	Don't Know	1(0.3)	1(0.0)
999	No Answer	5(1.4)	5(0.0)

[1] F8(YO17-YO21); multiple mentions allowed.   [2] Percent of Valium users at Time 1.

[3] Percent of mentions.

question at all four interviews (see Chapters 3 and 4 and Appendix N for descriptions of the coding procedures).

Respondents' most common decision rule was to take Valium when they felt tense or anxious (code 051); 35% of Valium users mentioned this reason at Time 1. This was lower than the percent of respondents who reported that they took Valium because of anxiety. The second most common decision rule was simply to take Valium at the prescribed times (code 801); 26% of Valium users mentioned this reason at Time 1. Presumably many of the anxious respondents used this decision rule. The third most common decision rule involved taking Valium when the individual had problems falling asleep (code 059); 21% of Valium users mentioned this reason at Time 1. Twelve percent followed regular rules such as taking it 3 times a day or every evening (code 802). Most other decision rules appeared to be more idiosyncratic and were only used by small numbers of respondents. Only 2% of respondents reported taking Valium when they were depressed (code 052), 5% reported taking it when they were in a stressful situation (code 602), and less than 1% reported taking Valium to "get high" (code 860).

Respondents' Reasons for Not Continuing to Take Valium

Interviewers brought with them to the second, third, and fourth interviews a list of the medications that respondents at the time of the previous interview had reported taking in the previous six weeks. If respondents did not mention one or more of these medications, they were reminded that they had reported taking it previously and were asked if they had taken it since the last interview. If they replied "no," then they were asked why they had not taken this medication since the last interview. Respondents' reasons for not continuing to take Valium are presented in Table 5.6 (see Chapters 3 and 4 and Appendix N for descriptions of the coding procedures).

As noted in Table 5.6, 82 to 87 respondents (depending on the wave) who had reported taking Valium at one interview did not report having taken Valium again before the subsequent interview. Of those respondents who had stopped taking the medication at Time 2, 40% reported that their problem, either physical or psychological, had gone away (codes 1-6 com-

Table 5.5
HOW RESPONDENTS DECIDE WHEN TO TAKE VALIUM[1]

Code	Reason	Time 1 (N=345)	Time 2 (N=296)	Time 3 (N=251)	Time 4 (N=241)
050	Mental disorders	4 (.6%)[2] (1.2%)[3]	6 (1.2%) (2.0%)	4 (1.0%) (1.6%)	4 (1.0%) (1.6%)
051	Tension, anxiety, nerves, "keyed up"	122 (19.4%) (35.4%)	89 (18.3%) (30.1%)	80 (19.7%) (31.9%)	70 (17.3%) (29.0%)
052	Depression, blues, sadness	6 (1.0%) (1.7%)	3 (0.6%) (1.0%)	7 (1.7%) (2.8%)	2 (0.5%) (.8%)
053	Fears, phobias, apprehension	4 (0.6%) (1.2%)	5 (1.0%) (1.7%)	3 (.7%) (1.2%)	2 (.5%) (.8%)
054	Upset or emotional	24 (3.8%) (6.7%)	29 (6.0%) (9.8%)	23 (5.7%) (9.2%)	24 (5.9%) (10.0%)
056	Withdrawal from Valium or dependence on Valium	0	1 (.2%) (.3%)	0	0
057	Withdrawal from other prescribed medication or dependence on other prescribed medication (e.g., Darvon, Tranxene)	1 (.2%) (.3%)	0	0	0
059	Sleep disorders, insomnia, any problems with falling to sleep	72 (11.4%) (20.9%)	74 (15.2%) (25.0%)	59 (14.5%) (23.5%)	62 (15.3%) (25.7%)
060	Diseases of the nervous system	1 (.2%) (.3%)	2 (.4%) (.7%)	4 (1.0%) (1.6%)	3 (.7%) (1.2%)

Table 5.5
HOW RESPONDENTS DECIDE WHEN TO TAKE VALIUM
(continued)

Code	Reason	Time 1 (N=345)	Time 2 (N=296)	Time 3 (N=251)	Time 4 (N=241)
062	Migraines	1 (.2%) (.3%)	1 (.2%) (.3%)	0	0
065	Diseases of the sense organs	0	0	1 (.2%) (.4%)	0
070	Diseases of the circulatory system	2 (.3%) (.6%)	1 (.2%) (.3%)	1 (.2%) (.4%)	0
072	Hypertension & high blood pressure	2 (.3%) (.6%)	1 (.2%) (.3%)	3 (.7%) (1.2%)	2 (.5%) (.8%)
073	Ischaemic heart disease, angina pectoris, myocardial infarction & heart attack	1 (.2%) (.3%)	1 (.2%) (.3%)	1 (.2%) (.4%)	1 (.2%) (.4%)
074	Stroke, brain hemorrhage, & cerebravascular disease	0	1 (.2%) (.3%)	0	0
080	Diseases of the respiratory system	0	0	1 (.2%) (.4%)	0
090	Diseases of the digestive system	1 (.2%) (.3%)	2 (.4%) (.7%)	0	0
091	Diseases of the tooth, jaws, and gums	1 (.2%) (.3%)	0	0	0

Table 5.5
HOW RESPONDENTS DECIDE WHEN TO TAKE VALIUM
(continued)

Code	Reason	Time 1 (N=345)	Time 2 (N=296)	Time 3 (N=251)	Time 4 (N=241)
092	Gastric, duodenal, & peptic ulcers & gastritis	0	1 (.2%) (.3%)	0	1 (.2%) (.4%)
093	Stomach disorders including indigestion, habitual vomiting (unless due to pregnancy), & acid stomach	3 (.5%) (.9%)	3 (.6%) (1.0%)	4 (1.0%) (1.6%)	2 (.5%) (.8%)
094	Colitis, ileitis, irritable bowel, constipation, & diarrhea	2 (.3%) (.6%)	0	0	1 (.2%) (.4%)
101	Diseases of the male or female genital organs	0	1 (.2%) (.3%)	0	0
102	Menopausal or post menopausal disorders or symptoms (e.g., cramps, or flushing IF due to these conditions)	1 (.2%) (.3%)	2 (.4%) (.7%)	0	0
130	Diseases of the musculoskeletal system & connective tissue	4 (.6%) (1.2%)	3 (.6%) (1.0%)	4 (1.0%) (1.6%)	6 (1.5%) (2.5%)
131	Pulled back, sore muscles, stiff muscles, sore back, sprains & strains of muscles & joints, & muscle spasms	14 (2.2%) (4.0%)	11 (2.3%) (3.7%)	13 (3.2%) (5.2%)	14 (3.5%) (5.8%)
160	Symptoms, signs, & ill-defined conditions	10 (1.6%) (2.9%)	4 (.8%) (1.4%)	5 (1.2%) (2.0%)	3 (.7%) (1.2%)

HOW RESPONDENTS DECIDE WHEN TO TAKE VALIUM

Table 5.5
(continued)

Code	Reason	Time 1 (N=345)	Time 2 (N=296)	Time 3 (N=251)	Time 4 (N=241)
162	Hallucinations	0	1 (.2%) (.3%)	0	0
165	Dizziness, giddiness, vertigo	4 (.6%) (1.2%)	3 (0.6%) (1.0%)	3 (0.7%) (1.2%)	1 (.2%) (.4%)
166	Lethargy, malaise, fatigue	2 (.3%) (.6%)	4 (.8%) (1.4%)	1 (.2%) (.4%)	3 (.7%) (1.2%)
167	Shaking	20 (3.2%) (5.6%)	8 (1.6%) (2.7%)	5 (1.2%) (2.0%)	7 (1.7%) (2.9%)
170	Symptoms involving nervous & musculoskeletal systems	1 (.2%) (.3%)	0	1 (.2%) (.4%)	0
171	Symptoms involving skin	1 (.2%) (.3%)	0	0	1 (.2%) (.4%)
172	Symptoms involving nutrition, metabolism, & development	1 (.2%) (.3%)	0	0	0
173	Symptoms involving head & neck	9 (1.4%) (2.6%)	5 (1.0%) (1.7%)	4 (1.0%) (1.6%)	3 (.7%) (1.2%)
174	Symptoms involving cardiovascular system	3 (.5%) (.9%)	2 (.4%) (.7%)	2 (.5%) (.8%)	2 (.5%) (.8%)

Table 5.5
HOW RESPONDENTS DECIDE WHEN TO TAKE VALIUM
(continued)

Code	Reason	Time 1 (N=345)	Time 2 (N=296)	Time 3 (N=251)	Time 4 (N=241)
175	Symptoms involving respiratory system	5 (.8%) (1.4%)	4 (.8%) (1.4%)	2 (.5%) (.8%)	5 (1.2%) (2.1%)
176	Symptoms involving digestive system	4 (.6%) (1.2%)	2 (.4%) (.7%)	2 (.5%) (.8%)	2 (.5%) (.8%)
180	Injury & poisoning	1 (.2%) (.3%)	0	0	0
501	Anger, temper, "pissed off"	8 (1.3%) (2.3%)	8 (1.6%) (2.7%)	1 (.2%) (.4%)	2 (.5%) (.8%)
502	To keep calm, relax, "keep cool"	19 (3.0%) (5.5%)	18 (3.7%) (6.1%)	11 (2.7%) (4.4%)	13 (3.2%) (5.4%)
503	Cry, want to cry	5 (.8%) (1.4%)	1 (.2%) (.3%)	0	2 (.5%) (.8%)
504	Boredom	1 (.2%) (.3%)	0	0	0
505	Low Self esteem, feelings of insecurity	1 (.2%) (.3%)	0	1 (.2%) (.4%)	0
506	Unspecified discomfort: uneasy feeling	9 (1.4%) (2.6%)	5 (1.0%) (1.7%)	3 (.7%) (1.2%)	6 (1.5%) (2.5%)

Table 5.5
HOW RESPONDENTS DECIDE WHEN TO TAKE VALIUM
(continued)

Code	Reason	Time 1 (N=345)	Time 2 (N=296)	Time 3 (N=251)	Time 4 (N=241)
601	Tried other things that didn't work, so trying the medication	6 (1.0%) (1.7%)	4 (.8%) (1.4%)	4 (1.0%) (1.6%)	3 (.7%) (1.2%)
602	Stressful situation (e.g., tragedy in family, financial problems, job stress, etc.)	17 (2.7%) (4.9%)	14 (2.9%) (4.7%)	8 (2.0%) (3.2%)	12 (3.0%) (5.0%)
603	Stressed but not clear if it is due to a situation, "can't cope" but source of problem is not specified	14 (2.2%) (4.0%)	4 (.8%) (1.4%)	5 (1.2%) (2.0%)	4 (1.0%) (1.6%)
604	Used to prevent an anticipated emotional state	7 (1.1%) (2.0%)	3 (.6%) (1.0%)	4 (1.0%) (1.6%)	6 (1.5%) (2.5%)
605	Used to prevent an anticipated situation	1 (.2%) (.3%)	3 (.6%) (1.0%)	1 (.2%) (.4%)	0
606	To cope with anticipated situation	11 (1.7%) (3.2%)	13 (2.7%) (4.4%)	10 (2.5%) (4.0%)	14 (3.5%) (5.8%)
701	Requested by health care professional (e.g., M.D., nurse, psychiatrist, counselor, psychologist)	4 (.6%) (1.2%)	2 (.4%) (.7%)	1 (.2%) (.4%)	2 (.5%) (.8%)
702	Requested by non-professional (e.g., spouse, friend, relative)	1 (.2%) (.3%)	2 (.4%) (.7%)	1 (.2%) (.4%)	0

Table 5.5
HOW RESPONDENTS DECIDE WHEN TO TAKE VALIUM
(continued)

Code	Reason	Time 1 (N=345)	Time 2 (N=296)	Time 3 (N=251)	Time 4 (N=241)
703	Requested by unspecified other	2 (.3%) (.6%)	0	0	0
801	As prescribed: either the box is checked or R says so	90 (14.3%) (26.1%)	63 (13.0%) (21.3%)	60 (14.8%) (24.0%)	51 (12.6%) (21.2%)
802	R follows regular rules (e.g., "every night before bed" "three times a day")	40 (6.3%) (11.6%)	36 (7.4%) (12.2%)	32 (7.9%) (12.7%)	40 (9.9%) (16.7%)
803	R takes as needed including "how I think I should take it"	62 (9.8%) (18.0%)	38 (7.8%) (12.8%)	28 (6.9%) (11.2%)	27 (6.7%) (11.2%)
850	Mentions concern about addiction	3 (.5%) (.9%)	0	1 (.2%) (.4%)	0
860	To get high	2 (.3%) (.6%)	2 (.4%) (.7%)	1 (.2%) (.4%)	0

1 F22 (YO22-YO26): multiple mentions allowed.

2 Percent of mentions.

3 Percent of Valium users mentioning this reason.

Table 5.6

FOR RESPONDENTS WHO TOOK VALIUM AT THE TIME OF THE PREVIOUS INTERVIEW BUT NOT AT THIS INTERVIEW, "WHY HAVEN'T YOU BEEN TAKING VALIUM SINCE YOUR LAST INTERVIEW?"

Code	Health Problem	Time 2 (N=82)	Time 3 (N=84)	Time 4 (N=87)
01	R's health or somatic problem(s) went away and R clearly indicates that the medication was responsible for its disappearance	0	0	1 (.8%)² (1.1%)³
02	R's health or somatic problem(s) went away	11 (11.1%) (13.4%)	14 (14.0%) (16.7%)	17 (13.8%) (19.5%)
04	Problem(s) have not come up recently but could come back-- may be health or social-psychological problem	6 (6.1%) (7.3%)	2 (2.0%) (2.4%)	18 (14.6%) (20.7%)
05	Under less stress	0	0	1 (.8%) (1.1%)
06	Don't need any more; unspecified problem(s) went away	16 (16.2%) (19.5%)	13 (13.0%) (15.5%)	17 (13.8%) (19.5%)
11	Addictive, habit-forming, dependence - R knows this from own use	2 (2.0%) (2.4%)	0	0
13	Addictive, habit-forming, dependence - R does not know this from own use or from use by family or friends	1 (1.0%) (1.2%)	2 (2.0%) (2.4%)	2 (1.6%) (2.3%)
14	Other undesirable side effects	13 (13.1%) (15.8%)	15 (15.0%) (17.9%)	12 (9.8%) (13.8%)
15	Believes drug was not effective, did not work well	5 (5.1%) (6.1%)	5 (5.0%) (5.9%)	7 (5.7%) (8.0%)
16	Heard negative/controversial reports in media	0	1 (1.0%) (1.2%)	0

129

Table 5.6

FOR RESPONDENTS WHO TOOK VALIUM AT THE TIME OF THE PREVIOUS INTERVIEW BUT NOT AT THIS INTERVIEW. "WHY HAVEN'T YOU BEEN TAKING VALIUM SINCE YOUR LAST INTERVIEW?":
(continued)

Code	Health Problem	Time 2 (N=82)	Time 3 (N=84)	Time 4 (N=87)
17	Psychopharmacological Calvinism: morally wrong to take drug	0	1 (1.0%) (1.2%)	0
18	R is pregnant	1 (1.0%) (1.2%)	0	0
21	Health professional instructed to stop	13 (13.1%) (15.8%)	15 (15.0%) (17.8%)	12 (9.8%) (13.8%)
23	Physician switched to a different drug for the same problem	9 (9.1%) (11.0%)	13 (13.0%) (15.5%)	7 (5.7%) (8.0%)
24	No faith in physician	1 (1.0%) (1.2%)	0	0
31	Using another medicine instead	11 (11.1%) (13.4%)	8 (8.0%) (9.5%)	8 (6.5%) (9.2%)
32	Using non-prescription drug instead	1 (1.0%) (1.2%)	0	1 (.8%) (1.1%)
33	Took care of problem by changing diet	0	0	4 (3.3%) (4.6%)
34	Using other behavioral coping	2 (2.0%) (2.4%)	0	3 (2.4%) (3.4%)
81	Cost: too expensive	0	0	1 (.8%) (1.1%)

130

Table 5.6

FOR RESPONDENTS WHO TOOK VALIUM AT THE TIME OF THE PREVIOUS INTERVIEW BUT NOT AT THIS INTERVIEW, "WHY HAVEN'T YOU BEEN TAKING VALIUM SINCE YOUR LAST INTERVIEW?"[1]
(continued)

Code	Health Problem	Time 2 (N=82)	Time 3 (N=84)	Time 4 (N=87)
82	Ran out of prescription	5 (5.1%) (6.1%)	8 (8.0%) (9.5%)	6 (4.9%) (6.9%)
84	Too hard to remember to take	0	1 (1.0%) (1.2%)	0
90	Didn't think it was necessary	0	0	2 (1.6%) (2.2%)
96	No reason: "just stopped"	1 (1.0%) (1.2%)	0	3 (2.4%) (3.4%)

[1]F51(YO32,YO33): multiple mentions allowed.
[2]Percent of mentions.
[3]Percent of Valium users who quit taking Valium.

131

bined). [28]   Sixteen percent reported that they had quit taking
Valium because they experienced undesirable side effects (code
14).   Six percent reported that they quit taking Valium because
they believed it was not effective (code 15).   Less than 4% of
these respondents mentioned discontinuing Valium use because of
a concern about addiction (codes 11 and 13 combined).   Sixteen
percent reported that a health professional had instructed them
to stop taking Valium (code 21).   Eleven percent said their
physician had told them to take a different medication (code
23), while another 13% said they had decided to take another
medication instead (code 31).

This information may be useful to physicians who prescribe
Valium.   For example, 21% of the respondents who quit taking
Valium did so either because of side effects or the belief that
the drug was ineffective.   Physicians might want to probe
patients for such concerns in follow-up visits.   By addressing
some of these concerns, they might be able to increase patient
compliance.

Health Status of Respondents

Physicians' diagnoses of respondents' conditions were not
obtained.   However, respondents were asked to report any health
problems they had (see Chapters 3 and 4 and Appendix N for
descriptions of the coding procedures).   Table 5.7 presents the
health problems mentioned by respondents (Valium users and nonusers) at all four interviews.   Only 8% of respondents reported
having no physical problems "these days" at the initial interview (code 996).   This number rose steadily so that by the
fourth interview 15% of respondents reported having no physical
problems. [29]

At Time 1 the most commonly mentioned physical ailment was
a pulled back or sore muscles (code 131); 18% of respondents
reported having this problem.   Eighteen percent reported having

---

[28] Time 2 percents are reported in the text.   As can be
seen from Table 5.6, Time 3 and Time 4 percentages are quite
similar.

[29] As noted in the section on stabilities in this chapter,
respondents also showed improvement on most of the indices of
affect, stress, and quality of life from Time 1 to Time 4.

Table 5.7

SELF-REPORTED HEALTH PROBLEMS OF RESPONDENTS'

Code	Health Problem	Time 1 (N=675)	Time 2 (N=675)	Time 3 (N=675)	Time 4 (N=675)
010	Infections & parasitic diseases	11 (.7%)² (1.6%)³	4 (.3%) (.6%)	9 (.6%) (1.3%)	17 (1.2%) (2.5%)
020	Neoplasms	18 (1.1%) (2.7%)	11 (.8%) (1.6%)	7 (.5%) (1.0%)	11 (.8%) (1.6%)
030	Endocrine, nutritional and metabolic diseases & immunity disorders	107 (6.5%) (15.8%)	80 (5.6%) (11.8%)	65 (4.6%) (9.6%)	71 (5.1%) (10.5%)
040	Diseases of the blood & blood forming organs	12 (.7%) (1.8%)	7 (.5%) (1.0%)	3 (.2%) (.4%)	6 (.4%) (.9%)
050	Mental disorders	48 (2.9%) (7.1%)	24 (1.7%) (3.6%)	21 (1.5%) (3.1%)	9 (.7%) (1.3%)
051	Tension, anxiety, nerves, "keyed up"	98 5.9% (14.5%)	78 (5.5%) (11.6%)	67 (4.8%) (9.9%)	79 (5.7%) (11.7%)
052	Depression, blues, sadness	18 (1.1%) (2.7%)	19 (1.3%) (2.8%)	22 (1.6%) (3.2%)	15 (1.1%) (2.2%)
053	Fears, phobias, apprehension	12 (.7%) (1.8%)	5 (.3%) (.7%)	5 (.4%) (.7%)	13 (.9%) (1.9%)
054	Upset or emotional	9 (.5%) (1.3%)	9 (.6%) (1.3%)	3 (.2%) (.4%)	9 (.7%) (1.3%)
055	Alcohol withdrawal or dependence or tremors, delerium tremens, agitation or restlessness associated with alcohol withdrawal or dependence	4 (.2%) (.6%)	1 (.1%) (.1%)	0	0

Table 5.7

SELF-REPORTED HEALTH PROBLEMS OF RESPONDENTS'
(continued)

Code	Health Problem	Time 1 (N=675)	Time 2 (N=675)	Time 3 (N=675)	Time 4 (N=675)
057	Withdrawal from other prescribed medication or dependence on other prescribed medication (e.g., Darvon, Tranxene)	3 (.2%) (.4%)	2 (.1%) (.3%)	0	0
058	Withdrawal from nonprescribed drug or dependence on non-prescribed drug (e.g., Heroin, PCP)	0	0	0	1 (.1%) (.1%)
059	Sleep disorders, insomnia, any problems with falling to sleep	11 (.7%) (1.6%)	10 (.7%) (1.5%)	14 (1%) (2.1%)	13 (.9%) (1.9%)
060	Diseases of the nervous system	27 (1.6%) (4.0%)	21 (1.5%) (3.1%)	17 (1.2%) (2.5%)	21 (1.5%) (3.1%)
061	Epilepsy	8 (.5%) (1.2%)	5 (.3%) (.7%)	7 (.5%) (1.0%)	8 (.6%) (1.2%)
062	Migraines	8 (.5%) (1.2%)	6 (.4%) (.9%)	5 (.4%) (.7%)	5 (.4%) (.7%)
063	Paraplegia & quadraplegia	4 (.2%) (.6%)	1 (.1%) (.1%)	1 (.1%) (.1%)	1 (.1%) (.1%)
065	Diseases of the sense organs	36 (2.2%) (5.3%)	31 (2.2%) (4.6%)	29 (2.1%) (4.3%)	25 (1.8%) (3.7%)
070	Diseases of the circulatory system	80 (4.8%) (11.8%)	72 (5%) (10.7%)	75 (5.3%) (11.1%)	48 (3.5%) (7.1%)
071	Arteriosclerosis & hardening of the arteries	4 (.2%) (.6%)	2 (.1%) (.3%)	0	1 (.1%) (.1%)

Table 5.7

SELF-REPORTED HEALTH PROBLEMS OF RESPONDENTS
(continued)

Code	Health Problem	Time 1 (N=675)	Time 2 (N=675)	Time 3 (N=675)	Time 4 (N=675)
072	Hypertension & high blood pressure	116 (7.0%) (17.2%)	98 (6.8%) (14.5%)	73 (5.2%) (10.8%)	96 (6.9%) (14.2%)
073	Ischaemic heart disease, angina pectoris, myocardial infarction & heart attack	32 (1.9%) (4.7%)	19 (1.3%) (2.8%)	21 (1.5%) (3.1%)	17 (1.2%) (2.5%)
074	Stroke, brain hemorrhage, & cerebravascular disease	10 (.6%) (1.5%)	8 (.6%) (1.2%)	8 (.6%) (1.2%)	6 (.4%) (.9%)
080	Diseases of the respiratory system	90 (5.4%) (13.3%)	110 (7.7%) (16.2%)	141 (10%) (20.9%)	120 (8.7%) (17.8%)
090	Diseases of the digestive system	38 (2.3%) (5.6%)	26 (1.8%) (3.8%)	20 (1.4%) (3.0%)	20 (1.4%) (3.0%)
091	Diseases of the tooth, jaws, and gums	15 (.9%) (2.2%)	8 (.6%) (1.2%)	9 (.6%) (1.3%)	11 (.8%) (1.6%)
092	Gastric, duodenal, & peptic ulcers & gastritis	32 (1.9%) (4.7%)	19 (1.3%) (2.8%)	20 (1.4%) (3.0%)	11 (.8%) (1.6%)
093	Stomach disorders including indigestion, habitual vomiting (unless due to pregnancy), & acid stomach	27 (1.6%) (4.0%)	16 (1.1%) (2.4%)	35 (2.5%) (5.2%)	25 (1.8%) (3.7%)
094	Colitis, ileitis, irritable bowel, constipation, & diarrhea	29 (1.8%) (4.3%)	14 (1%) (2.1%)	14 (1%) (2.1%)	21 (1.5%) (3.1%)
100	Diseases of the genitourinary system	24 (1.5%) (3.5%)	21 (1.5%) (3.1%)	23 (1.6%) (3.4%)	22 (1.6%) (3.2%)

Table 5.7

SELF-REPORTED HEALTH PROBLEMS OF RESPONDENTS
(continued)

Code	Health Problem	Time 1 (N=675)	Time 2 (N=675)	Time 3 (N=675)	Time 4 (N=675)
101	Diseases of the male or female genital organs	35 (2.1%) (5.2%)	24 (1.7%) (3.6%)	30 (2.1%) (4.4%)	17 (1.2%) (2.5%)
102	Menopausal or post menopausal disorders or symptoms (e.g., cramps, or flushing IF due to these conditions)	13 (.8%) (1.9%)	9 (.6%) (1.3%)	4 (.3%) (.6%)	5 (.4%) (.7%)
110	Complications of pregnancy, childbirth & the puerperium	13 (.8%) (1.9%)	14 (1%) (2.1%)	5 (.4%) (.7%)	5 (.4%) (.7%)
120	Diseases of the skin & subcutaneous tissue	17 (1.0%) (2.5%)	14 (1%) (2.1%)	10 (.7%) (1.5%)	10 (.7%) (1.5%)
130	Diseases of the musculoskeletal system & connective tissue	123 (7.4%) (18.2%)	128 (8.9%) (19.0%)	134 (9.6%) (19.9%)	120 (8.7%) (17.8%)
131	Pulled back, sore muscles, stiff muscles, sore back, sprains & strains of muscles & joints, & muscle spasms	124 (7.5%) (18.4%)	105 (7.3%) (15.6%)	125 (8.9%) (18.5%)	100 (7.2%) (14.8%)
132	Bursitis, tendonitis, swelling due to either of these	6 (.4%) (.9%)	5 (.3%) (.7%)	9 (.6%) (1.3%)	9 (.7%) (1.3%)
140	Congenital anomalies	6 (.4%) (.9%)	3 (.2%) (.4%)	2 (.1%) (.3%)	3 (.2%) (.4%)
160	Symptoms, signs, & ill-defined conditions	12 (.7%) (1.8%)	16 (1.1%) (2.4%)	16 (1.1%) (2.4%)	21 (1.5%) (3.1%)
161	Coma, stupor, unconsciousness	0	2 (.1%) (.3%)	0	0

136

Table 5.7

SELF-REPORTED HEALTH PROBLEMS OF RESPONDENTS:
(continued)

Code	Health Problem	Time 1 (N=675)	Time 2 (N=675)	Time 3 (N=675)	Time 4 (N=675)
163.	Blackout, fainting, collapse. & syncope	1 (.1%) (.1%)	0	1 (.1%) (.1%)	4 (.3%) (.6%)
164	Convulsions (except epilepsy)	0	0	1 (.1%) (.1%)	1 (.1%) (.1%)
165	Dizziness, giddiness, vertigo	18 (1.1%) (2.7%)	15 (1%) (2.2%)	8 (.6%) (1.2%)	13 (.9%) (1.9%)
166	Lethargy, malaise, fatigue	31 (1.9%) (4.6%)	45 (3.1%) (6.7%)	44 (3.1%) (6.5%)	36 (2.6%) (5.3%)
167	Shaking	6 (.4%) (.9%)	3 (.2%) (.4%)	4 (.3%) (.6%)	2 (.1%) (.3%)
170	Symptoms involving nervous & musculoskeletal systems	5 (.3%) (.7%)	4 (.3%) (.6%)	3 (.2%) (.4%)	5 (.4%) (.7%)
171	Symptoms involving skin	14 (.8%) (2.1%)	17 (1.2%) (2.5%)	15 (1.1%) (2.2%)	19 (1.4%) (2.8%)
172	Symptoms involving nutrition, metabolism, & development	15 (.9%) (2.2%)	7 (.5%) (1.0%)	6 (.4%) (.9%)	13 (.9%) (1.9%)
173	Symptoms involving head & neck	47 (2.8%) (7.0%)	71 (5%) (10.5%)	60 (4.3%) (8.9%)	49 (3.5%) (7.2%)
174	Symptoms involving cardiovascular system	9 (.5%) (1.3%)	8 (.6%) (1.2%)	7 (.5%) (1.0%)	8 (.6%) (1.2%)
175	Symptoms involving respiratory system	27 (1.6%) (4.0%)	41 (2.9%) (6.1%)	39 (2.8%) (5.8%)	55 (4%) (8.1%)

Table 5.7

SELF-REPORTED HEALTH PROBLEMS OF RESPONDENTS'
(continued)

Code	Health Problem	Time 1 (N=675)	Time 2 (N=675)	Time 3 (N=675)	Time 4 (N=675)
176	Symptoms involving digestive system	12 (.7%) (1.8%)	22 (1.5%) (3.2%)	10 (.7%) (1.5%)	24 (1.7%) (3.6%)
177	Symptoms involving urinary system	0	3 (.2%) (.4%)	0	3 (.2%) (.4%)
180	Injury & poisoning	49 (3.0%) (7.2%)	37 (2.6%) (5.5%)	35 (2.5%) (5.2%)	32 (2.3%) (4.7%)
190	Surgery, dialysis	80 (4.8%) (11.8%)	32 (2.2%) (4.7%)	27 (1.9%) (4.0%)	24 (1.7%) (3.6%)
691	Tried other things that didn't work, so trying the medication	1 (.1%) (.1%)	0	0	0
996	No physical problems or diseases	57 (3.5%) (8.4%)	79 (5.5%) (11.7%)	93 (6.6%) (13.8%)	102 (7.4%) (15.1%)
997	Other	0	0	1 (.1%) (.1%)	0

¹A3, A4, & A8(YOO9-YO12); multiple mentions allowed.
²Percent of mentions.
³Percent of respondents.

138

other types of musculoskeletal problems (code 130) such as arthritis, neuritis, and bone and joint disorders. Seventeen percent of respondents reported having hypertension (code 072). Twelve percent reported having disorders referable to the circulatory system (code 070) such as varicose veins, hemorrhoids, phlebitis, and heart murmurs. Sixteen percent of respondents mentioned endocrine or metabolic disorders (code 030) such as thyroid, goiter, and pituitary disorders or diabetes, vitamin deficiencies, obesity, and malnutrition. Fourteen percent of respondents mentioned being tense or anxious (code 051). Thirteen percent of respondents mentioned having problems referable to the respiratory system (code 080) such as the common cold, tonsillitis, pneumonia, influenza, asthma, and allergies. Twelve percent of respondents mentioned recently undergoing surgery or dialysis (code 190). Other physical problems were quite uncommon. For example, only 3% mentioned having a tumor or growth (code 020), 5% reported having heart disease (code 073), and 5% reported having ulcers (code 092).

As noted earlier, most respondents were recruited into this study because they had recently filled a prescription for some medication. It is likely, therefore, that these respondents had more health problems than do most Americans. Consequently, the information in Table 5.7 was presented primarily to provide descriptive information about the health status of these respondents. Although subjective ratings of health were used in later bivariate and multivariate analyses, these self-reports of specific illnesses were not because of their unknown validity and because the number of respondents in most categories was too small for analysis.

Comparison of the Health of Valium Users and Nonusers

Table 5.8 presents a comparison of the self-reported current health problems of respondents who had taken Valium within six weeks of the initial interview and respondents who had not. Valium users were about twice as likely as nonusers to report being tense or anxious. More Valium users than nonusers reported having disorders referable to the nervous or circulatory systems, hypertension, heart disease, gastric disorders, problems related to the musculoskeletal system, and

Table 5.8

SELF-REPORTED HEALTH PROBLEMS OF VALIUM USERS AND NONUSERS AT TIME 1

Code	Health Problem	Valium users (N=345)	Non-Valium users (N=330)
010	Infections & parasitic diseases	4 (.4%)[1] (1.2%)[2]	7 (1.0%) (2.1%)
020	Neoplasms	13 (1.4%) (3.8%)	5 (.7%) (1.5%)
030	Endocrine, nutritional and metabolic diseases & immunity disorders	47 (5.0%) (13.6%)	60 (8.4%) (18.2%)
040	Diseases of the blood & blood forming organs	8 (0.9%) (2.3%)	4 (.6%) (1.2%)
050	Mental disorders	27 (2.9%) (7.8%)	21 (2.9%) (6.4%)
051	Tension, anxiety, nerves, "keyed up"	67 7.2% (19.4%)	31 (4.3%) (9.4%)
052	Depression, blues, sadness	9 (1.0%) (2.6%)	9 (1.3%) (2.7%)
053	Fears, phobias, apprehension	7 (.7%) (2.0%)	5 (.7%) (1.5%)
054	Upset or emotional	9 (1.0%) (2.6%)	0
055	Alcohol withdrawal or dependence or tremors, delerium tremens, agitation or restlessness associated with alcohol withdrawal or dependence	2 (.2%) (.6%)	2 (.3%) (.6%)

140

Table 5.8

SELF-REPORTED HEALTH PROBLEMS OF VALIUM USERS AND NONUSERS AT TIME 1 (continued)

Code	Health Problem	Valium users (N=345)	Non-Valium users (N=330)
057	Withdrawal from other prescribed medication or dependence on other prescribed medication (e.g., Darvon, Tranxene)	2 (.2%) (.6%)	1 (.1%) (.3%)
059	Sleep disorders, insomnia, any problems with falling to sleep	9 (1.0%) (2.6%)	2 (.3%) (.6%)
060	Diseases of the nervous system	20 (2.1%) (5.8%)	7 (1.0%) (2.1%)
061	Epilepsy	7 (.7%) (2.0%)	1 (.1%) (.3%)
062	Migraines	6 (.6%) (1.7%)	2 (.3%) (.6%)
063	Paraplegia & quadraplegia	3 (.3%) (.9%)	1 (.1%) (.3%)
065	Diseases of the sense organs	22 (2.3%) (6.4%)	14 (2.0%) (4.2%)
070	Diseases of the circulatory system	57 (6.1%) (16.5%)	23 (3.2%) (7.0%)
071	Arteriosclerosis & hardening of the arteries	2 (.2%) (.6%)	2 (3.2%) (.6%)
072	Hypertension & high blood pressure	70 (7.5%) (20.3%)	46 (6.4%) (13.9%)
073	Ischaemic heart disease, angina pectoris, myocardial infarction & heart attack	24 (2.6%) (7.0%)	8 (1.1%) (2.4%)

Table 5.8

SELF-REPORTED HEALTH PROBLEMS OF VALIUM USERS AND NONUSERS AT TIME 1 (continued)

Code	Health Problem	Valium users (N=345)	Non-Valium users (N=330)
074	Stroke, brain hemorrhage, & cerebravascular disease	6 (.6%) (1.7%)	4 (.6%) (1.2%)
080	Diseases of the respiratory system	37 (3.9%) (10.7%)	53 (7.4%) (16.1%)
090	Diseases of the digestive system	20 (2.1%) (5.8%)	18 (2.5%) (5.4%)
091	Diseases of the tooth, jaws, and gums	8 (.9%) (2.3%)	7 (1.0%) (2.1%)
092	Gastric, duodenal, & peptic ulcers & gastritis	21 (2.2%) (6.1%)	11 (1.5%) (3.3%)
093	Stomach disorders including indigestion, habitual vomiting (unless due to pregnancy), & acid stomach	17 (1.8%) (4.9%)	10 (1.4%) (3.0%)
094	Colitis, ileitis, irritable bowel, constipation, & diarrhea	19 (2.0%) (5.5%)	10 (1.4%) (3.0%)
100	Diseases of the genitourinary system	11 (1.2%) (3.2%)	13 (1.8%) (3.9%)
101	Diseases of the male or female genital organs	18 (1.9%) (5.2%)	17 (2.4%) (5.2%)
102	Menopausal or post menopausal disorders or symptoms (e.g., cramps, or flushing IF due to these conditions)	10 (1.1%) (2.9%)	3 (.4%) (.9%)
110	Complications of pregnancy, childbirth & the puerperium	4 (.4%) (1.2%)	9 (1.3%) (2.7%)

Table 5.8

SELF-REPORTED HEALTH PROBLEMS OF VALIUM USERS AND NONUSERS AT TIME 1 (continued)

Code	Health Problem	Valium users (N=345)	Non-Valium users (N=330)
120	Diseases of the skin & sub-cutaneous tissue	8 (.9%) (2.3%)	9 (1.3%) (2.7%)
130	Diseases of the musculoskele-tal system & connective tissue	70 (7.5%) (20.3%)	53 (7.4%) (16.1%)
131	Pulled back, sore muscles, stiff muscles, sore back, sprains & strains of muscles & joints, & muscle spasms	73 (7.8%) (21.2%)	51 (7.1%) (15.4%)
132	Bursitis, tendonitis, swelling due to either of these	4 (.4%) (1.2%)	2 (.3%) (.9%)
140	Congentinal anomalies	5 (.5%) (1.4%)	1 (.1%) (.3%)
160	Symptoms, signs, & ill-defined conditions	6 (.6%) (1.7%)	6 (.8%) (1.8%)
163	Blackout, fainting, collapse, & syncope	1 (.1%) (.3%)	0
165	Dizziness, giddiness, vertigo	14 (1.5%) (4.0%)	4 (.6%) (1.2%)
166	Lethargy, malaise, fatigue	16 (1.7%) (4.6%)	15 (2.1%) (4.5%)
167	Shaking	4 (.4%) (1.2%)	2 (.3%) (.6%)
170	Symptoms involving nervous & musculoskeletal systems	1 (.1%) (.3%)	4 (.6%) (1.2%)

Table 5.8

SELF-REPORTED HEALTH PROBLEMS OF VALIUM USERS AND NONUSERS AT TIME 1 (continued)

Code	Health Problem	Valium users (N=345)	Non-Valium users (N=330)
171	Symptoms involving skin	6 (.6%) (1.7%)	8 (1.1%) (2.4%)
172	Symptoms involving nutrition, metabolism, & development	7 (.7%) (2.0%)	8 (1.1%) (2.4%)
173	Symptoms involving head & neck	24 (2.6%) (7.0%)	23 (3.2%) (7.0%)
174	Symptoms involving cardiovascular system	6 (.6%) (1.7%)	3 (.4%) (.9%)
175	Symptoms involving respiratory system	18 (1.9%) (5.2%)	9 (1.3%) (2.7%)
176	Symptoms involving digestive system	5 (.5%) (1.4%)	7 (1.0%) (2.1%)
180	Injury & poisoning	25 (2.7%) (7.2%)	24 (3.4%) (7.3%)
190	Surgery, dialysis	46 (4.9%) (13.3%)	34 (4.8%) (10.3%)
601	Tried other things that didn't work, so trying the medication	1 (.1%) (.3%)	0
996	No physical problems or diseases	11 (1.2%) (3.2%)	46 (6.4%) (13.9%)

[1]A3, A4, & A8(YO09-YO12); multiple mentions allowed.
[2]Percent of mentions.
[3]Percent of respondents.

144

pulled or sore muscles. Nonusers were more likely than Valium users to report disorders of the respiratory system (code 80), but Valium users were more likely than nonusers to mention respiratory symptoms (code 175). Valium users were about four times less likely than nonusers to report having no physical problems or diseases. In sum, the self-reported health of Valium users appeared to be poorer than the health of nonusers at Time 1. [30]

Use of Valium with Other Prescribed Drugs

Users and nonusers of Valium during the six weeks prior to an interview were compared to determine if they differed in the number of other prescribed drugs they took during that same period. When examining these comparisons, recall that differences between Valium users and nonusers were intentionally biased by respondent recruitment procedures (see Chapter 3). Nonusers were selected in part because they had no antianxiety drugs, antidepressants, antipsychotics, or antihistamines on their pharmacy records during the respondent intake period (although virtually all of them had filled a prescription for some medication). Thus, Valium users would be expected to take more drugs, particularly of these types. In fact, Valium users were found to take more prescribed drugs of almost all types than nonusers.

Table 5.9 shows the average number of different prescribed drugs used by respondents sometime in the six weeks prior to each interview. The table provides two different averages. The first excludes Valium, and the second (in parentheses) excludes all antianxiety drugs, antidepressants, antipsychotics, and antihistamines. Valium-using respondents mentioned about 3.0 drugs other than Valium, and nonusers mentioned about 1.8 drugs, averaging across all waves. Thus, Valium users reported about 1.2 more drugs than nonusers. When antianxiety drugs, antidepressants, antipsychotics, and antihistamines were excluded from these analyses, Valium-using respondents still mentioned about one more drug, on the average, than nonusers.

---

[30] As reported in Chapter 3, the selection criteria used for nonusers of Valium may have biased the results in this direction.

Table 5.9

AVERAGE NUMBER OF DIFFERENT PRESCRIBED DRUGS USED BY
VALIUM USERS AND NONUSERS IN THE SIX WEEKS PRIOR TO
EACH INTERVIEW (EXCLUDING VALIUM)[1]

	Valium Users in the Prior 6 Weeks	Nonusers of Valium in the Prior 6 Weeks
Wave 1	2.71 (2.06)	1.77 (1.23)
Wave 2	2.97 (2.25)	1.82 (1.27)
Wave 3	3.14 (2.39)	1.81 (1.29)
Wave 4	3.08 (2.37)	1.77 (1.29)

Note: Differences between Valium users and nonusers were
intentionally biased by respondent recruitment procedures.
Thus, averages in parentheses were computed excluding antianxiety drugs, antidepressants, antipsychotics, and
antihistamines--the drugs which nonusers of Valium were
required not to have on their pharmacy records in order to
be included in the study. See "Methods" Chapter 3 for
details.

[1]Although the total N for each wave was 675, there was a
shift of respondents from the Valium group to the non-
Valium group from the beginning to the end of the study.
This shift occurred as some respondents stopped taking
Valium.

Table 5.10 shows the percentages of Valium users (in the
six weeks prior to Wave 1) and nonusers who took particular
types of prescribed drugs.[31] This table provides percentages
of all prescribed drugs other than Valium, and of all drugs excluding antianxiety drugs, antihistamines, antidepressants, and
antipsychotics (in parentheses). The table uses the drug effect coding scheme described in Chapter 4 and in Appendix Q.
The first two columns of the table show that a higher propor-

[31]Data comparing Valium users and nonusers from each of
the other three waves were also examined and found to be basically consistent with Wave 1 data. Thus, primarily data from
Wave 1 are presented.

tion of Valium users took at least one other prescribed drug of almost every type in the six weeks prior to Wave 1. The largest difference is in the case of drugs having effects similar to that of Valium; use of such drugs was reported by 63% of Valium users, but only 34% of nonusers.

Columns three and four of Table 5.10 show the percentages of drugs mentioned having each of the five effects. For example, 41% of all drugs (other than Valium) mentioned by Valium-using respondents at Wave 1 were coded as having CNS depressant-like effects; 33% of all drugs mentioned by non-users had such effects. The similarity of most of these percentages suggests that the distribution of drugs having these five effects is similar within Valium-using and non-using subgroups, even though the actual number of other drugs and the percentage of respondents using other drugs were greater in the Valium-using group.

The percentages in parentheses, which exclude the drug types used in respondent recruitment, reflect similar patterns of use to those discussed above. The percentages dropped about equally in Valium-using and nonusing groups. This suggests that the drugs listed in a person's pharmacy record do not necessarily reflect the drugs that the person actually takes in the following weeks; if nonusers did not take such drugs, percentages for nonusers would not have decreased when drugs used for respondent selection were removed from the analyses. This is not surprising, given that (a) there was some lag time between examination of the pharmacy record and the actual interview, during which respondents could have obtained a new prescription, (b) respondents may have taken "old" prescriptions, from some time prior to the pharmacy record intake period, and (c) respondents could have obtained a prescription from another pharmacy. This does not make the nonusers an unsuitable comparison group, as long as these differences are kept in mind and appropriate controls are made.

The percentages of Valium users and nonusers who took at least one drug intended for psychoactive effect was also examined. This analysis was broken down into two drug groups at Wave 1: prescription psychotropics (benzodiazepines other than

147

Table 5.10

USE OF DRUGS OTHER THAN VALIUM BY PHARMACEUTICAL EFFECT (WAVE 1)[1]

Drug Effect	Percent of Respondents Mentioning at Least One Drug Having Specified Effect Below		Percent of Drugs Mentioned Having Specified Effect Below[2]	
	Valium Users[3]	Non-Users[3]	Valium Users[3]	Non-Users[3]
Effect Similar to that of Valium	63% (50%)	34% (25%)	41% (34%)	33% (26%)
Effect Opposite to that of Valium	21% (19%)	14% (12%)	10% (11%)	11% (12%)
Effects Both Similar and Opposite to that of Valium	14% (8%)	11% (5%)	6% (4%)	8% (5%)
Effects Neither Similar nor Opposite to that of Valium (i.e., neutral)	51% (51%)	38% (38%)	39% (46%)	38% (47%)
Unknown Effect	10% (10%)	14% (12%)	5% (6%)	10% (11%)

Note: Differences between Valium users and nonusers were intentionally biased by respondent recruitment procedures. Thus, percentages in parentheses were computed excluding antianxiety drugs, antidepressants, antipsychotics, and antihistamines. These are drugs which nonusers of Valium were required not to have on their pharmacy records in order to be included in the study. See "Methods" Chapter 3 for details.

[1] Percentages based on frequency of use in the 6 weeks prior Wave 1. The other three waves had very similar percentages.

[2] The frequencies on which these numbers are based varies depending on the subgroup. For example, among the 345 respondents reporting the use of Valium at some time during the 6 weeks prior to Wave 1 (called "Valium users" in the table), there were 858 separate drugs mentioned (other than Valium). Of these, 84 (10%) were drugs expected to have an effect opposite to that of Valium. Note that only 71 respondents reporting use of Valium at some time in the previous 6 weeks is 345, and the number of nonusers is 330. At Wave 4 these numbers are 242 and 433, respectively.

[3] At Wave 1, the number of respondents reporting use of Valium at some time in the previous 6 weeks is 345, and the number of nonusers is 330. At Wave 4 these numbers are 242 and 433, respectively.

Valium, anti-depressants, anti-psychotics, anti-anxiety drugs, sedative/hypnotics, barbiturates and stimulants) and prescription analgesics (coronary vasodilators, opiate alkaloids and synthetics derivatives, and nonopiate analgesics). Among respondents who used Valium at some time in the last six weeks, 10.7% also took at least one prescribed psychotropic other than Valium, compared to 16.7% among nonusers. This is a statistically significant difference ($p < .02$). The comparable figures for analgesics are 39.1% for Valium users and 16.1% for nonusers, also a significant difference ($p < .01$). When psychotropics, analgesics, and street drugs (all having psychoactive properties) are combined, the comparable figures are 49.9% for Valium users and 31.5% for nonusers, again a significant difference ($p < .01$). (For statistics specifically on use of street drugs, see the next section.)

The data presented thus far describe use of drugs over the six weeks prior to the interview. This is because no detailed information was obtained on most prescribed drugs (i.e., those not on the interview follow-up list) regarding use in the week prior to each interview. Only general information about use in the six weeks prior to each interview was obtained for these "unlisted" drugs. As can be seen in Appendix O, however, information regarding use in the last week (but not necessarily simultaneous use) was obtained on 72% of all mentions of prescribed drugs having some effect similar to that of Valium (at Wave 1). This was because these drugs were on the questionnaire follow-up list (presented in Appendix I, Section F, p. 33).

Forty percent of respondents at Wave 1 who took Valium in the last week also took at least one other drug during that period having some CNS depressant-like effects (49% at Wave 4); 25% of nonusers at Wave 1 took at least one drug having such an effect (22% at Wave 4). The zero-order correlation between Valium use and use of CNS depressant-like drugs in the last week was .17 at Wave 1. [32]

---

[32] Valium users in the last week were compared to nonusers only with respect to their use of prescribed drugs having CNS depressant-like effects. Use of other classes of drugs in the

149

How much of this use of other drugs by Valium users occurred during times when they were not taking Valium? How does that amount of use compare to use of these drugs by people who were not Valium users? To answer these questions, respondents reporting use of Valium sometime in the last six weeks but not in the last week were compared to respondents reporting no Valium use. Twenty-two percent of nonusers and 39% of Valium users reported use of at least one other drug having a CNS depressant-like effect in the last week (at Wave 4 these percentages were 19% and 43%, respectively).[33] Thus it appears that use of these other drugs in the last week was greater among the Valium-using respondents than among the nonusers, regardless of whether Valium was actually taken in the last week.

The above analyses can not indicate specifically whether the other drugs were frequently used simultaneously with Valium, even if they were both used at some time during the same week. These analyses do suggest that respondents who used Valium also tended to use more prescribed drugs of other kinds. These results support other findings reported in the sections of this chapter dealing with the "Portrait of Valium Users" and the upcoming section "Searching for Spurious Effects" which suggest that people who use Valium are likely to be less healthy, and consequently use more medication than nonusers. The above results are fairly stable across the four waves of the study.

Use of Valium with Alcohol, Cigarettes,
Caffeine, and Street Drugs

Analyses similar to those presented above were also performed to compare Valium users to nonusers on their consumption of alcohol, cigarettes, caffeine, and street drugs (collectively referred to hereafter as "other substances"). These

---

last week (e.g., having stimulant or neutral effects) was too infrequent for meaningful analysis (see Appendices O, Q, and "Measuring Use of Medications" in Chapter 4).

[33] Comparisons were made only with respect to the use of drugs having CNS depressant-like effects in the last week because that category was the only one with a sufficient number of drug mentions (see previous footnote).

analyses were also performed separately for males and females because national surveys reveal that males tend to consume more alcohol, street drugs, and cigarettes than females (Fishburne, et al., 1979).

Table 5.11 depicts such comparisons for use of Valium and other substances in the last week. The table shows both a comparison of average use and a comparison of percentages of respondents reporting at least one use of each of the other substances. [34] For example, at Wave 1, respondents using Valium at some time in the last week drank an average of 5.7 alcoholic drinks in the same week; nonusers drank an average of 6.1 drinks. This difference is not statistically significant. Also, 52% of Valium users and 66% of nonusers reported drinking alcohol at least once in the last week. A statistical significance test applied to the latter percentages shows that Valium users were significantly less likely ($p < .01$) to have had one or more drinks in the week prior to the Wave 1 interview than nonusers. The zero-order correlation between use of Valium and alcohol in the week prior to Wave 1 was .01 (n.s.).

Valium users in the week prior to Wave 1 reported smoking significantly more cigarettes on the average than did nonusers. Valium users were also significantly more likely to have smoked at least once. In addition, the zero-order correlation between milligrams of Valium used and cigarettes smoked in the week prior to Wave 1 was low, but positive and statistically significant ($r = .14$, $p < .01$).

Valium users did not differ significantly from non-users in their use of caffeinated drinks or of street drugs. Zero-order correlations between Valium use and caffeine and street drug use were essentially zero.

At Wave 4 of the study, most of these basic differences still existed, although substance use had decreased somewhat for both groups, and the statistical significance of the differences was less or absent. Again, the general trend of respondents becoming healthier during the course of the study

---

[34] These figures are very similar to those found in a national sample by Fishburne, et al. (1979).

Table 5.11

AVERAGE USE OF ALCOHOL, CIGARETTES, CAFFEINE, AND STREET DRUGS IN THE LAST 7 DAYS:
VALIUM USERS IN THE LAST 7 DAYS VS. NONUSERS AT WAVE 1 AND AT WAVE 4.[2]

Variable		WAVE 1			WAVE 4		
		Mean	Standard Deviation	Percent of Respondents Greater Than Zero	Mean	Standard Deviation	Percent of Respondents Greater Than Zero
Number of Alcoholic Drinks in the last 7 days (Y412)	Valium users	5.7	14.2	52%**	4.7	7.5	47%**[3]
	Non-users	6.1	11.9	66%	4.5	7.7	60%
Number of Cigarettes Per Day in the Last 7 Days (X641)	Valium users	12.7**	17.1	47%*	10.9*	15.8	44%
	Non-users	9.0	14.4	38%	8.2	13.0	38%
Milligrams of Caffeine Per Day in the Last 7 days (Y411)	Valium users	421	658	82%	404	546	81%
	Non-users	465	536	87%	396	447	82%
Number of Uses of Street Drugs in the Last 7 Days (Y616)	Valium users	0.1	0.7	4%	0.1	1.1	2%
	Non-users	0.1	0.9	3%	0.1	0.7	3%

Note: Statistically significant (p ≤ .05) sex differences are noted when they occur.

* For a difference of this magnitude between Valium users and nonusers, p ≤ .05.

**For a difference of this magnitude between Valium users and nonusers, p ≤ .01.

[1]"Valium users" in this table are those respondents who took Valium in the last 7 days. Nonusers are respondents who did not take Valium at any of the four waves. The number of Valium users is 258 at Wave 1, and 189 at Wave 4. The number of nonusers is 308 at both waves.

[2]The t-test of independent means and chi-square statistics were used to compute significance levels of differences between means and percents respectively.

[3]Statistically significant difference only for females. This sex difference occurred only at Wave 4. Although the difference for males was not statistically significant, it was in the same direction.

152

is supported by their decreased use of affect-modifying substances.

Even though Table 5.11 depicts use of Valium and other substances over the last week, a question is still unanswered: Were Valium users consuming these other substances at the same time (or on the same days) that they took Valium, or did they use Valium and the other substances at different times? This study was not designed to deal explicitly with this question. Nevertheless, data from respondents about their pattern of Valium use over the six weeks prior to each interview provided an opportunity to explore some aspects of the question. Table 5.12 compares respondents who used Valium "every day or every other day" during the six weeks prior to each interview with the same respondents from Table 5.11 who never took Valium during the four waves of the study--a more extreme split between the two groups than in the earlier table. Although this would still provide no certainty that Valium use was simultaneous with use of the other substances, the likelihood of overlap on a given day would be increased.

Daily or almost daily Valium users consumed slightly less of most of these substances than Valium users as a whole. Thus, differences between Valium users and nonusers became slightly more pronounced (see Table 5.12), but only for alcohol consumption. Average use of alcohol in the last week, as well as the percentage of respondents who drank at least once, dropped both at Wave 1 and at Wave 4. The statistical significance of differences at Wave 1 remained the same as it was in Table 5.11, but at Wave 4 the differences increased. Thus, it appears that Valium users were particularly less likely to drink alcohol when they were daily users.

Another question regarding use of Valium and other substances was also explored: If Valium users are prone to take affect-modifying substances to make them feel better, do they take more such substances during times when they are not using Valium? This could be true even though they may reduce use of such substances during the times when they are actually taking Valium (as suggested above with alcohol). Table 5.13 presents data on respondents who used Valium at some time in the six

Table 5.12

AVERAGE USE OF ALCOHOL, CIGARETTES, CAFFEINE, AND STREET DRUGS IN THE LAST 7 DAYS: DAILY VALIUM USERS IN THE LAST 7 DAYS VS. NONUSERS AT WAVE 1 AND AT WAVE 4[1,2]

Variable		WAVE 1			WAVE 4		
		Mean	Standard Deviation	Percent of Respondents Greater Than Zero	Mean	Standard Deviation	Percent of Respondents Greater Than Zero
Number of Alcoholic Drinks in the last 7 days (Y412)	Valium users	4.8	15.7	48%**	2.4**	5.2	38%**
	Non-users	6.1	11.9	66%	4.7	7.5	60%
Number of Cigarettes Per Day in the Last 7 Days (X641)	Valium users	12.8**	17.2	47%	11.4*	16.1	45%
	Non-users	9.0	14.4	38%	8.2	13.0	38%
Milligrams of Caffeine Per Day in the Last 7 days (Y411)	Valium users	487	832	83%	401	557	79%
	Non-users	465	536	87%	396	447	82%
Number of Uses of Street Drugs in the Last 7 Days (Y616)	Valium users	0.04	0.4	1.4%	0.1	0.6	0.8%
	Non-users	0.1	0.9	2.9%	0.1	0.7	2.6%

Note: No statistically significant ($p \leq .05$) sex differences were found in this table.

* For a difference of this magnitude between Valium users and nonusers, $p \leq .05$.

**For a difference of this magnitude between Valium users and nonusers, $p \leq .01$.

[1] "Valium users" in this table are those respondents who took Valium in the last 7 days and who took Valium "every day or every other day" during the last six weeks. Nonusers in this table are those respondents who did not take Valium at any of the four waves. The number of Valium users is 140 at Wave 1, and 118 at Wave 4. The number of nonusers is 308 at both Wave 1 and at Wave 4.

[2] The t-test of independent means and chi-square statistics were used to compute significance levels of differences between means and percents respectively.

weeks prior to an interview but <u>not</u> in the prior seven days, and compares them to respondents who did not use Valium at all in the course of the study. This table is structured similarly to Table 5.11.

Use of cigarettes and caffeinated drinks is almost identical in Tables 5.11 through 5.13: Valium users tended to smoke more cigarettes than nonusers, and the two groups did not differ with respect to use of caffeinated drinks. Thus, the Valium users appeared to smoke more cigarettes and consume about the same amount of caffeine as nonusers, regardless of whether they were actually taking Valium during the same week. In other words, these habits appeared to be relatively stable, regardless of Valium use. Similar patterns exist within Wave 4, although mean levels were lower and statistical significance of differences was not achieved within Wave 4 (a pattern also observable in Table 5.11).

The picture is slightly different for alcohol and street drug consumption for Valium users who did not use Valium in the seven days prior to a particular wave (see Table 5.13). At Wave 1, although no statistically significant differences were found between Valium users and nonusers on the whole, female Valium users appeared to be consuming significantly more alcohol on the average (during a week when <u>not</u> taking Valium) than female nonusers. Valium users of both sexes reported a higher mean level of street drug use than did nonusers. Also, more female Valium users reported at least one use of a street drug in the last week (during a week when <u>not</u> taking Valium) than female nonusers. Similar but statistically non-significant trends existed for males. By Wave 4 these results changed, with Valium and non-Valium groups being virtually identical with respect to their use of alcohol. Also at Wave 4, differences in the average use of street drugs applied only to males, and no significant difference existed in the number of respondents using a street drug one or more times. [35]

---

[35] The number of street drug users in this study is quite small, so caution is urged regarding the reliability and generalizability of this finding. For example, the 8.1% of Valium users who reported use of at least one street drug in the last week at Wave 1 only represents 7 respondents; the 2.7%

Table 5.13

AVERAGE USE OF ALCOHOL, CIGARETTES, CAFFEINE, AND STREET DRUGS IN THE LAST 7 DAYS: VALIUM USERS IN THE LAST 6 WEEKS (BUT NOT IN THE LAST 7 DAYS) VS. NONUSERS AT WAVE 1 AND AT WAVE 4 [1,2]

Variable		WAVE 1			WAVE 4		
		Mean	Standard Deviation	Percent of Respondents Greater Than Zero	Mean	Standard Deviation	Percent of Respondents Greater Than Zero
Number of Alcoholic Drinks in the last 7 days (Y412)	Valium users	9.2[3]*	25.7	57%	4.2	6.6	57%
	Non-users	6.1	11.9	66%	4.7	7.5	60%
Number of Cigarettes Per Day in the Last 7 Days (XG41)	Valium users	12.6*	16.2	50%*	11.1	16.3	37%
	Non-users	9.0	14.4	38%	8.2	13.0	38%
Milligrams of Caffeine Per Day in the Last 7 days (Y411)	Valium users	483	685	89%	381	437	74%
	Non-users	464	536	87%	396	447	82%
Number of Uses of Street Drugs in the Last 7 Days (Y616)	Valium users	0.4*	1.4	8.3%[3]	0.8[4]	5.5	3.9%
	Non-users	0.1	0.9	2.9%	0.1	0.7	2.6%

Note: Statistically significant (p ≤ .05) sex differences are noted when they occur.

* For a difference of this magnitude between Valium users and nonusers, p ≤ .05.

[1] "Valium users" in this table are those respondents who took Valium at some time during the six weeks prior to the interview, but not in the last 7 days. Nonusers are respondents who did not take Valium at any of the four waves. The number of Valium users is 71 at Wave 1, and 51 at Wave 4. The number of non-users is 308 at both Wave 1 and Wave 4.

[2] The t-test of independent means and chi-square statistics were used to compute significance levels of differences between means and percents respectively.

[3] Statistically significant difference for females only, but see footnote 11.

[4] Statistically significant difference for males only, but see footnote 11.

Thus, there appeared to be a slight tendency for female Valium users to use more alcohol during times (a) when they were not using Valium, and (b) when their levels of stress and negative affect were highest (i.e., at Wave 1 as opposed to Wave 4). When levels of negative affect and stress were lower (i.e., at Wave 4), no differences between Valium-using and non-using groups appeared. If mental health and stress were controlled, the small differences which exist at Wave 1 would likely disappear. Sex differences appeared to account for most of the differences in street drug use in Table 5.13. Nevertheless, as noted above, the frequency of such use brings even these small differences into question.

In summary, these analyses showed that Valium-using respondents drank less alcohol during times when they were using Valium. These findings may be due to compliance with the recommended medical regimen (i.e., not mixing Valium and alcohol). Such an effect could also be due to Valium users experiencing a decreased need for alcohol, or nonusers using alcohol instead of other affect-modifying substances such as Valium. There was a slight tendency for female Valium users to drink more alcohol during times when they were not taking Valium but when they may have had particularly stressful or unhappy life conditions. Valium users tended to smoke more cigarettes than nonusers, but there were no differences in consumption of caffeinated drinks. Analyses of street drug use suggest little evidence of differences between Valium users and nonusers.

Professional Counseling and Valium Use

It has sometimes been suggested that the use of tranquilizers in conjunction with psychotherapy may be an effective combination for treating anxiety. To see how many respondents received professional counseling in conjunction with Valium use in this study, respondents were asked if they had received any kind of therapy or counseling from a minister, a psychologist, a psychiatrist, a marriage counselor, or any other kind of

---

of nonusers represents only 9 respondents. When examined by sex, these numbers became even smaller.

therapist. At the first interview respondents were asked if they had received such counseling at any time during the previous year. At subsequent interviews they were asked if they had received counseling since the last interview.

Of the 345 Valium users at Time 1, 28% (98 respondents) reported having seen a therapist or counselor during the past year. Of these 98 respondents, almost half (47) also reported seeing a counselor at least one time during the 6-week periods prior to interviews 2 through 4. There were 27 Time 1 Valium users (8%) who did not report seeing a counselor during the year prior to the first interview but did indicate they had seen a counselor at least once after the first interview. Only 6% of Time 1 Valium users reported seeing a counselor at all four interviews, and 64% did not report seeing a counselor or therapist at any of the four interviews.

Across all four waves the types of counselors most frequently seen were psychiatrists, psychologists, and ministers. Of the 200 mentions of professional counselors seen, 40% were psychiatrists, 23% were psychologists, 12% were ministers, and the remaining 25% were an assortment of social workers, marriage and family counselors, other physicians, and other types of therapists.

An additional factor potentially related to the effectiveness of therapy was the counselor's supportiveness as perceived by the Valium user (cf., Uhlenhuth, et. al., 1969). In this study perceived supportiveness was assessed with a 2-item index comprised of questions asking how much time was available with the counselor to discuss everything the respondent wanted to talk about, and how "warm or cold" the counselor was with people. On the average and across all four waves, Valium users who received professional counseling rated their therapists as very supportive (4 on a scale from 1 to 5). Respondent ratings of support from counselors were the same (within rounding) as the ratings made by all Valium users of the support from their prescribing physicians. Both physicians and counselors were rated on identical dimensions.

Attitudes Regarding the Use of Valium and Minor Tranquilizers

The patient's own attitudes toward a medication can be an important determinant of its effectiveness, hence the concern for including placebos in double-blind trials of drugs. This study examined two sets of attitudes regarding tranquilizers: attitudes about their efficacy and appropriateness in general, and attitudes about Valium's helpfulness for the respondent in particular. This distinction is important because a person's attitudes regarding the use of tranquilizers by people in general might differ from one's attitude toward his or her own use of tranquilizers or Valium in particular.

At Time 4 all respondents were asked about their attitudes toward tranquilizers in general. An index of these questions covered the extent to which the respondent believed that tranquilizers generally prevented versus helped people work through problems and regain control of their lives. The index also asked about beliefs regarding the safety of tranquilizers and about the position that it is better to use willpower than tranquilizers to solve one's problems (a concept originally termed "psychopharmacologic Calvinism" by Klerman in 1972). Item analyses led to the development of an overall index of favorable/unfavorable attitude toward tranquilizers which included questions about the morality as well as the efficacy of use. Overall, about half the respondents had a favorable attitude and the other half an unfavorable attitude toward the use of tranquilizers (an average of 2.5 on a 4-point scale). About 6% were strongly opposed to tranquilizer use, about 43% were moderately opposed, about 43% were moderately in favor, and about 8% were strongly in favor. There was a significant difference in the percentage of Time 4 Valium users versus non-users endorsing each point on this index. A favorable attitude was expressed by 72% of Valium users, but only by 39% of non-users.

At Times 1 through 4 Valium users were asked about their perceptions of the helpfulness to them of Valium specifically. The index included items dealing with the extent to which the medication made the person feel better, increased control over emotions, and increased ability to deal with problems in life. Results showed that Valium users considered Valium to be help-

159

ful, with ratings being almost identical at all four waves (a mean of about 3.5 where 1 = low endorsement and 4 = high endorsement; the standard deviation was about .75 at all four waves). On the whole, these findings suggested that Valium-taking individuals generally believed in the efficacy of Valium.

Summary of Portrait of Valium Users

In this study Valium was prescribed most often by physicians in general practice or internal medicine. Osteopaths and psychiatrists were the next most likely to prescribe Valium. These findings are consistent with data drawn from national studies.

Most Valium users found their prescribing physician supportive. The small percent who made use of the services of therapists or counselors also found them similarly supportive.

The most commonly prescribed dosages of Valium per day ranged from 10-20 mg. As has been found elsewhere, on the average respondents tended to take less rather than more milligrams of Valium than were prescribed, a pattern of use sometimes described as conservative. About 1/3 of the Valium users took Valium "only once in a while" whereas about half the Valium users reported taking Valium "every day or every other day the whole time" during the 6-week period prior to the interview.

The large majority (83%) of persons taking Valium reported taking it within the seven days preceding each interview, and the majority of Valium users (59%) took some Valium during each of the 6-week periods prior to each of the four interviews. Nevertheless, there was a considerable range of dosages and patterns of use across and within the 6-week periods between interviews. Users of Valium generally considered the drug to be helpful.

Valium users tended to drink less alcohol than nonusers, particularly during weeks when they used Valium daily or every other day. Valium users also tended to smoke more cigarettes than nonusers. There was little evidence of differences with regard to caffeine or street drug use. While Valium users tended to take more prescribed drugs of all other kinds than nonusers, this difference was probably largely due to the intentional bias in recruitment procedures for the two groups.

Bivariate Analyses

Overview

This section presents a set of analyses that were performed as necessary but preliminary steps to using more complex multivariate longitudinal methods. These steps were needed, in part, to make sure that certain statistical assumptions (i.e., linearity, additivity) were valid. The section begins by describing analyses that were applied to determine the best measures of Valium use for the study. Then there is a summary of the checks that were made to see if any of the bivariate relationships were curvilinear. If curvilinear relationships exist, analyses that assume simple linearity, such as correlational analyses, will underestimate the total amount of relationship between the pair of variables. One needs to identify such situations and make appropriate adjustments, if necessary, prior to interpreting results.

Next, the text describes an examination of the stability of means, standard deviations, and relationships among variables from Time 1 and Time 4. Evidence of instability could indicate that certain processes linking variables were changing from wave to wave of data collection.

A set of correlational analyses appear next which examine the extent to which relationships among pairs of variables (such as between Valium and anxiety) changed in magnitude depending on whether the variables were measured at the same point in time (no lag or zero lag) or were measured at different points in time (lagged relationships). These analyses searched for evidence that there was an optimum lag or lags for detecting effects of one variable on another (such as for detecting the effects of Valium on quality of life).

Finally we examine two types of effects that may change the relationships that variables have with one another or may change the interpretation of those relationships--spurious effects and moderator effects. Spurious effects resulting from

161

other variables can cause a relationship to look stronger or weaker than would be the case if these effects were controlled. Moderators can influence relationships so that they are of different magnitude in one subgroup than in another subgroup. Both of these types of effects are explained in more detail below.

Which Measures of Valium Should Be Used?

Milligram-weighted versus unweighted measures. Was the number of milligrams per Valium pill an important component of Valium use in this study? To answer this question, two types of measures of Valium use were constructed: measures weighted by the milligrams consumed and unweighted versions which assessed only the number of pills taken. [36] These two types of measures were constructed for each of several different indicators of Valium use. Zero-order correlations between milligram-weighted and unweighted measures ranged from .84 to .86. Thus, the two types of measures were very similar, but not identical.

Then milligram-weighted and unweighted measures were each examined to determine their correlations with a set of ten other measures representative of a variety of constructs in the study. Those other measures included anxiety, quality of life-as-a-whole, social support, performance at work and in the personal life, quality of life of the personal other, control, stress, and coping by using a positive approach. In about 80% to 90% of the cases the milligram-weighted measures correlated more highly than unweighted measures with these other variables. The differences in correlations ranged from about .01 to .08. Although the differences in correlations were small, and the number of Valium pills consumed explained most of the variance in interpersonal and social factors, the number of milligrams per Valium pill also appeared to be relevant. Thus, the milligram-weighted measures of Valium were used for most analyses presented in this report.

---

[36] The latter measures were early versions of measures of Valium use over the seven days or six weeks prior to Wave 1, and had not been weighted by milligrams per pill.

Pattern of use. Did the weekly pattern with which people took Valium explain additional variance in people's behaviors and emotions, above and beyond the effect of the number of milligrams they consumed? This question was addressed by examining respondents' reports of their pattern of Valium use in the week prior to each interview; response choices were "every day the whole week," "every day except one," "a few days," "just one day the whole week," or "none at all." Multiple Classification Analysis (MCA), a regression-like technique (cf., Andrews, Morgan, Sonquist, & Klem, 1973), was used to examine main and interaction effects of Valium use and pattern of use during the week prior to Wave 1. The dependent variables in these analyses were anxiety and quality of life-as-a-whole at Waves 1 and 2.

Evidence of interaction effects would suggest that pattern of use had an effect for some levels of Valium use, but not for others. Two findings are of particular interest: (a) the pattern of use variable accounted for only trivial amounts of variance in anxiety and quality of life beyond the effects of milligrams of Valium, and (b) there were no significant interaction effects between pattern of use and milligrams of Valium.

Any use versus nonuse. Is it possible that the quantity of Valium taken was less important than whether respondents took Valium at all? In other words, could any dosage have the same effect compared to not taking Valium at all? Three analyses were conducted to answer this question. For each, a simple dichotomous measure of Valium use (yes, took Valium, or no, did not take Valium) was created, for each of the 6-week periods prior to each interview.

A correlation matrix was generated which contained the dichotomous measure of Valium at 14 different timepoints and 79 other major indices, most of which were measured midway through the study (e.g., stress, quality of life, social support, affects, performance, and control at Wave 2). This matrix was compared to another matrix that was identical, except that it used the continuous measure of Valium (i.e., the milligram-weighted version discussed above). A comparison of the 1,106 pairs of correlations between Valium-taking and major indices

(14 x 79 = 1,106) showed that in no cases were the correlation coefficients for members of each pair different by more than .16. Most differences were close to zero. Only six of the differences were as large as .10. Of these six, four involved attitudes about the helpfulness of Valium (for which the continuous measure showed slightly stronger relationships than the dichotomous measure). These analyses indicated that, for nearly all of the basic correlational relationships of interest in this study, whether one used the dichotomous or continuous measures of Valium made no difference.

Another set of analyses further investigated the potential value of a yes/no measure of Valium use. One analysis examined whether the measure of use would have stronger effects for people who were under high rather than low stress. This could be the case if people decided to take or not take Valium depending on how much stress they were experiencing. To examine this issue, an analysis was conducted in which separate correlation matrices were computed for high and low stress subgroups (based on the "Multiple Stress" measure). About 85 respondents were in each group. Results were the same as above: continuous and dichotomous measures did not differ substantially or systematically in their relationships with other variables.

In a final examination of the dichotomous measure of Valium use, structural equation analysis was used to examine the effects of Valium on anxiety and quality of life. Relationships among the concepts were nearly identical to those from a similar analysis using continuous Valium measures, although the "fit" of the model was somewhat worse. (see description of Model A under "Multivariate Modeling" below.) [37]

As a result of these investigations, the continuous milligram-weighted measure was selected for most analyses. It is used throughout this report.

---

[37] As for use versus nonuse of Valium in a large number of interactions, the reader is referred to the section below on "Valium as a Moderator of the Stress-Strain Relationship."

Therapeutic dose. There is debate about how much Valium must be taken in order to derive benefit from it. After discussing the issue among the project staff and with several pharmacy experts, 30 mg of Valium per week was selected as a minumum therapeutic dose and 280 mg per week was selected as a maximum therapeutic dose. This does not constitute a recommendation for usage. These cutoff points were selected to test whether respondents taking more or less than one arbitrary indicator of therapeutic dose per week would differ with respect to the effects of Valium.

Valium-using respondents were separated into two groups: those using a therapeutic dose of Valium in the week prior to an interview, and those using a nontherapeutic dose. Then correlations among a set of about 80 major indices were compared for the two subgroups. The two groups did not differ significantly. (See Appendix T for a more detailed description of this analysis.)

Check for Curvilinear Relationships

This study has focused on relationships, both bivariate and multivariate, to draw conclusions about the social-psychological causes and consequences of Valium-taking. The statistical methods commonly used to examine such relationships are correlational and require the assumption that variables are related in a linear fashion. Because many of the analyses in this study were correlational, specific checks were made on the appropriateness of the linearity assumption.

Measures of Valium use and several indices representing all of the primary variables in the study were interrelated using two different statistics: (a) Pearson product-moment correlation coefficients, and (b) eta coefficients. When squared, either coefficient indicates the percentage of variation in one variable which is associated with variation in another variable. However, the correlation coefficient indicates association only of a linear form, whereas the eta coefficient indicates all association between two variables including both linear and curvilinear components. Thus, the difference between these squared coefficients indicates the percentage of variance which is due to a curvilinear association

165

between two variables and which would, therefore, be lost in correlational analyses.

Both correlation and eta coefficients were computed for a set of primary variables to test their associations at various lags (e.g., one variable measured at one interview and the other variable measured at a different interview). Because of its central importance in the study, Valium use was related to 20 other primary variables; some of these primary variables were also related to each other. Some comparisons involved a zero lag (e.g., where both variables were measured at the same interview); others involved a lag of one (e.g., where the measure of one variable was taken at one interview and the other variable at an adjacent interview); other comparisons involved lags of two and three interview periods.

Of 184 comparisons between the correlation and eta coefficients, only seven showed more than a 1% difference in the accounted for variance. The largest of these differences was slightly less than 2% of the variance accounted for. These results suggested that none of the primary variables were curvilinearly related to one another. Thus, the linearity assumption necessary for correlational analyses was met.

Stabilities in Means, Standard Deviations and Relationships Over Time

Means, standard deviations, and correlations at Time 1 and Time 4 were compared for the 675 respondents interviewed at all four timepoints. Did mean levels of anxiety, for example, remain stable over time? Did the amount of variability in anxiety remain stable over time? Did the magnitude of relationships, such as between anxiety and Valium use, remain constant over time? These are the types of questions this analysis addressed. In this analysis 53 variables were examined including affect, quality of life, social support, social conflict, coping and defense, control, stress, performance, psychotherapy, and attitudes about tranquilizers, and use of alcohol, caffeine, and Valium.

Means. Of the 53 pairs of means examined, 31 (58%) differed significantly between Time 1 and Time 4. In general, respondents' lives seemed to improve between Time 1 and Time 4.

Respondents' levels of anger, anxiety, depression, somatization, and general negative affect were all significantly higher at Time 1 than at Time 4. Respondents' quality of life in the self, personal life, sleep, life as a whole, and cognitive domains were all significantly lower at Time 1 than at Time 4. Both informational social support and social conflict were significantly higher at Time 1 than at Time 4. Use of the coping techniques of "positive approach" and "help from others" decreased significantly over time. The amount of internal control respondents had and wanted over their emotions significantly increased, while the amount of control respondents thought others had over their personal lives significantly decreased. The amount of control respondents thought chance had over their personal lives, and the amount of chance control respondents wanted over their personal lives, both significantly decreased. Three out of four stresses decreased significantly (role conflict in work life, role ambiguity in personal life, and negative life events). Levels of one stressor (role ambiguity in work life) increased significantly. Levels of self-rated technical and social performance in the work life decreased significantly. The number of respondents in therapy decreased. Finally, use of both alcohol and Valium decreased significantly.

In sum, respondents showed improvement on a wide variety of measures from Time 1 to Time 4. Respondents reported worse conditions over time for only a few variables, notably increased role ambiguity and decreased performance in the work domain. Given that respondent selection was based on having recently filled a prescription, it is not surprising that respondents' lives appeared to be at a low point at Time 1 and showed improvement by Time 4. At Time 1 many respondents apparently had health problems which caused them to see a physician and fill a prescription as part of the medical treatment. Presumably by Time 4 these problems were disappearing either because medical treatment had been effective, because patients had adapted to the problem(s), because a natural course of abatement had taken place or any combination of these.

167

Standard Deviations. Most standard deviations were smaller at Time 4 than at Time 1. However, except for a few cases, these differences were quite small (typical Time 4 standard deviations were 90% of Time 1 standard deviations). The standard deviations for the caffeine and alcohol measures were much smaller at Time 4 than at Time 1. (Time 4 standard deviations were 50-80% of Time 1 standard deviations.)

Relationships. The magnitudes of the correlations among these 53 variables at Time 1 were compared with those at Time 4. Fifteen percent of the differences between Time 1 and Time 4 correlations were significant at the p<.05 level. [38] There was a tendency for correlations with measures of affect to be stronger at Time 1. In contrast there was a trend for correlations with quality of life variables to be stronger at Time 4. Most of these differences were small, however, and are unlikely to influence interpretation of the findings.

Bivariate Relationships at Various Lags

Purpose and nature of the analyses. Given that nearly all variables were measured at four waves, and that the retrospective "calendar" portion of the interview provided measures of a few variables (Valium-taking, anxiety, quality of life-as-a-whole) for each of 24 weeks, it was possible to examine relationships that reflected conditions at different timepoints. For example, the study lends itself to seeing how Valium-taking relates to levels of anxiety at any of many different weeks prior to the Valium-taking, and also to anxiety at many different weeks after the Valium-taking. These are called "lagged" relationships. Exploring relationships at various lags is important because it can provide hints about what might be reasonable time intervals required for the effects of something (such as Valium-taking) to show up and about the most promising time intervals to use in subsequent analyses. [39]

---

[38] Because many variables in the study are interrelated, it is not safe to assume that random fluctuations would produce only 5% statistically significant differences at the p<.05 level.

[39] Observing that a particular interval shows the strongest relationships does not prove that that is the causal interval.

168

A few words about terminology and a simple hypothetical example will clarify the later presentation of results. The time interval (in weeks) between the two variables being related is the _lag_ of the relationship. A lag-0 ("lag-zero") relationship is one in which two variables refer to the same time; sometimes this is called a "simultaneous" or "concurrent" relationship. Positive lags refer to situations in which the assumed effect comes _after_ the assumed cause; negative lags indicate the reverse order. For example, if Valium-taking is the assumed cause and anxiety is the assumed effect, a lag 3 relationship would show how Valium-taking related to anxiety 3 weeks later.

In a study such as this there are usually multiple estimates of any particular lagged relationship, and the relationship reported is the mean value of _all_ _possible_ estimates. [40] For example, linking Valium-taking at Week 1 to anxiety at Week 4 provides one estimate of the lag 3 relationship. Using data from weeks 2 and 5 provides another estimate; so do data from Weeks 3 and 6; and so on up to Weeks 21 and 24, which is the end of the series. In this instance, we would report the mean of 21 separate relationships as our best estimate of the lag 3 relationship.

Figure 5.2 shows lagged relationships for some _hypothetical_ data and suggests the general trends one would expect to see if Valium-taking were to be associated with long-term reductions in anxiety. In Figure 5.2 the magnitude of hypothetical relationship between Valium-taking and anxiety is shown on the vertical axis and the lag interval appears on the horizontal axis. Note that when anxiety _precedes_ Valium-taking (negative lags, on the left of the plot) the relationships are

---

Kessler and Greenberg (1981) present a technical discussion on why this is the case.

[40] Averaging over all the estimates is a reasonable procedure when one is observing a stable system--e.g., when the relationships over a 3-week lag in June are about the same as over a 3-week lag in December. Although we observed a modest tendency for relationships to increase as respondents' experience with the study lengthened, the increase was not large enough to lead us to reject the stability assumption.

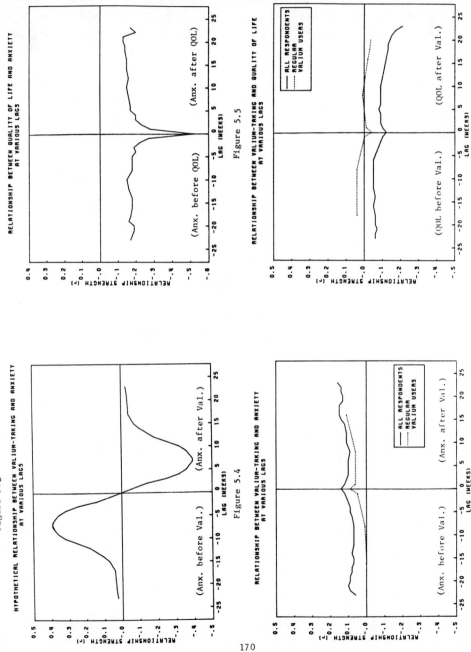

Figure 5.2

HYPOTHETICAL RELATIONSHIP BETWEEN VALIUM-TAKING AND ANXIETY
AT VARIOUS LAGS

(Anx. before Val.)   (Anx. after Val.)

Figure 5.4

RELATIONSHIP BETWEEN VALIUM-TAKING AND ANXIETY
AT VARIOUS LAGS

ALL RESPONDENTS
REGULAR VALIUM USERS

(Anx. before Val.)   (Anx. after Val.)

Figure 5.3

RELATIONSHIP BETWEEN QUALITY OF LIFE AND ANXIETY
AT VARIOUS LAGS

(Anx. before QOL)   (Anx. after QOL)

Figure 5.5

RELATIONSHIP BETWEEN VALIUM-TAKING AND QUALITY OF LIFE
AT VARIOUS LAGS

ALL RESPONDENTS
REGULAR VALIUM USERS

(QOL before Val.)   (QOL after Val.)

170

hypothesized to be positive--reflecting the idea that more anxious people later take greater amounts of Valium. Note also that the relationships are hypothesized to be negative when anxiety follows Valium-taking (positive lags, right side of the plot)--reflecting the idea that taking Valium is followed by reduced anxiety. However, these are hypothetical data and are presented only to describe the format of the figures that follow.

Two kinds of analyses were used to explore lagged relationships. The first used the 24 weeks of retrospective data to link Valium-taking, anxiety, and quality of life-as-a-whole. The second kind of analysis looked--more broadly but in less depth--at how Valium-taking related at various time intervals to about 80 other variables.

Results for Quality of life-as-a-whole and anxiety.

Figure 5.3 shows the mean estimates of the relationship between quality of life-as-a-whole and anxiety at various lags. [41] As can be seen, all relationships are negative (as expected); there is a sharp peak at lag 0 (r=-.52; "peaks" point downward for negative relationships), and a symmetrical and rapid decline in the magnitude of the relationships on both sides of lag 0; when lags reach 4-6 weeks, the relationships between life quality and anxiety are in the -.1 to -.2 range and do not decline much below that as lags get longer. Although not shown in the figure, virtually identical results were obtained when the relationships were computed only for regular Valium users (i.e., people who took some Valium during the 6-week period preceding each of the interviews).

Everything here is in accord with the idea that factors which influence evaluations of life quality concurrently influence anxiety. The only (mild) surprise is that

---

[41] The measures of quality of life-as-a-whole and of anxiety are single-item measures taken directly from the "calendar" portion of the interview. These measures include varying amounts of retrospection (0-6 weeks), but the retrospection effect, if any, will not influence these results because it has been spread out over the different lags by the averaging process described in the text.

relationships do not erode back to zero at long lags. This is
likely the result of some weak methodological effect.

Results   for   Valium-taking   and   anxiety.   Lagged
relationships for Valium-taking and anxiety are shown in Figure
5.4. [42] Two sets of relationships are shown: one based on all
675 respondents who completed four waves of data collection,
the second for the 217 of these who were regular Valium users--
defined as people who used some Valium during the 6-week period
preceding each of the data collections. In the figure one can
see that: (1) The relationship is always positive, regardless
of the lag and regardless of whether anxiety precedes or follows Valium-taking--i.e., higher amounts of anxiety go with
higher amounts of Valium, and vice versa; (2) the relationship
is always weak--never more than .16; (3) the regular Valium
users show even weaker relationships than the total group of
respondents; (4) slight peaks in the relationship occur at lag
0 and when anxiety follows Valium-taking by relatively long
periods (16-23 weeks); and (5) there is a tendency for the
relationship to be slightly stronger when anxiety follows
Valium-taking than when anxiety precedes Valium-taking, particularly among the subgroup of respondents who were regular
Valium users.

The pattern of results for Valium-taking and anxiety is
clearly very different from the hypothetical pattern presented
in Figure 5.2. Why is this? The persistent, but weak, positive relationship evident in Figure 5.4 is examined from a
variety of perspectives in later portions of this chapter and
shown, in the section on multivariate modeling, to be explainable by the persistence of certain factors (stress levels,
health status, etc.) that relate to both anxiety and Valium-
taking. The gentle rise in the relationship as the measurement
of anxiety changes from 16 weeks before Valium-taking to 16
weeks after Valium-taking is not yet understood--but never be-
comes strong enough to be important.   The absence of sharp

---

[42] The measure of Valium-taking is the adjusted bracketed
pills per week measure described in Chapter 4.   The anxiety
measure is as described in the preceding footnote.

peaks at particular lags suggests that there is no one lag interval that is much better for analysis than others.

Results for Valium-taking and quality of life-as-a-whole. The results for this pair of variables, shown in Figure 5.5, are very similar to those just discussed for the relationship between Valium-taking and anxiety, except that the sign of the relationship is reversed (as expected).[43] All relationships are weak (never exceeding -.21); the regular Valium users show even weaker relationships than the total group of respondents; there are very slight downward peaks at lag 0 and at the longest positive lags--18-23 weeks; and there is a slight tendency for the relationship to become more negative (or less positive) as one moves from negative to positive lags.

As will be seen in the sections of this chapter that discuss multivariate analyses, the persistent negative relationships that appear when all respondents are analyzed together can be attributed to stabilities in factors that relate to life quality and Valium-taking (e.g., stress and health, again). And, as with anxiety and Valium, the absence of sharp peaks here leaves open the choice of lag intervals for use in future analysis.

Results for Valium-taking and many major variables. This analysis examined the relationships between the amount (milligrams) of Valium taken during the week prior to a given interview and about 80 major variables used in the study, including measures of affect, life quality, social support, social conflict, coping and defense, control, sources of stress, performance, attitudes about Valium and tranquilizers, education, income, receipt of therapy, and use of caffeine, alcohol, cigarettes, and other psychoactive drugs.[44] Because of the large number of concepts involved, and because most of them had been measured only at the four main data collections (not on a week-by week basis), this analysis was less detailed than those

---

[43] The measures used in Figure 5.5 are the same as those described in the preceding footnotes.

[44] These measures include most of the scales described in Chapter 4.

described previously. Here, Valium-taking at 14 different timepoints during the study was related to the other variables, all of which were measured at week 12 of the study (i.e., the week of the second interview). This provided one estimate of each relationship at the following lags: -12, -10, -7, -6, -4, -2, -1, 0, +1, +2, +5, +6, +8, and +11. (The negative lags indicate that phenomena occurred before Valium-taking; positive lags, after Valium-taking.) Although less detailed, the analysis did provide a broad scan over more than a thousand relationships. It let us see how Valium-taking related to most of the important concepts of the study at a variety of positive and negative lags spanning the most likely time intervals for finding substantively important results.

Results were clear and can be easily summarized. With just a few exceptions, all relationships were very weak, and there were no sharp peaks associated with particular lags. There were mild tendencies, consistent with what what was reported above, for relationships to be slightly stronger when computed for positive lags (i.e., when Valium-taking preceded the other variable) than for zero or negative lags. The strongest relationships involved Valium-taking and attitudes about tranquilizers, and even here relationships reached only about .35. The next highest relationships (all positive in the middle .20's) involved Valium-taking and anxiety, [45] depression, somatic complaints, feelings of being "upset" (negative affect), evaluations of poor health, and the number of other CNS depressant-type drugs being taken. These, however, were the peak relationships between Valium-taking and these concepts, and at most lags the relationships were somewhat weaker. Most relationships in this analysis were under .20. In short, despite a broad scan, there seemed to be no strong relationships between Valium-taking and any of the other concepts, at any of a wide range of lags.

---

[45] In this analysis, the anxiety measure is the score on the Hopkins Symptom Checklist scale. The fact that this relationship between Valium-taking and anxiety is a little higher than the .16 peak relationship cited earlier is probably attributable to the use of different measures of anxiety and Valium-taking, and--as noted in Chapter 4-- the somewhat higher

In a further exploration of these relationships, these analyses were repeated using a different measure of Valium-taking. Instead of milligrams-per-week, a simple no-yes scale based on whether the person reported taking any Valium during the prior seven days was used. Changing the measure of Valium-taking basically did not alter the results reported above.

Conclusions. The conclusions one can draw from the results reported in this section were straightforward. Anxiety and quality of life were strongly, oppositely, and simultaneously related to each other. Valium-taking, however, showed only very weak relationships to anxiety, life quality, and virtually all other phenomena as they were measured in this study; and these relationships did not vary much according to the lag interval or according to which measure of Valium-taking was examined.

These simple relationships indicated that (a) regardless of the length of the lag, and (b) regardless of whether Valium use was antecedent to, concurrent with, or following the measurement of anxiety and quality of life, Valium use was associated with higher rather than lower anxiety, and lower rather than higher quality of life. One interpretation of these results, as suggested by multivariate analyses in later sections of this report, is that such effects were due to the stabilities of stress and health problems in people's lives. Controlling for such stabilities produced quite a different set of results and conclusions, which are described later.

Searching for Spurious Effects

Sometimes a meaningful relationship between two variables may be obscured by some third variable. A relationship between two variables may appear stronger or weaker than it would be if the effect of the third variable was removed. A classic example of such an effect is the relationship between verbal ability and height among young people. Of course, height doesn't cause verbal ability--their positive relationship is due to the effects of a third variable: aging or maturation

---

reliability of the anxiety scale as compared to the single-item "calendar" measure.

processes. Because verbal ability increases with age, and because height increases with age among young people, verbal
ability and height also increase together; this is a spurious
relationship which is decreased when the effects of the third
variable are removed.

Valium use might have spurious relationships with various
outcomes if, for example, (a) stress or (b) use of other drugs
were associated with the outcomes. For example, the negative
relationship between Valium use and quality of life could be
spurious if stress simultaneously increases Valium use and
decreases quality of life. As another example, the positive
relationship between Valium use and depression could be
spurious if people who use other drugs also tend to be people
who both use Valium and are depressed (e.g., because they are
sick). To examine these hypotheses, correlations were computed
between Valium use and 45 indices (including measures of Hopkins affects, quality of life, social support, conflict,
coping, performance, and control). These correlations were
computed for all respondents and then for subgroups high on
Multiple Stress, low on Multiple Stress, high on use of other
drugs having effects similar to that of Valium, low on use of
such drugs, high on use of drugs having effects opposite to
that of Valium, and low on use of such drugs.[46] With respect
to the above hypotheses, if the relationship between Valium use
and a particular outcome were in fact attributable to stress or
to use of other drugs, there should be a substantial decrease
or reversal of the relationship in both subgroups, when compared to all respondents as a whole. Many relationships
decreased slightly, but none decreased (or increased) substantially. Thus, it appeared that neither stress nor use of other
drugs substantially affected the relationship between Valium
use in the last seven days and other variables measured in this
study.

---

[46] These correlations were computed at Wave 1 and Wave 4 with
Multiple Stress as the potential confounding variable, and at
Wave 4 with the two variables measuring use of other drugs as
potential confounding variables.

Given that clinical trials have shown Valium to reduce anxiety, it seemed possible that the positive bivariate relationship between Valium use and anxiety in the last seven days (r=.30) might be spurious. The relationship between Valium use and 46 indices in the study at Time 1 (including measures of Hopkins Checklist affects, quality of life, social support, coping, control, stress, performance, and use of other drugs) was examined to test for such a spurious effect. The relationship between Valium and anxiety was examined after each one of the other variables was statistically controlled or "partialled out." None of these 46 variables was found to be producing a positive relationship and obscuring a negative relationship between Valium and anxiety.[47] Controlling for the effects of two variables, somatic complaints and perceived health, did result in a substantial decrease in the positive relationship between Valium and anxiety (each individually reducing the .30 relationship to .15). When the effects of these variables were removed simultaneously, the relationship dropped to .12--it did not however become a negative relationship. Thus, while the .30 relationship could be reduced, no important spurious effects attributable to variables we had measured appeared to be altering the basic low positive relationship between Valium and anxiety.

Potential Moderators of the Relationship Between Valium Use and Outcome Measures

Moderators are variables which change the relationship between two other variables. For example, if Valium has a stronger effect on anxiety in one age group than in another age group, then age is said to be a moderator of the relationship between Valium use and anxiety. Moderator effects are described statistically as interaction effects among three or more variables such as among anxiety, Valium use, and age.

There are two major reasons for searching for moderators in this study. One reason is that the discovery of moderators

---

[47] This same procedure was used to look for suppressor variables which, when their effects were removed, might increase the positive relationship between Valium and anxiety. No such variables were found.

would identify conditions under which a minor tranquilizer was more or less effective in producing a specified effect. Such information is of both applied and theoretical value. Second, the discovery of moderators may explain why nonmoderated relationships fail to appear. For example, for the set of respondents as a whole there might be no relationship between Valium-taking and performance. But it is possible that for some subgroup of respondents, e.g., those who are receiving high levels of social support, there is a relationship (either positive or negative) between Valium-taking and performance.

How should potential moderators be selected? It is not practical to search for potential moderating effects of all the variables in this study. We selected as potential moderators (a) those variables for which reasonable hypotheses could be generated and (b) demographic variables which might represent the accumulated effects of a number of underlying variables.

What methods and criteria should be used to detect moderator effects? One can search for two basic forms of evidence of an interaction (Arnold, 1982). One of these would be evidence that the linear correlation between two variables of interest, such as between Valium use and performance, is different for one group than for another. For example, if the correlations were .35 in the group reporting high social support and .06 in the group reporting low social support, this would be evidence of an interaction (assuming the difference between the two correlations is statistically significant). This method assumes that the distributions of scores on the two variables in the relationship to be potentially moderated are similar and that only the slope of the association of these two variables differs from one subgroup to another. If this assumption is not met, correlations in different subgroups may be different merely because there is different variation in one or both of the variables in the subgroups. (We did check for this potential problem in our data but no adjustments were necessary.)

A second method of searching for interactions is to examine the differences in the mean levels of an outcome variable. If the effects of one variable on mean levels of an out-

178

come variable are different for different levels of a third variable, this is evidence of an interaction. For example, if the effects of Valium versus no Valium on mean levels of performance were different for males and females, this would demonstrate an interaction.

Since we were interested in relationships more than mean levels, we used correlations to test for moderator effects. Moderator effects were examined by comparing subgroup correlations. High and low subgroups were formed on each potential moderator (e.g., high social support and low social support) using extreme splits. [48] At least 100 respondents were included in each subgroup except in the case of a few moderators (e.g., therapeutic dose, reason for taking Valium); in no case did moderator group size drop below 65. [49] Significance tests were computed for the differences between the correlations found for high and low subgroups. Moderator variables were measured at Time 3. Valium use was measured at all four timepoints and 49 outcome variables were measured at Time 4 (see Table 5.14 for the list of outcome variables and moderators). This choice of timepoints allows examination of Valium use preceding and following both the moderator variable and the outcome variables.

A number of criteria were used to determine if an interaction appeared to be of substantive interest. Correlations had to differ significantly between groups. The variances for the two groups had to be similar on the predictor and dependent variables. Effects which replicated at several points in time were given more credence because of their stability. Similarly, effects which were repeated among related variables were given more credence. For example, if the relationship between Valium use, technical performance, and a moderator were comparable to those for Valium use, social performance, and the same moderator, the results were considered better validated.

---

[48] Median splits were considered but rejected because the inclusion of more moderate scores may mask effects which would be found with extreme splits like those which were used.

[49] Sample size of 65 refers to the majority of pairs of variables. Variables which were relevant only for working respondents have a smaller sample size and must be viewed with caution.

There were 6,820 analyses conducted which involved a hypothesized moderator, predictor, and dependent variable (49 outcome variables, 35 moderators, and one predictor (Valium-use) included at four timepoints). Approximately 14% of these tests were significant at the p<.05 level. [50] While some theoretically plausible moderator effects were found, the magnitude of these effects was usually small and most findings did not replicate consistently across waves. Furthermore, three of the most promising moderator variables were examined in subgroup multivariate models. Results of these analyses are described in the section on multivariate models, which concludes that these moderators proved not to have much actual effect on the relationships among Valium-taking, anxiety, and life quality. This leads us to suspect that other modifier effects which were found are also likely to have quite small impacts. Consequently, these findings are not presented in the main body of the report but can be found in Appendix T. While we did not feel that the pattern of results was consistent enough or strong enough to warrant interpretation, they may provide hypotheses which can be tested in future research.

---

[50] Because a number of the outcome variables were intercorrelated, the various significance tests were not independent.

Table 5.14

MODERATOR AND OUTCOME VARIABLES EXAMINED IN MODERATOR ANALYSES

Moderator Variables Examined

sex of respondent
race
age
informational social support
esteem social support
social conflict
social support from physician who prescribed Valium
social performance in personal life
role ambiguity in personal life
role ambiguity in work life
role conflict in work life
negative life events and conditions
perceived quality of health
internal control misfit in personal life
internal control misfit over emotions
control by others misfit in personal life
control by others misfit over emotions
control by chance misfit in personal life
control by chance misfit over emotions
perceived chance control in personal life
religious beliefs
positive approach on life
reinterpretation of negative events
seeking help from others
alcohol
CNS depressant-like ("+ effect") medications
CNS stimulant-like ("- effect") medications
therapy/counseling
attitudes about tranquilizers
anxiety
anxiety/depression ratio
taking Valium for reasons related to anxiety (2 versions)
compliance
therapeutic dose

Outcome Variables

anxiety
depression
quality of life (QOL) self
QOL personal life
QOL work life

Table 5.14

MODERATOR AND OUTCOME VARIABLES EXAMINED IN MODERATOR ANAYLSES
(Continued)

QOL life as-a-whole
QOL positive affect
QOL negative affect
QOL cognition
QOL of personal other
QOL of work other
perceived quality of health
informational social support
esteem social support
social conflict
religious beliefs
positive approach on life
reinterpretation of negative events
seeking help from others
role conflict in work life
role ambiguity in work life
role ambiguity in personal life
negative life events and conditions
technical performance in work life
social performance in work life
technical performance in personal life
social performance in personal life
Valium users' perceptions of Valium's helpfulness
attitudes about tranquilizers
caffeine
alcohol
perceived internal control in personal life
perceived internal control over emotions
perceived control by others in personal life
perceived control by others over emotions
perceived control by chance in personal life
perceived control by chance over emotions
desired internal control in personal life
desired internal control over emotions
desired control by others in personal life
desired control by others over emotions
desired control by chance in personal life
desired control by chance over emotions
internal control misfit in personal life
internal control misfit over emotions
control by others misfit in personal life
control by others misfit over emotions
control by chance misfit in personal life
control by chance misfit over emotions

Valium Use as a Moderator of the Stress-Strain Relationship

As noted in Chapter 1, psychologists have considered many concepts, such as social support and perceived control, as moderators of the relationship between stress and strain. We hypothesized that the use of Valium might also moderate the relationship between stress and strain. Individuals who take Valium might feel less strain while under stress because of the effects of the medication.

A number of subgroup analyses were conducted to examine this hypothesis. Each of these analyses is described in the following sections.

Analysis I. Respondents were divided into two groups: those who had taken Valium within the week prior to the Time 1 interview and those who had not. The relationship between 13 different stressors[51] and 16 different outcomes (strains)[52] were computed separately for Valium users and for nonusers. These relationships were computed for all four possible combinations of stress and strain at Time 1 and Time 2 (i.e., stress at Time 1, strain at Time 1; stress at Time 2, strain at Time 1, etc.).

A number of these stress-strain relationships were significantly different comparing Valium users and nonusers.[53] These effects were categorized into two types: buffering effects (i.e., the positive relationship between stress and

---

[51]The stressors were social conflict, negative life events, role ambiguity in work life, role ambiguity in personal life, role conflict in work life, misfit on internal control over personal life and emotions, misfit on control by others over personal life and emotions, misfit on control by chance over personal life and emotions, multiple stress, and highest stress (see Chapter 4 for a description of these measures).

[52]The outcome measures were anxiety, depression, negative affect, positive affect, life quality in the domains of health, self, life-as-a-whole, cognition, work-life, and personal-life, technical and social performance in the personal and work life, alcohol use, and caffeine use.

[53]Twelve percent of the correlations were significantly different. While this is higher than the 5% expected by chance, a number of the stresses and outcome measures were intercorrelated so it is likely that more than 5% could be expected to be significant due to chance.

strain was _lower_ for Valium users than for nonusers) and exacerbating effects (i.e., the positive relationship between stress and strain was _higher_ for Valium users than for nonusers). The ratio of buffering to exacerbating effects was two to one. In every case in which the difference in the relationships between stress and anxiety for Valium users and nonusers reached statistical significance, the magnitude of the positive relationship was less for Valium users than for nonusers. In 22 out of the 25 relationships between stress and measures of life quality which were significantly different between Valium users and nonusers, the negative relationship between stress and quality for life was lower for Valium users than for nonusers. Valium use was also a frequent buffer of the relationship between stress and alcohol use. In every case, the relationship between stress and alcohol use was slightly negative for Valium users (i.e., the greater the stress, the less the alcohol use), while for nonusers the relationship was slightly positive (i.e., the greater the stress, the greater the alcohol use). The exacerbating effects of Valium occurred most frequently when the outcome measure was performance. That is, stress was more highly related to poor performance for Valium users than for nonusers. Most of the significant differences occurred when both stress and strain were measured at Time 1.

Analysis II. The analyses reported in Analysis I were repeated with Valium use assessed at Time 3 and stress and strain measured at Times 3 and 4. As before, buffering effects of Valium were more common than exacerbating effects, but fewer relationships were significantly different than were found at Time 1.

Analysis III. As described in earlier sections of this chapter, Valium users reported higher levels of stress and strain than did nonusers. Also, levels of stress and strain were higher for all respondents at Time 1 than at later waves. To ensure that the differences in the stress-strain relationships between Valium users and nonusers found at Time 1 were not due to their different stress levels, Analysis I was repeated only for Valium users and nonusers who reported experiencing at least some stress.[54] The results were comparable to those found in Analysis I.

Analysis IV. We hypothesized that the effects of Valium use on the stress-strain relationship might differ for daily and nondaily users of Valium. Nondaily users might be more likely than daily users to take Valium in response to acute stress and consequently their Valium use might have a larger effect on the stress-strain relationship. To test this hypothesis, the analyses conducted for Analysis I were repeated separately for daily and nondaily users of Valium at Time 1. There were more significant moderating effects for nondaily users than for daily users. Although the majority of these effects showed weaker stress-strain relationships for nondaily Valium users than for nonusers (i.e., buffering), there were exceptions. Most notably, nondaily users frequently exhibited a stronger negative relationship between stress and performance at work and in personal life than did nonusers.

Conclusions. There was some evidence that Valium moderated the relationship between stress and strain. In most cases the relationship between stress and strain was weaker for Valium users than nonusers but there were cases in which the reverse was found. The effects were not consistent enough (e.g., they did not always replicate across waves and there was only partial evidence for a "specificity" hypothesis[55]) to alter the overall conclusion that Valium has little effect, either positive or negative, on outcomes such as life quality.

---

[54]Respondents had to have a score of at least "3" on the Multiple Stress index which had a low point of "1" and a high point of "7." Eighty-seven respondents who had been included in Analysis I were omitted from Analysis III because their stress level was below this criterion.

[55]The specificity hypothesis states that stresses and strains will be most related when they are maximally relevant conceptually to one another. There was evidence that moderating effects were most likely to occur when the stress and strain being examined were maximally relevant to each other. For example, role ambiguity in one's personal life and performance in the personal life are relevant to each other because they are both in the personal life domain. However, even when only relevant stress-strain relationships were examined, the number of moderating effects was modest and there was no obvious explanation of when they did and did not occur.

185

There were, however, enough effects to suggest that this represents a promising direction for future research.

Summary of Bivariate Analyses

Relationships among Valium use, anxiety, and quality of life were examined both cross-sectionally and across all the possible lags of the approximately 24 weeks of data collection. Anxiety and quality of life were strongly, simultaneously, and oppositely related to one another (high anxiety was associated with low quality of life). Valium use showed only weak relationships with anxiety, quality of life and many other phenomena, including the well-being of significant others, regardless of the lag. These weak associations tended to be in the direction of higher Valium use being associated with poorer outcomes. Multivariate analyses, described below, suggested that these associations were largely due to stabilities of health problems and stress among the users of Valium.

These relationships were observed after it had been determined that there was no curvilinearity in the data and that there were no spurious effects that might obscure the relationships. Variances of measures and correlations across the four waves of the study were quite stable over time although means on a large number of variables changed in the direction of improvement over time (e.g., higher quality of life, lower anxiety).

A search of 6,820 potential moderator effects did not alter the basic bivariate relationships. The moderators included gender, perceived control, perceived supportiveness of the physician, and many other variables assessed in the study.

Analyses were also conducted to determine if Valium use moderated the effects of stress on strain. Valium use was somewhat more likely to weaken the effects of stress on strain than to exacerbate those effects. However, these findings are viewed only as suggestive of avenues for future research because they did not consistently replicate across waves of the study.

Multivariate Analyses

Overview

Making use of the findings from the bivariate analyses, this section presents a number of analyses which generally involved three or more variables. The first of these was longitudinal multivariate modeling. The theory behind this technique is presented along with findings from tests of more than 20 models. As a follow-up analysis, there was an examination of the effects of changes in Valium use on changes in other variables. These analyses were done to see if results would be different when change scores instead of absolute levels of the variables were used.

In a third analysis, to see what effects Valium use has on highly anxious persons, highly anxious Valium users were compared to equally anxious nonusers on mean values of anxiety, depression, quality of life, performance, and a number of other variables.

Multivariate Modeling: Theory and Method

Chapters 1 and 2 of this report describe the full range of concepts and hypotheses that guided the design of the study. The analyses reported here take a few of the most important concepts and estimate their empirical linkages using the relatively new technique of structural modeling. This technique should provide the best available information on causal relations. The analyses begin with just three concepts--Valium-taking, anxiety, and quality of life-as-a-whole--and then expand to include three additional concepts--perceived health, stress, and performance in personal life.

The basic theory explored here is simple. Anxiety was expected to reduce assessments of life quality and increase Valium-taking; and Valium-taking was expected to reduce anxiety.

The more complex analysis keeps the basic theory and adds the following: perceived health was expected to have direct effects on stress, anxiety, Valium-taking, performance, and life quality; stress was expected to have direct effects on anxiety and perceived health; anxiety was expected to have a

187

direct effect on performance; and performance was expected to have direct effects on anxiety and quality of life. In general, perceived health and stress were regarded as concepts near the beginning of the causal sequence, anxiety and Valium-taking as intermediate concepts, and performance and life quality as "outcomes." However, there was no expectation that earlier concepts in this sequence would wholly determine the later concepts; allowance was made for other unspecified concepts to have some influence on every concept.

For addressing interests in the social effects of Valium, the primary focus is on the direct effect of Valium-taking on anxiety and the subsequent effects of anxiety on performance and the quality of life. Our theory assumes that if Valium, a chemical substance with psychoactive properties, is going to have an influence on a person's performance and life quality, that influence will occur through Valium's effects on the person's anxiety levels. The results from clinical drug trials support this assumption although they do not preclude more direct effects on various outcomes.

The analysis technique used to estimate the effects each concept had on the others was structural modeling as implemented in the LISREL (Linear Structural Relationships) computer program by Joreskog and Sorbom (1978). This is an approach that estimates a set of direct causal effects of one factor on another (the factors representing theoretical concepts) in accord with a prespecified theory while taking account of several kinds of measurement errors in the assessment of the concepts. This technique, although relatively new, represents an important advance in analysis methodology because it combines, in a single estimation operation, concerns for both the measurement aspects of the data and the theoretical linkages of the concepts. This technique has attracted a great deal of attention in the past decade and has proven to be well suited for handling a wide variety of data, including longitudinal data with multiple measures of concepts, as in the present study. Because recent and extensive reviews and expositions of the LIS-REL methodology have been published by Bentler (1980), Joreskog and Sorbom (1978), Maruyama and McGarvey (1980), Joreskog and

Sorbom (1977), and others, only a brief overview of the logic of the technique will be presented here.

A LISREL analysis begins with the variances and covariances (or correlations) among a set of measures, and a prespecified model that indicates how various factors are presumed to influence the measures and one another. The LISREL estimation algorithm then computes the variance of each factor and the strength of each hypothesized linkage so the predicted variances and covariances (or correlations) among the measures will come as close as possible to what was actually observed. The results let one see how strongly each factor would affect each other factor, directly and indirectly, if the world actually worked as one's model specifies. The results also indicate how well the model can account for the data. Although the technique involves the simultaneous estimation of many parameters under a variety of constraints, the basic logic is similar to that of any other multivariate statistical technique (e.g., multiple regression) that seeks a set of parameters that will optimally reproduce a set of data.

As with any sophisticated operation, there are a variety of things that merit attention before one should believe the final results. The measures must be suitable for the computations of variance and covariance and for modeling in an essentially additive linear system. The model itself must be theoretically reasonable in the light of what is known or suspected about the concepts. The final parameter estimates must be within the range of permissible values and must do a good job of reproducing the observed covariance structure of the measures. We believe the results described below meet each of these criteria to at least a reasonable extent and that the essential conclusions would not be changed by refinements in either the measures or the models.

This belief is founded on: (1) the extensive scale development work reported in Chapter 4 and widespread experience (e.g., Labovitz, 1970) that scales of this type provide reasonable estimates of parametric statistics; (2) a demonstration, described earlier in this chapter, that curvilinearity is not a problem for the types of concepts incorporated in our models; (3) the theoretical reasonableness of the model and the reported parameter estimates; (4) the fact that all parameter estimates fell within permissible ranges (e.g., 0 to +1 for estimates of variances and validities); (5) the adequate fit of the models for data sets of the size analyzed here (as assessed by the chi-square-per-degrees-of-freedom ratio and the magnitude of discrepancies between observed and predicted relationships among the measures);[56] (6) the variety of alternative models, each one only modestly different from the ones shown here, that have been explored (as described below), and the finding that the parameter on which we primarily focus here--the linkage from Valium-taking to anxiety--changed very little; (7) an extensive scan for interaction effects associated with Valium-taking and anxiety which showed that marked interactions were not present among these variables; (8) the variety of subgroups of respondents that have been run to check some of the most likely interactions, and the finding that the Valium-taking-to-anxiety links were largely unaffected and consistently replicated other analyses;[57] and (9) our experience that models incorporating simple no-yes measures of Valium use showed essentially identical results to models employing the more quantitative pills-per-week or milligrams-per-week measures. In short, although the models shown below are not perfect, we believe they are satisfactory and provide a useful insight into the dynamics of Valium-taking, anxiety, life quality, perceived health, stress, and performance. This is particularly true for the results obtained for Waves 2, 3, 4--i.e., after the impacts of these

---

[56]For the two specific models (A and B) described below these figures were as follows: Model A: df= 217, χ^2= 1026.9, χ^2/df=4.73, χ^2/df/N= .0071, maximum residual= -.298, mean absolute residual= .021. Model B: df= 1176, χ^2= 3469.3, χ^2/df= 2.95, χ^2/df/N= .0044, maximum residual= .246, mean absolute residual= .041.

[57]These special subgroups analyses included: only Valium users, only people who changed in their use of Valium during the study, only people who took therapeutic doses of Valium (defined as 30-280 mg per week), only people who took no CNS stimulant-like drugs at any wave, and only people who did take CNS stimulant-like drugs at all four waves of the study.

phenomena at an earlier time (i.e., at Wave 1) have had a chance to be reflected in the results.[58]

Results--Model A. Figure 5.6 presents results from one version of what will be designated as "Model A." This model involves linkages among three main concepts--anxiety, Valium-taking, and quality of life-as-a-whole--each measured at four points in time, three purely methodological factors that help to account for small amounts of correlated measurement error, and 24 observed measures (two measures for each of the three major concepts at each of four timepoints). As is conventional in such diagrams, rectangles represent measures,[59] ovals represent factors (which stand for concepts as labelled), one-headed arrows represent direct causal influences, and two-headed arrows represent simple relationships that remain unanalyzed with respect to causal direction or origin. The numbers on the one-headed arrows represent the strength of the causal impact and show the amount by which the result variable would change (in standard deviation units) if the causal variable changed by one standard deviation unit when all other causes, if any, remained constant. The numbers on the two-headed arrows are covariances. The numbers at the ends of short arrows represent the variances of the residuals--i.e., the sources not explicitly accounted for elsewhere in the model that influence a measure or a factor.[60]

---

[58]Experts on modeling will recognize a technical problem in specifying the model that leads us to be suspicious of the Wave 1 results. We had two choices: The Wave 1 factors could be treated as exogenous, but then it would be difficult to include a full set of first-order serial covariations among measurement errors; alternatively, the Wave 1 factors could be treated as endogenous, but then we could not achieve both identification and reflection of correlations among the variables due to their previous impact on one another. We tried estimating the models both ways, and observed that it made virtually no difference in the results for Waves 2, 3, and 4.

[59]Rectangles are labelled only at Wave 1; an identical set of measures was used at each succeeding wave.

[60]All versions of Model A (and also B) presented in this report incorporate an arbitrary standardization such that the variances of all measures and all factors have been set to 1.0. This ensures that parameters can be easily interpreted (as described in this paragraph). To ensure that the three minor

191

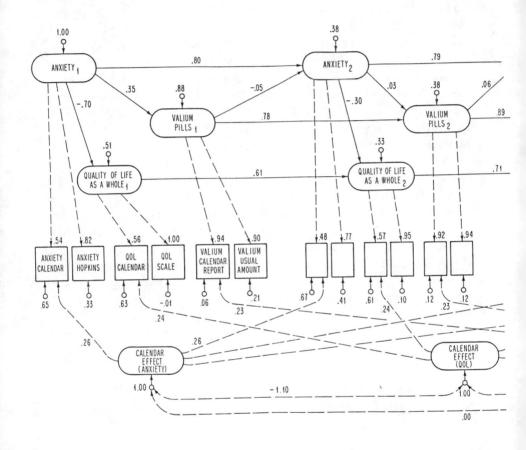

Figure 5.6

Model A: Anxiety, Valium-taking, and quality of life.

(Note: First-order serial covariations among the residuals for the non-calendar measures are omitted from the figure but were part of the model.)

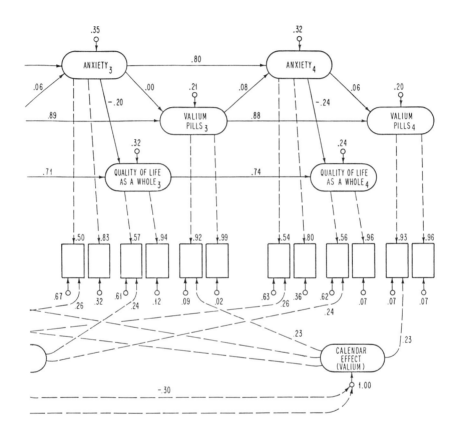

Figure 5.6 (continued)

In Model A two measures are used to represent each concept. It is assumed that respondents' scores on the Hopkins Anxiety scale and their answers to the single-item question about anxiety in the "calendar" portion of the interview reflect their anxiety levels--but not necessarily perfectly or to the same degree. Similarly, their scores on the quality of life-as-a-whole scale and their answers to the life quality question in the "calendar" portion of the interview are expected to reflect (again, not perfectly or equally) their true feelings about life-as-a-whole. Valium-taking is represented by answers to the Valium pills-per-week item in the "calendar" portion of the interview (adjusted to span a full week, as described in Appendix P) and by an independent estimate of Valium-taking based on reports of the usual number of pills consumed per day in conjunction with information about when each respondent most recently took Valium.

In addition to the direct effects that the main substantive factors were expected to have on the measures, Model A allows for certain measurement errors. Three minor factors, each labelled "calendar" effects, represent stable differences among respondents in the way they responded to the "calendar" questions on anxiety, life quality, and Valium-taking, respectively. In addition, Model A allows for three sets of first-order serial covariations among the measurement errors in the the (non-calendar) measures of anxiety, life quality, and Valium-taking (not shown in Figure 5.6).[61] Although the attention to measurement errors and their correlations significantly improved the fit of the models, and hence increased our confidence in the results, none of the correlations among measurement errors is large enough to be of much substantive importance.

measurement-error factors (described below) represented the intended correlated error concepts, and that unique parameter estimates could be obtained, all linkages from each of these factors to the measures were constrained equal.

[61]These allow the model to reflect any stable differences that may exist among respondents in the way they responded to each of these measures, but any such effects are required to be statistically independent of the "calendar" measurement ef-

Before discussing the most important results in Figure 5.6, it is helpful to observe the general magnitude of the links between each of the main factors and their respective measures. As noted in Chapter 4, each of these may be interpreted as an estimate of construct validity. The fact that the anxiety and quality of life scales have higher estimated validities than the comparable single-item measures is exactly what should occur, and the substantial level of all the factor-measure linkages gives confidence that the factors closely represent the intended concepts.

With regard to the effects of Valium, the most important result shown in Figure 5.6 is the very low direct effect that Valium-taking is estimated to have on anxiety about six weeks later. (The values are .06 and .08 for links from Waves 2 to 3 and 3 to 4, where we have the greatest confidence.) This means that, even after allowing for imperfections in the measures, variations in Valium-taking recorded at one wave of the study accounted for less than one percent of the variation in anxiety recorded approximately six weeks later. This is, clearly, a trivially small amount. Furthermore, because any effect of Valium-taking on subsequent life quality must, according to this model, pass through anxiety, it is also evident that Valium-taking has virtually no systematic indirect effect-- either beneficial or detrimental--on subsequent life quality.

Other linkages between the factors in the model shown in Figure 5.6 are also of interest. In Waves 2, 3, and 4, one sees a direct effect of anxiety on concurrent life quality (-.24 to -.30, a direction and a magnitude that both seem reasonable);[2] a very weak positive effect of anxiety on concurrent Valium-taking (.00 to .06); and strong stability effects from wave to wave for each of the main concepts--about .88 for Valium-taking, about .80 for anxiety, and in the low .70's for life quality.

---

fects. These nine covariations were all very low (range= -.04 to +.06, median= .02).

[2]Recall that in the examination of bivariate lagged relationships reported earlier in this chapter there was clear

The low effect of Valium-taking on later anxiety was a surprise to us when it first emerged, and more than 20 versions of Model A were run to see whether alternative assumptions about the causal dynamics of these concepts would alter the basic conclusion that Valium-taking had virtually no effects on either anxiety or life quality six weeks later. None of the models that did not have to be rejected, because of much worse fit or totally unreasonable values of other parameters, supported a different conclusion. Among the more interesting variants of Model A were versions that substituted a simultaneous Valium-to-anxiety link in place of the lagged linkage shown in Figure 5.6 (values were .10 to .12 for this new link, and all other parameters stayed about the same), and a version that added a direct Valium-to-later-life-quality link (which came out a trivial .03 while all other parameters remained about the same). As noted in the earlier discussion on reasons for confidence in these results, the model shown in Figure 5.6, and some others as well, were also run on selected subgroups of respondents for whom we thought the effects of Valium might be most pronounced. The results for these groups also showed trivially low effects of Valium on anxiety and life quality six weeks later.

Model A, although useful for examining the effects of Valium-taking on subsequent anxiety and life quality, involves only three concepts and hence is conceptually rather thin. There is no explanation included in the model for why people have the anxiety levels they do, and only very partial explanations for why they assess life quality or take Valium as they do. Although all these variables show substantial stabilities over time, there is not much hint as to why these stabilities occur. In order to arrive at a better explanation, particularly for the persistent weak positive relationship between Valium-taking and anxiety observed at all possible lag intervals (as reported in the section of this chapter on lagged bivariate relationships), it seemed appropriate to introduce into the analysis some concepts which are theoretically an-

---

evidence that feelings of anxiety and assessments of life quality were concurrent concepts.

tecedent in the causal chain to the variables in Model A. It was also desirable, we thought, to include another outcome variable in addition to assessments of life quality. Accordingly, Model A was expanded by the addition of three more concepts to produce what will be called "Model B."

Results--Model B. Figure 5.7 shows the form and parameter estimates for Model B. The basic structure is the same as Model A, except that the anxiety-to-anxiety stability links have been removed. Added are perceived health and stress as new factors early in the causal chain and an additional outcome variable, performance in personal life, near the end of the causal chain.[63]

The measures for anxiety and life quality are the same in Model B as they were in Model A. The Valium measures are similar in source, but include an accounting of the milligram strength of the Valium respondents were taking.[64] The perceived health concept is represented by three separate subjective health measures (the components of the health life quality scale, see Chapter 4), the stress concept by two measures ("Highest stress" and "Multiple stress," described in Chapter 4), and the performance in personal life concept by two measures (the scales of technical and social performance in personal life described in Chapter 4).[65]

---

[63]In estimating Model B, the same equality constraints described for Model A in a preceding footnote were imposed.

[64]The milligram-weighted measures are probably our best measures of Valium-taking but had not been constructed when Model A was first run. The difference between the pills-per-week measures and the milligrams-per-week measures is small (probably because most people took the same size pills) and do not significantly affect the results.

[65]In contrast to the situation for anxiety, life quality, and Valium-taking, where the several measures used to represent a concept can be seen as alternative measures of exactly the same underlying concept, the several measures of perceived health, of stress, and of personal-life performance are more appropriately viewed as measures of distinctive but related concepts. The factor in the model, then, takes its meaning from the functional overlap among the separate concepts. For example, two related concepts were distinguished in personal life performance, technical performance and social performance; the meaning of the performance factor will be whatever these

197

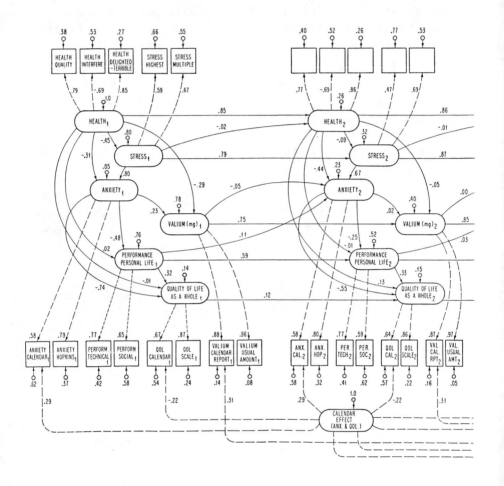

Figure 5.7

Model B: Health, stress, anxiety, Valium-taking, quality of life, and performance.

(Note: First-order serial covariations among the residuals for the non-calendar measures are omitted from the figure but were part of the model.)

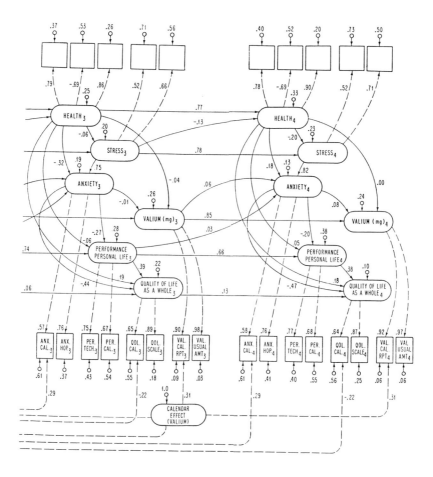

Figure 5.7 (continued)

As in Model A, Model B includes several minor measurement-error factors (experience with Model A suggested only two were actually needed) to handle persistent individual differences in the way respondents interpreted the "calendar" portion of the interview, and first-order serial covariations among other measurement errors[a]. As in Model A, the measurement error apparatus improves the fit of the model and increases confidence in the main results but is of little substantive importance in its own right.

The key result from Model B in Figure 5.7 is, as was the case in Model A, the linkage between Valium-taking and subsequent anxiety. At Waves 2, 3, and 4, this parameter ranges from .00 to +.06. This would imply that Valium-taking accounts for less than one-half of one percent of the variation in anxiety six weeks later. Since it is through anxiety that we hypothesize that Valium will have its (indirect) effects on subsequent performance and quality of life, it follows that there is no indirect effect of Valium on either of these outcomes.

The other linkages among the main factors are also of substantive interest and support the overall reasonableness of the model. One can see that perceived health has modest impacts in expected directions on stress, anxiety, and life quality (averaging across Waves 2-4 these are, respectively, -.12, -.31, and .17); that stress has a major impact on concurrent anxiety (average= .75) and a very slight impact on later perceived health (average= -.07); that anxiety has a very weak impact on concurrent Valium-taking (average= .03), as was the case in Model A, and much stronger impacts on performance and life quality (average= -.24 and -.49, respectively); and that performance has a moderate impact on concurrent life quality (average= .37).

---

two concepts share. Furthermore, the factor-to-measure links are interpretable as factor loadings but not as construct validity coefficients.

[a]To simplify figure 5.7, these serial covariations are not shown. The model includes 30 such parameters, and all were low (median = .102, maximum = .199).

One of the interesting differences between Models A and B is the difference in the stability coefficients for anxiety and life quality. Both are low (or absent) in Model B;[67] both were substantial in Model A. The explanation would seem to be that Model B includes two antecedent concepts--perceived health and stress--which are themselves highly stable and which link to anxiety, and through anxiety to life quality. Given the presence of these two rather stable concepts in the model, subsequent levels of anxiety and life quality can be largely accounted for without the expedient of merely attributing them to previous levels of themselves. (Because Valium-taking and performance in personal life are much less well explained by causally antecedent concepts, substantial stability parameters still appear for them.)

Conclusions. One of the "lessons" of these analyses is the importance of considering the stability of antecedent causal phenomena. We believe it is the failure to take account of these phenomena that produces the consistent, positive bivariate relationship between Valium-taking and subsequent anxiety, and the consistent negative bivariate relationship between Valium-taking and life quality. These relationships appear in the data of this study and elsewhere in the real world and have been observed and commented upon by many evaluators of Valium. However, when antecedent causal factors which are reasonably stable, such as perceived health and stress, are considered (explicitly as in Model B, or implicitly as in Model A), the apparently "detrimental" effects of Valium-taking essentially vanish. This suggests the original relationships were spurious effects of perceived health and stress and not due to the direct effects of Valium-taking.

Correlations among Changes in Valium, Anxiety, and Life Quality

Purpose and nature of the analysis. One of the central questions being addressed in this report is whether taking

---

[67]The low values for the life quality stability links is a direct estimation. The anxiety stability links are absent because experience with modifications of Model B showed more meaningful results when this link was set to zero. (How the anxiety stability links were handled in Model B, however, had virtually no impact on the estimated effects of Valium.)

Valium produces a subsequent "long-range" (e.g., six weeks later) reduction in anxiety and improvement of life quality. The analyses presented in previous sections have addressed this question by relating the level of Valium use to subsequent levels of anxiety and life quality. An alternative approach to this question involves examining how changes in Valium-taking relate to changes in anxiety and quality of life. For example, one might ask how increases in Valium use from the first to the second interview are related to changes in anxiety over that same 6-week period and over other intervals (e.g., from the second to the third interview or from the first to the third interview). Furthermore, although change scores present a number of problems (e.g., reduced reliability), they have an interesting advantage over the raw scores from which they were computed: constant factors that influence respondents' answers over time (generating either true stabilities or correlated measurement errors) are cancelled out when the raw scores are subtracted from one another. Thus, change scores are free of such constant factors leaving only "true" change and random noise in the change measures.

To see if analyses of change measures might produce substantially different results from those presented above, change scores were constructed for reported Valium use, anxiety, and quality of life-as-a-whole during the seven days preceding each interview. Each change score was a simple difference: a measurement at a later interview minus a measurement at an earlier interview. Thus, increases in a variable over time produced positive change score values, while decreases produced negative change score values. For each of the three major concepts, six change scores were computed: three involved changes over approximately six weeks (interviews 2-1, 3-2, and 4-3); two involved changes over approximately 12 weeks (interviews 3-1 and 4-2); and one involved changes over approximately 18 weeks (interviews 4-1).

These change scores were then intercorrelated using data for the 675 respondents who participated in all four interviews. For each pair of concepts (e.g., Valium use and anxiety), this produced three estimates of a simultaneous

202

relationship involving a 6-week change (e.g., how changes in Valium use between interviews 1 and 2 related to changes in anxiety between those waves); two estimates of a simultaneous relationship involving 12-week changes (i.e., interviews 3-1 and 4-2); and one estimate of a simultaneous relationship involving an 18-week change (interviews 4-1). There were also four estimates of 6-week lagged relationships (e.g., two with Valium use preceding anxiety and two with anxiety preceding Valium use). These correlations indicated, for example, how change in Valium use between interviews 1 and 2 related to change in anxiety between interviews 2 and 3. There were also two estimates of 12-week lagged relationships (e.g., one with Valium use preceding anxiety and one with anxiety preceding Valium use).

Results. Table 5.15 shows the correlations between changes in Valium-taking and changes in anxiety for the various intervals over which change was measured and the lags between change scores being correlated. Average correlations were tabulated when there was more than one estimate for a given change interval and lag. Tables 5.16 and 5.17 are comparable for Valium-taking and life quality and for anxiety and life quality, respectively. Several points can be made about these results: (a) The simultaneous relationships were all about the same regardless of whether changes were measured over 6-week, 12-week, or 18-week intervals. (b) The lagged relationships tended to be smaller than the simultaneous ones (with the possible exception of Valium-taking and life quality). (c) All relationships were low; the highest were produced by simultaneous changes in anxiety and life quality and were only in the low .20's. (d) The lagged relationships between changes in Valium use and changes in anxiety were low and nearly equal regardless of whether Valium use preceded or followed anxiety.

To summarize, the lagged-change-score approach did not produce strong results or ones that would suggest alternative interpretations of the data. Consistent with results from other types of analyses presented above, the simultaneous (i.e., no lag) relationships between change scores tended to be slightly stronger than the lagged relationships. However, all

203

Table 5.15

CORRELATIONS OF CHANGES IN VALIUM-TAKING AND ANXIETY

Change Intervals:	Lags:	Change in Anxiety precedes Change in Valium		Simultaneous	Change in Valium precedes Change in Anxiety	
		12 wks[1]	6 wks[2]	0 wks[3]	6 wks[4]	12 wks[5]
6-week changes		-.01	-.03	+.09*	-.03	-.03
12-week changes				+.08*		
18-week changes				+.08*		

*p< .05 (under conventional statistical assumptions)

[1]This correlation was based on the changes in Valium use from Time 1 to 2 with changes in Anxiety from Time 3 to 4.

[2]This is the average of correlations for changes in Valium use from Time 1 to 2 with changes in Anxiety from Time 2 to 3, and for changes in Valium use from Time 2 to 3 with changes in Anxiety from Time 3 to 4.

[3]This is the average of correlations for simultaneous changes (i.e., over the same time interval) for 6-week intervals (Time 1 to 2, Time 2 to 3, and Time 3 to 4), for 12-week intervals (Time 1 to 3 and Time 2 to 4), and for one 18-week interval (Time 1 to 4).

[4]This is the average of correlations for changes in Anxiety from Time 1 to 2 with changes in Valium use from Time 2 to 3, and for changes in Anxiety from Time 2 to 3 with changes in Valium use from Time 3 to 4.

[5]This correlation was based on changes in Anxiety from Time 1 to 2 with changes in Valium use from Time 3 to 4.

Table 5.16

CORRELATIONS OF CHANGES IN VALIUM-TAKING AND QUALITY OF LIFE (QOL)

Change Intervals:	Lags:	Change in QOL precedes Change in Valium		Simultaneous	Change in Valium precedes Change in QOL	
		12 wks[1]	6 wks[2]	0 wks[3]	6 wks[4]	12 wks[5]
6-week changes		-.05	+.07	-.06	-.07	+.08*
12-week changes				-.06		
18-week changes				-.11*		

*p< .05 (under conventional statistical assumptions)

[1] This correlation was based on the changes in Life quality from Time 1 to 2 with changes in Valium use from Time 3 to 4.

[2] This is the average of correlations for changes in Life Quality from Time 1 to 2 with changes in Valium use from Time 2 to 3, and for changes in Life Quality from Time 2 to 3 with changes in Valium use from Time 3 to 4.

[3] This is the average of correlations for simultaneous changes (i.e., over the same time interval) for 6-week intervals (Time 1 to 2, Time 2 to 3, and Time 3 to 4), for 12-week intervals (Time 1 to 3 and Time 2 to 4), and for one 18-week interval (Time 1 to 4).

[4] This is the average of correlations for changes in Valium use from Time 1 to 2 with changes in Life quality from Time 2 to 3, and for changes in Valium use from Time 2 to 3 with changes in Life quality from Time 3 to 4.

[5] This correlation was based on changes in Valium use from Time 1 to 2 with changes in Life quality from Time 3 to 4.

Table 5.17

CORRELATIONS OF CHANGES IN ANXIETY AND QUALITY OF LIFE (QOL)

Change Intervals:	Lags:	Change in Anxiety precedes Change in QOL		Simultaneous	Change in QOL precedes Change in Anxiety	
		12 wks[1]	6 wks[2]	0 wks[3]	6 wks[4]	12 wks[5]
6-week changes		+.06	+.05	-.22*	+.12*	-.05
12-week changes				-.23*		
18-week changes				-.25*		

*p< .05 (under conventional statistical assumptions)

[1]This correlation was based on the changes in Anxiety from Time 1 to 2 with changes in Life quality from Time 3 to 4.

[2]This is the average of correlations for changes in Anxiety from Time 1 to 2 with changes in Life quality from Time 2 to 3, and for changes in Anxiety from Time 2 to 3 with changes in Life quality from Time 3 to 4.

[3]This is the average of correlations for simultaneous changes (i.e., over the same time interval) for 6-week intervals (Time 1 to 2, Time 2 to 3, and Time 3 to 4), for

Several points can be made about these results: (a)

[4]This is the average of correlations for changes in Life quality from Time 1 to 2 with changes in Anxiety from Time 2 to 3, and for changes in Life quality from Time 2 to 3 with changes in Anxiety from Time 3 to 4.

[5]This correlation was based on changes in Life quality from Time 1 to 2 with changes in Anxiety from Time 3 to 4.

the relationships were rather weak and should be interpreted cautiously.

Changes in Stress, Strain, and Performance among the Highly Anxious: A Comparison of Valium Users and Nonusers

An ideal experiment on the effects of Valium use would randomly assign persons to take Valium or to take a placebo. There would be steps to ensure that the Valium and placebo groups took their medicine between pre-tests and post-tests. And persons would be admitted for participation only if their levels of anxiety warranted clinical intervention. Although this study is not such an experiment, analyses reported in this section attempted to approximate as many of these conditions as possible in some special subgroups.

Two sets of analyses were performed comparing selected groups of Valium users' and nonusers' levels of anxiety and potential social effects. Comparisons were made across the four waves of the study. The nonusers were selected to have approximately the same Wave 1 scores on the Hopkins Anxiety Scale as the Valium users with whom they were being compared. Furthermore, respondents in these analyses were restricted to those whose mean level of anxiety fell within ranges typically found at pretest in clinical trials. The levels of anxiety for the respondents are described below.

In one set of analyses, the users of Valium were those who reported taking Valium daily or almost every day from the six weeks preceding Wave 1 through Wave 2 (hereafter called "daily users"). These daily users tended to take 5 to 10 mg of Valium per day, a regimen within the limits recommended in the package insert for Valium. A course of daily use for six weeks is not unusual in a trial. Clinical studies show that optimum change in anxiety is reached within six weeks, and often within two weeks (see Chapter 1 for citations). In other important regards, however, this group could not approximate a group in a clinical trial. There was no random assignment to treatment and no double-blind condition. There was no appropriate period of drug "washout" prior to entering the study. Within these limitations, the analyses of daily users might be viewed as a search for any potentially undesirable effects of daily or near-daily continuous use over a period of approximately 12 weeks.

The second set of selected users of Valium were new users. New users were defined as persons who started taking Valium for the first time at some point within the six weeks preceding Wave 1, a period covered by data from the calendar. The new users, in a sense, had a washout period in that they reported having no prior use of Valium. The nonusers of Valium, compared with both sets of Valium users, were restricted to persons who had taken no Valium in the period from six weeks prior to Wave 1 through Wave 2.

All respondents in these analyses had to have a score on the Hopkins Anxiety Scale of at least 1.7 (levels as low as 1.75 have been used in published clinical trials although levels around 2.25 at pretest are more common). The mean level and distribution of anxiety were determined for each set of Valium users at Wave 1. Then nonuser control groups were randomly selected such that their mean and distribution on anxiety matched the users' distribution as closely as possible. As a result there were no significant differences in mean anxiety between daily users and their nonuser controls and between new users and their nonuser controls. The mean levels of Hopkins anxiety for the daily and nonusers were about 2.30 and 2.25, respectively. For the new users and their nonusers the mean anxiety scores were 1.90. New users tended as a group to have lower levels of Wave 1 anxiety than daily users.

Results from the structural equation modeling analyses, described in an earlier section, suggested that anxiety and use of Valium might both be influenced by stresses including poor subjective health. In a trial with random assignment these influences would have been randomized between the drug and nondrug groups, but not so here. To obtain a clearer picture of the effects of Valium without the potentially confounding effects of stress, statistical controls were introduced for any differences between the Valium and nonValium groups in stress and perceived health. Such control was achieved by using a procedure known as analysis of covariance (Hays, 1973). With this procedure it was possible to examine the means on outcome variables of interest, such as anxiety or performance, after making adjustments for any differences in the means that might have been due to differences in stress and perceived health between the Valium and nonValium groups. Each time a potential outcome variable was examined at each of the four waves, controls were introduced for the stresses assessed at that same wave.

Figures 5.8a through 5.33b present the results. Only a selected number of outcome variables were examined, chosen for their ability to represent the large number of measures in the study. The "a" series of the figures compares approximately 36 daily Valium users with 51 nonuser controls, all of whom met the above mentioned criteria for inclusion in these particular analyses. Following the same procedures, the "b" series of the figures compares 19 new users with 46 nonuser controls.[68]

Each graph shows the mean level of a particular dependent variable for the Valium and nonValium group at each point in time. Each mean is adjusted for measures of stress and perceived health. Where one of the covariates is itself the dependent variable, it was omitted as a covariate in the analyses.

Anxiety and other emotions. For users and nonusers of Valium there was a drop in the initially high level of anxiety from Wave 1 to Wave 2 (Figures 5.8a and b). Then anxiety stabilized from Wave 2 through Wave 4. The curves of Hopkins anxiety over the four waves were similar and were never differed significantly between the users and nonusers. Consequently, there was no evidence of any effect of Valium use on anxiety. These findings essentially parallel those obtained from the structural equation analyses described earlier.

The trends with regard to depression and anger (Figures 5.9a through 5.10b) were similar to those for anxiety, and the users and nonusers did not differ significantly ($p > .05$) at

---

[68]The sample sizes vary slightly as a function of missing data for these analyses.

Waves 1 through 4.⁶⁹ Consequently, there was no evidence that daily use or new use either exacerbated or reduced levels of anxiety, depression, and anger.

Caffeine, cigarettes, and alcohol. There were no significant differences between users and nonusers of Valium in the consumption of caffeine or cigarettes (Figures 5.11a through 5.12b). Alcohol consumption (Figures 5.13a and b) presented a somewhat different picture, but only with respect to daily users of Valium. At all four waves, daily users reported consuming less alcohol (about 1 to 1.5 drinks per week) than did nonusers of Valium (about 4.5 to 6.5 drinks per week).⁷⁰

The higher levels of alcohol consumption among the nonusers, even excluding nondrinkers, would not be labelled excessive according to accepted research standards (for example, Cahalan, et al., 1969). Consequently, if one viewed the behavior of taking Valium as a substitution for use of alcohol, it could not be said that Valium substitutes for excessive levels of alcohol consumption. To determine if the level of drinking among anxious nonusers was higher, separate analyses were made to examine the amount of drinking among nonusers who were less anxious than those in these analyses. The two groups of nonusers, highly anxious and all others, did not differ significantly in their levels of reported alcohol consumption.

The finding that daily users, but not new users of Valium, drank significantly less alcohol than nonuser controls is open to at least two distinct interpretations. One is that daily users may be avoiding alcohol because of previous adverse experience of combining alcohol with this medication--an ex-

---

⁶⁹In some of these analyses, the curves for the nonusers in the graphs for daily users and new users may differ slightly. The differences are due variation from one random sampling to the other. Given that the control respondents were randomly resampled anew for the new user analysis, there are about 21 cases that overlap.

⁷⁰These mean levels rose to about 8 to 9 drinks per week for nonusers, and 4 to 7 drinks per week for daily users when persons drinking no alcohol in the last seven days were excluded.

perience which new users have not had. A second interpretation is suggested however by the finding that new users indeed consistently drank less alcohol than nonuser controls, though this difference was not significant as was the case for daily users compared to nonusers. It is possible that new users, like daily users, avoided use of alcohol on days when they took Valium, but drank on other days in the same period of time; thus the effect of avoiding alcohol in this group would emerge only weakly in the analysis, as it did. The latter interpretation would be consistent with the possibility that both groups of users--daily users and new users--chose to avoid alcohol at times when they were taking Valium, perhaps because they were complying with medical admonitions against combining alcohol with this medication.

Stress. There were no marked differences between Valium users and nonusers with respect to change over time in the indices of Multiple Stress and Highest Stress. The Multiple Stress index (Figures 5.14a and b) showed a drop in stress from Waves 1 to 2 for all groups. This drop continued beyond Wave 3 only for Valium users. Daily users had significantly lower scores on Multiple Stress than nonusers at Wave 4 and there was a similar but nonsignificant trend for new users. There is no obvious reason why such a difference between users and nonusers should have appeared only at Wave 4. The replication of the pattern in both daily and new users, however, suggests that the finding may deserve further investigation.

The Highest Stress Index (Figures 5.15a and b) showed no consistent pattern of change for either group of users or nonusers of Valium. Recall that this index can tap a qualitatively different form of stress at each wave for each person (see the description of this variable in Chapter 4). Consequently, the curves could reflect an instability inherent in the concept.

Another aspect of stress is perceived lack of control. Perceived control that others have over one's emotions showed patterns from Waves 1 to 4 that were similar for the users and nonusers of Valium (Figures 5.16a and b). Perceived control that others had over the focal respondent's personal life also

211

varied across the four waves in the same manner for users and nonusers of Valium (Figures 5.17a and b).

A measure of goodness of fit between desired and perceived control by self over one's personal life was also examined. The measure of fit allows for the possibility that people differ in whether they have less than, more than, or the amount of control they desire. There were no differences in the patterns of change between users and nonusers of Valium (Figures 5.18a and b). Average person-environment fit improved for all these subgroups over the four waves of the study.

Quality of performance. Quality of performance was examined in these analyses of highly anxious persons only in the personal life domain. There were too few respondents in the work domain for this analysis.

The highly anxious daily users did not differ from matched nonusers in their levels of either perceived technical or social performance at any of the four waves (Figures 5.19a and 5.20a). New users did not differ significantly from matched nonusers on technical performance, although the new users reported higher levels of social performance at Waves 1 and 3 compared to the nonusers (Figures 5.19b and 5.20b).

This difference in quality of social performance at Wave 1 may have accounted for the later difference at Wave 3. This interpretation is supported by an additional analysis. When Wave 1 quality of performance was added as a covariate (that is, statistically controlled), differences in quality of performance between new and nonusers became nonsignificant at Wave 3.

Ratings of the quality of performance of the users and of nonusers of Valium were available from the significant others in personal life (Figures 5.21a through 5.22b). There were no significant differences between users versus nonusers in the ratings received from their personal others at any of the four waves.

Quality of life. The daily users had consistently poorer self-reported health than equally anxious nonusers, although the differences diminished to nonsignificance by Wave 4

212

(Figures 5.23a and b). In further analyses, controlling for perceived quality of health at Wave 1, the differences at Waves 2 and 3 disappeared; this suggests that the consistently poorer health reported by the daily users reflected chronic health problems.

New users, by contrast to daily users, tended to report better perceived health than their nonuser comparison group. However, the difference was significant only at Wave 4.

The poorer perceived health of Valium users compared to nonusers, noted earlier in this chapter, apparently predated the beginning of the study (for example, proportionately more Valium users than nonusers reported taking medicines for high blood pressure). The relatively better perceived health of the highly anxious new users could have occurred because they may have experienced anxiety that was associated primarily with non-health stresses. If so, they would appear in better health than the nonusers, who were intentionally selected because they received a prescription medicine which was not indicated for emotional problems (and who, therefore, might have had health-related problems). Hence, new users might not have appeared healthier than an equally anxious nonuser group selected from the community at large rather than from pharmacy clients who were under medical treatment.

There were no differences between daily and nonusers of Valium in quality of personal life across all four waves (Figure 5.24a). At Wave 1, new users reported significantly lower quality of personal life than did nonusers, but there were no significant differences at Waves 2 through 4 (Figure 5.24b).

Quality of life with regard to self was consistently higher for new users than for the nonusers; this difference reached significance only at Wave 3 (Figure 5.25b). In contrast, daily users generally had lower levels of quality of life with regard to self than nonuser controls (Figure 5.25a). These findings parallel the pattern reported above for perceived health.

213

Quality of life-as-a-whole showed no significant differences between users and nonusers of Valium (Figures 5.26a and b). The new users changed from having a lower quality of life-as-a-whole than nonusers at Wave 1, to a higher one at Waves 3 and 4, but the differences were never significant.

For the positive and negative affects and for cognitive components of life-as-a-whole (Figures 5.27a through 5.29b), daily users did not differ from nonusers. New and daily users as well as nonuser controls tended to show reduction in mean negative affect from Wave 1 to Wave 4. New users also tended to show an increase in the positive and cognitive components of life quality from Wave 1 to Wave 4. By Wave 4, new users had significantly lower levels of negative affect, and significantly higher levels of positive affect and of the cognitive component of quality of life-as-a-whole, than nonusers.

The higher levels of self-rated life quality among new users compared to nonusers might be explained in terms of their levels of performance. Earlier it was noted that the new users tended to report higher levels of social performance. This pattern of findings suggests two interpretations of the results.

One interpretation is that new users, even before they took Valium, may have been better at coping and performing. If so, when experiencing high levels of anxiety, they might have sought Valium as well as have engaged in a number of other coping activities. Such coping could have improved life quality independent of the effects of Valium use.

A second possible interpretation is that use of Valium improved quality of performance, which, in turn, improved quality of life. Quality of social performance in personal life was positively correlated with quality of life. For example, at Wave 1 social performance correlated with quality of personal life .34 (df= 673, p< .001).

When statistical controls for measures of performance were introduced, they eliminated the significant differences between users and nonusers with regard to measures of quality of life. However, such analyses may control out the effect of the Valium

214

as well as any inherent coping ability in persons predisposed to use Valium. This conundrum cannot be resolved with this analytic approach. The measures of performance and quality of life developed in this study can, however, be used in experimental designs to evaluate these hypotheses.

If new users have better inherent abilities to perform socially compared to daily users (Figures 5.20a and b), this could account for daily users remaining at lower levels of quality of life than new users. If they lacked coping resources, daily users would be unable to overcome stresses in their lives, and would continue to take Valium on a regular basis to cope with chronic anxiety. Alternatively, daily users may have had the misfortune to have encountered stresses which are more resistant to control, such as the stress of a chronic illness or a chronically ill member of the family.

Significant others' ratings of the quality of life of the users and nonusers of Valium were available for the personal life domain (Figures 5.30a and b). There was no difference between daily users and nonusers in the ratings they received across the four waves. New users, however, were consistently rated as having lower quality of personal life than nonusers, and the difference reached statistical significance at Wave 4. This finding contradicts the pattern of results found for the several self-ratings of new users and nonusers. The explanation of the contradiction is unclear especially in view of the fact that the personal others did rate the performance of new users as relatively high.

Mental health of the personal other. Personal others of users and nonusers of Valium did not differ on a reduced version of the Hopkins Anxiety Scale (see Appendix M) at any of the four waves (Figures 5.31a and b). With regard to depression (Figures 5.32a and b), personal others of daily users, compared to personal others of nonusers, had significantly different levels of the reduced version of the Hopkins Depression measure only at Wave 4, when their depression was higher (see Appendix M). The difference for daily users at Wave 4 appears to be the result of two changes. One was a continuing reduction in depression among the nonusers' personal others. The other change was a Wave 4 increase in depression among the daily users' personal others. There is no one apparent reason for the latter change at Wave 4 and not at the prior waves.

New users' personal others had consistently higher levels of depression than the nonusers' significant others across all four waves. The differences, however, reached significance only at Wave 2. The personal other's quality of personal life was also examined in these analyses. There were no significant differences between the personal others of users and nonusers regarding quality of personal life (Figures 5.33a and b).

Summary

Users and nonusers of Valium with matched, relatively high levels of anxiety were compared with regard to stresses, strains, quality of performance, quality of life, and the well-being of their personal others. These analyses statistically controlled for differences between users and nonusers with regard to levels of stress and health.

Two sets of analyses of covariance were performed. One set restricted Valium users to daily users (persons who used Valium from six weeks preceding Wave 1 through Wave 2 on a daily or near daily basis). The other analysis restricted Valium users to new users (persons who began taking Valium for the first time sometime during the six weeks preceding Wave 1).

At the outset of this section, a number of differences were noted between the respondents included in these analyses and those in a typical clinical trial. Daily users had used Valium before entering the study and had no washout period. At best, therefore, analyses of daily users were a search for undesirable effects of at least 12 weeks of continuous use for that group. For new users the analyses examined the effects of initial use of Valium and could be seen as equivalent to including a washout period for prior Valium use.

The analyses found little evidence that use of Valium affected stress, strain, performance, or quality of life in either an adverse or beneficial way. However, daily users were likely to consume less alcohol than nonusers. This may be either because of compliance with medical admonitions to avoid

216

drug interaction effects, or because Valium substituted for alcohol. The study lacks sufficient data to select between these two interpretations, both of which could have been operating.

New users, compared to nonusers, also tended to show more improvement in some indicators of life quality (particularly, negative affect, positive affect, and cognitive components). No such differences were observed for these indicators when daily users and their matched nonusers were compared. It was noted that the apparent benefit among new users could be due to the medication. It could also be due to some inherent coping capability which caused them to seek Valium and, at the same time, make use of a number of other coping techniques for dealing with anxiety-provoking situations. At this time, both explanations are plausible.

With regard to perceived health, daily users were more likely than new users to rate their health as poor when compared to nonusers. The perceived health differences appear to be antecedent and/or coincident with the use of Valium rather than resulting from it. The differences were present from the outset of the study and appeared to represent chronic conditions or chronic risk of poor health. The data suggest that new users are less likely than daily users to have accompanying health problems. New users may be more likely to be taking Valium for reasons independent of physical health problems.

All of the findings must be viewed with caution because of the small numbers of respondents in these specially constructed groups. Perhaps the greatest value of such findings is to suggest directions for further research in clinical trials and in other types of designs.

Analyses of covariance restricted to respondents with initially high Wave 1 scores on the Hopkins Anxiety Scale. The "a" series of figures compares Daily users and nonusers whose Wave 1 mean Hopkins Anxiety Scores were 2.3 and 2.25, respectively.

The "b" series of figures compares new users and nonusers whose Wave 1 mean Hopkins Anxiety Scores were both 1.90. See the accompanying text for definitions of "daily," "new," and "nonusers." Means are adjusted for concurrent levels of stress and perceived health (Quality of Life-Health), except where stress or perceived health is a dependent variable. In such cases, analyses of a dependent variable never included that variable as a covariate. If significance levels are not noted, group differences are nonsignificant at all four waves.

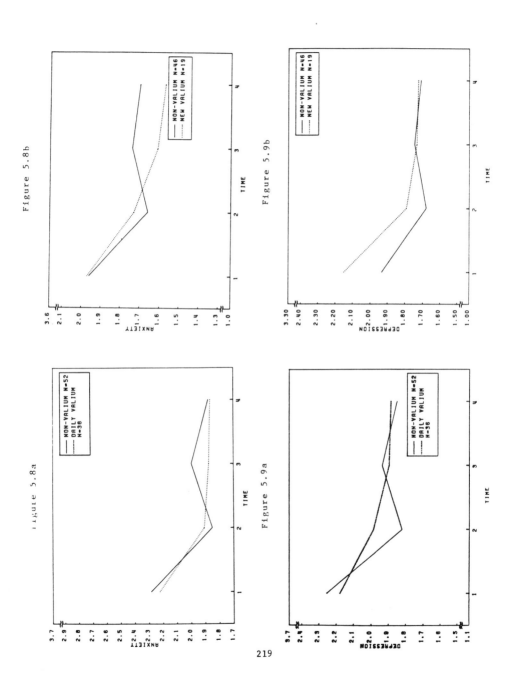

Figure 5.8b

Figure 5.8a

Figure 5.9b

Figure 5.9a

219

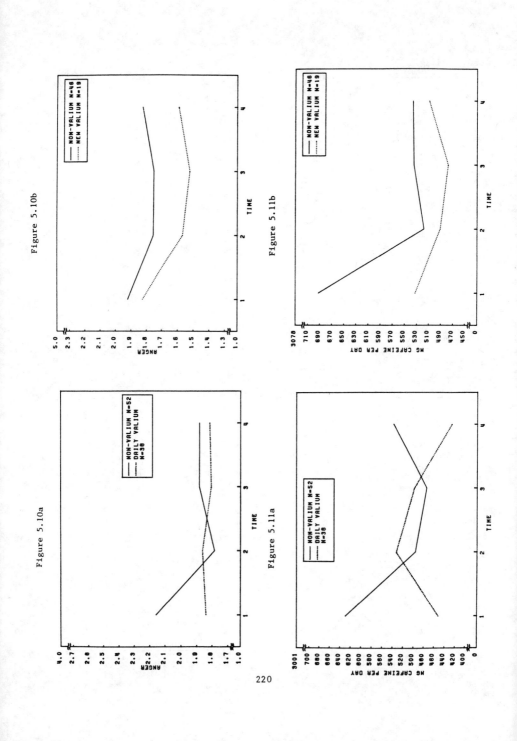

Figure 5.10a

Figure 5.10b

Figure 5.11a

Figure 5.11b

220

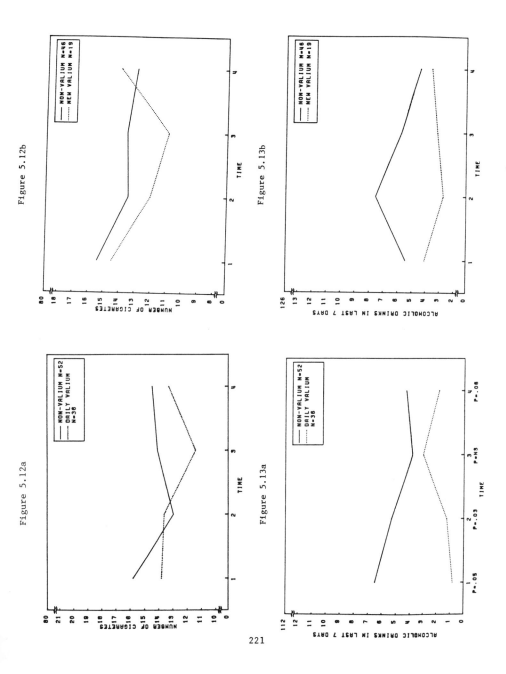

Figure 5.12a

Figure 5.12b

Figure 5.13a

Figure 5.13b

221

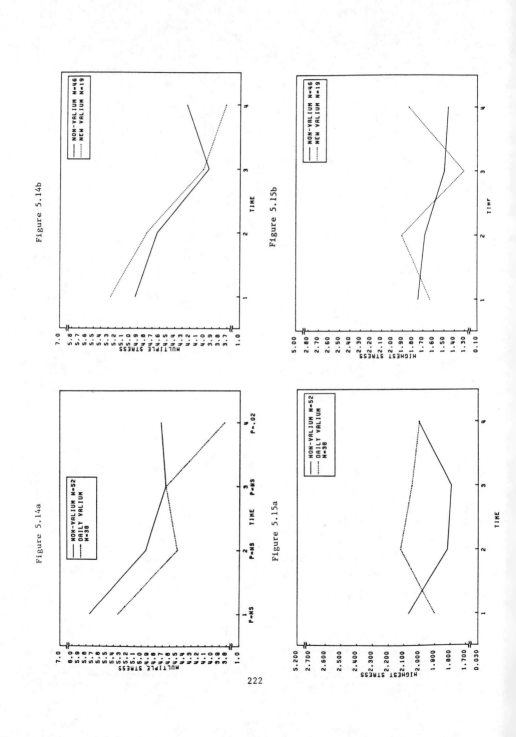

Figure 5.14b

Figure 5.14a

Figure 5.15b

Figure 5.15a

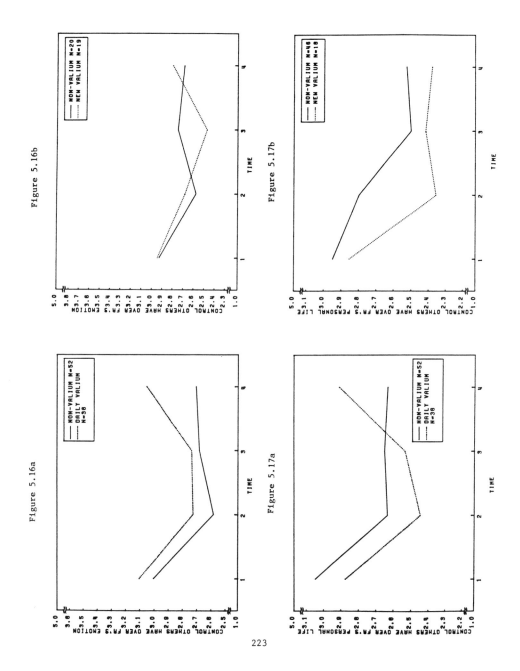

Figure 5.16a

Figure 5.16b

Figure 5.17a

Figure 5.17b

223

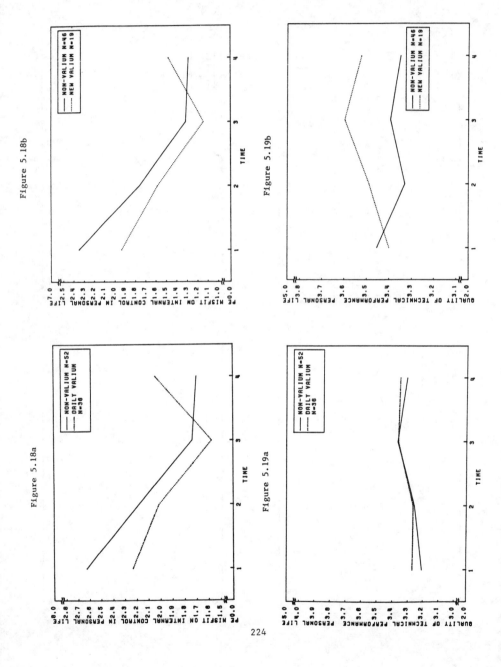

Figure 5.18a

Figure 5.18b

Figure 5.19a

Figure 5.19b

Figure 5.20a

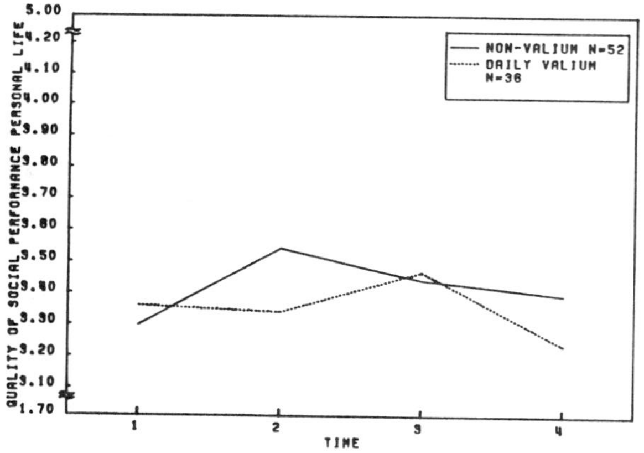

Figure 5.20b

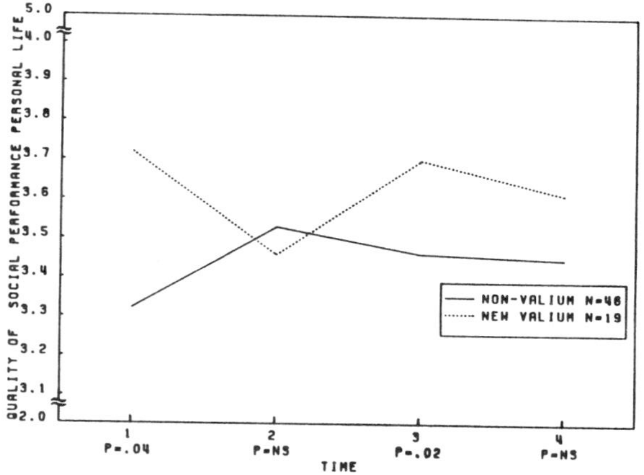

Figure 5.21a

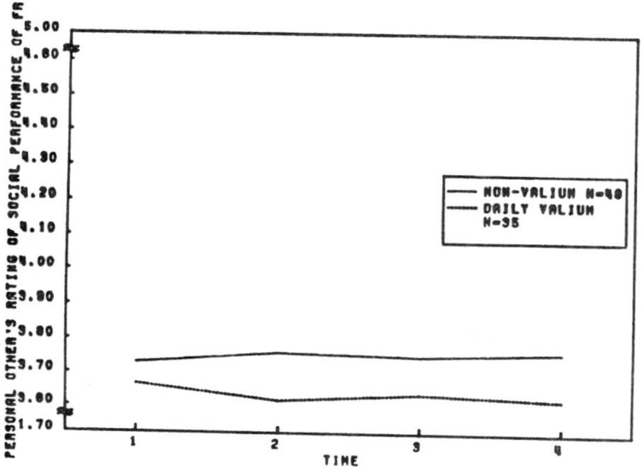

Figure 5.21b

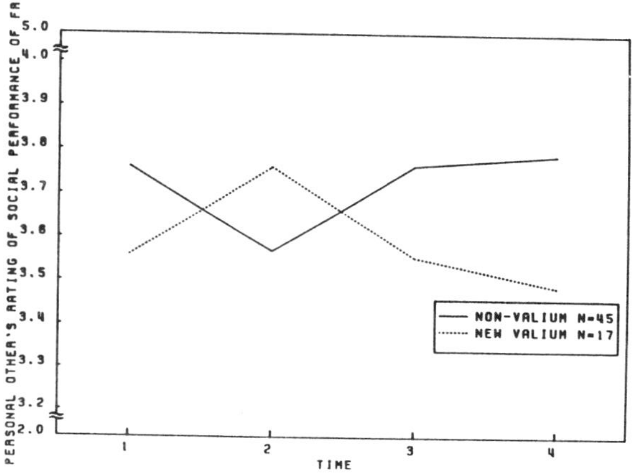

225

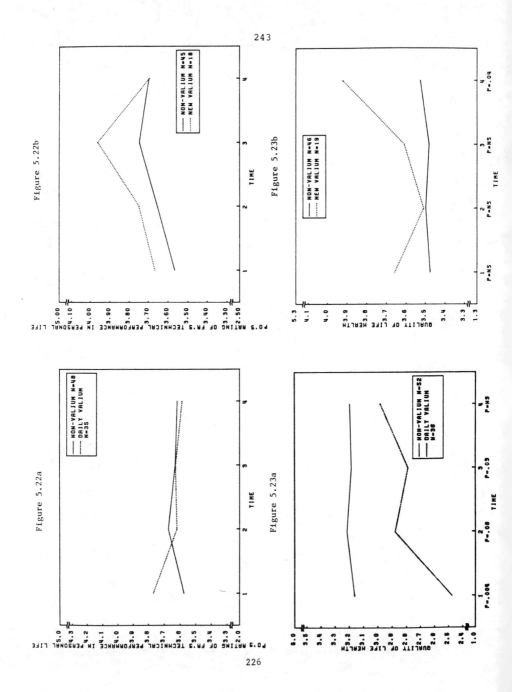

Figure 5.22b

Figure 5.23b

Figure 5.22a

Figure 5.23a

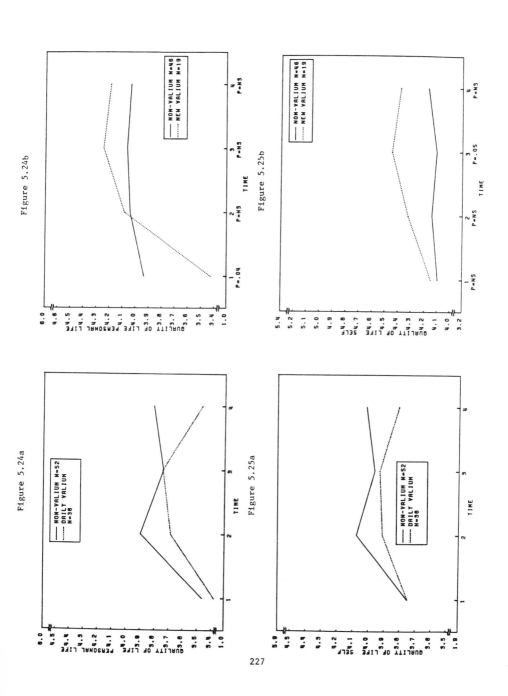

Figure 5.24a

Figure 5.24b

Figure 5.25a

Figure 5.25b

227

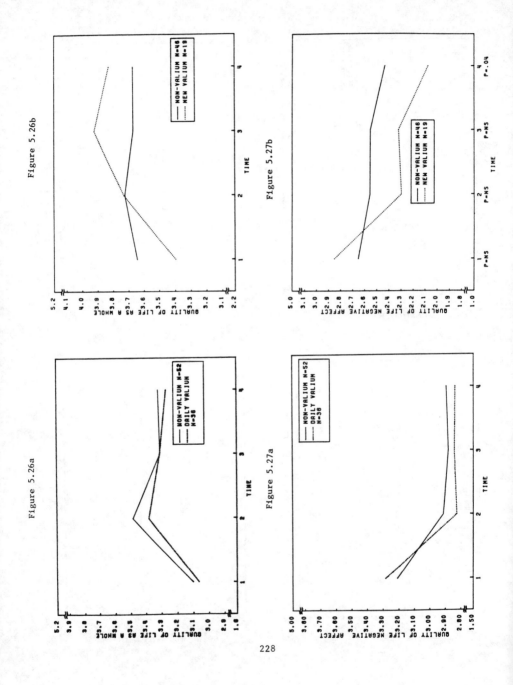

Figure 5.26b

Figure 5.27b

Figure 5.26a

Figure 5.27a

228

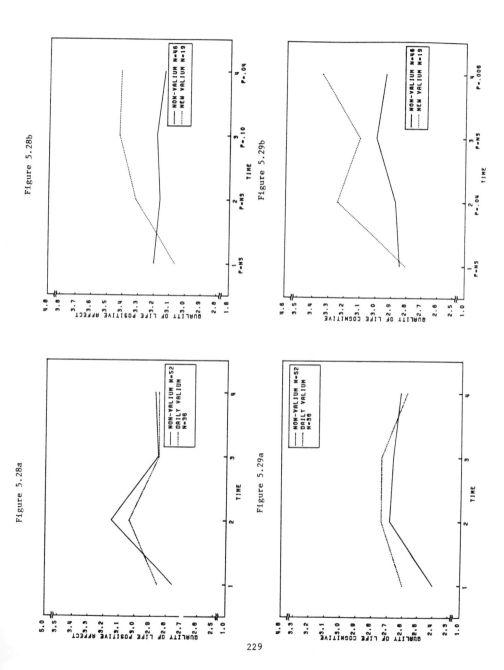

Figure 5.28b

Figure 5.28a

Figure 5.29b

Figure 5.29a

229

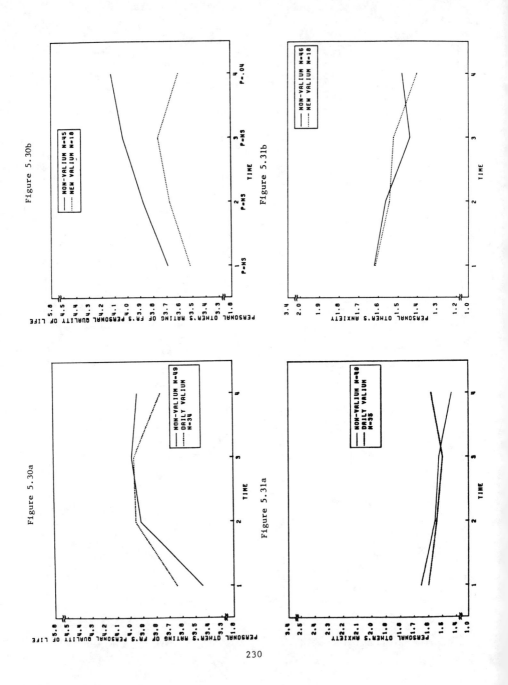

Figure 5.30b

Figure 5.31b

Figure 5.30a

Figure 5.31a

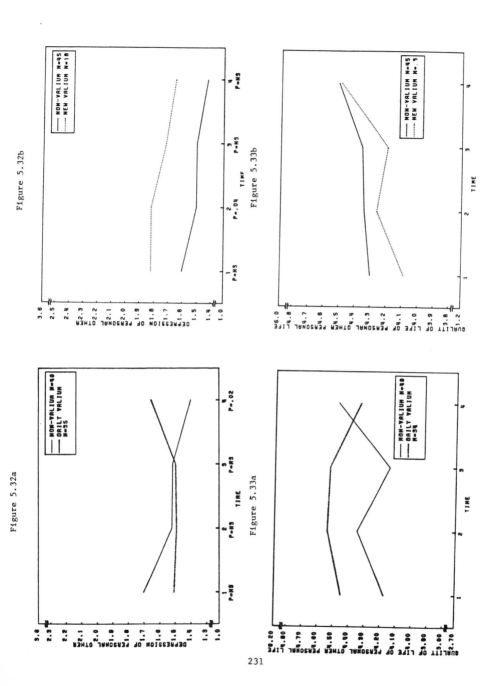

Figure 5.32b

Figure 5.33b

Figure 5.32a

Figure 5.33a

231

Summary of Multivariate Analyses

A variety of multivariate analyses suggested that Valium had no notable detrimental or beneficial effects on quality of life, performance, or a large number of other variables. The use of structural equation modeling showed that the weak cross-sectional associations of increased Valium use with high levels of anxiety and low levels of quality of life approached zero when controls were applied for stabilities in the stress and perceived health problems of users of Valium. Lagged change-score analyses were also performed, and they failed to uncover any relationships which were contrary to these findings.

Analysis of covariance was performed to compare daily or near-daily users of Valium with nonusers, and to compare new users with nonusers, all of whom had initial levels of anxiety found at entry in typical drug trials. These analyses controlled for initial differences between the users and nonusers of Valium in perceived health and stress. Means on a variety of potential social effects were examined at all four waves. These analyses also confirmed the absence of any harmful or beneficial effects of use of Valium on either the Valium user or the personal other. It is noteworthy that daily users consumed significantly less alcohol than nonusers, an effect that may reflect appropriate use of alcohol when taking Valium and/ or substitution of Valium for alcohol as a mood-modifying substance. Although there were a few other significant results, the small numbers of respondents in these analyses require that the findings should be interpreted with caution, but may be viewed as suggestive for lines of future research.

Within-person Analyses of Valium-taking, Anxiety, and Quality of Life

Research Questions

Several important questions are answered by the analyses reported in this portion of the chapter: For a typical individual, how does the amount of Valium taken at different times during the study relate to concurrent (or preceding or subsequent) levels of anxiety and life quality? Are there some individuals for whom Valium shows "beneficial" results--in the sense that Valium-taking tends to be followed by lower levels of anxiety and/or higher levels of life quality? Are there other individuals for whom Valium shows "detrimental" results or no results at all? If there are such individuals, are there any systematic differences between people who show "beneficial" effects, people who show "detrimental" effects, and people who show no effects?

Nature of the Analysis

The analyses reported in this portion of the chapter are distinctively different from those reported elsewhere. Most analyses in this report begin by examining variation across respondents, e.g., seeing how the variation across respondents in Valium-taking relates to variation in life quality, either simultaneously or some weeks after the Valium-taking. However, the analyses reported here begin with variation across weeks in the life of a given individual. The relationship between week-to-week variation in Valium-taking and week-to-week variations in anxiety and in quality of life was examined for each of the approximately 300 focal respondents who showed any changes on these phenomena.[1]

This kind of analysis is unusual in survey research because the necessary number of data points for each individual is rarely available. However, the "calendar" portions of the four sequential interviews conducted for this study provide a series of approximately 24 weekly reports on Valium-taking, anxiety, and quality of life-as-a-whole, and these are the data that were used.[2]

Using this information, Pearson product-moment correlation coefficients (r's) were computed between (a) Valium-taking and anxiety and (b) Valium-taking and life quality, separately for each individual. For each pair of concepts, nine r's were computed--one for each of the following lags: -9, -6, -3, -1,

---

[1] Cattell (1952) denotes the usual analysis that examines variation among people as an "R-type" analysis, and the within-person across-time analysis used here as a "P-type" analysis. An example of previous research which has used "P-type" analysis can be seen in Conway, Vickers, Ward, and Rahe, 1981.

[2] The Week 1 Valium-taking measure was adjusted to reflect a full 7-day span of time, as described in Chapter 4.

233

0, 1, 3, 6, 9.[73] Thus, for example, we can examine how the week-by-week variation in Valium-taking relates to the week-by-week variation in anxiety when anxiety precedes Valium-taking by three weeks (lag -3), when the anxiety is concurrent with Valium-taking (lag 0), and when the anxiety follows Valium-taking by one week (lag 1). Similarly, relationships between Valium-taking and life quality can be examined at the same nine time intervals.

Within-person Relationships for the "Typical" Individual

Table 5.18 presents the values of the within-person, over-time relationships between Valium-taking and anxiety when averaged across all the focal respondents for whom they were computed. At lag 0 (when concurrent Valium-taking and anxiety are related) the average correlation was positive and low (.17)--i.e., there was a modest tendency for higher anxiety to be linked with greater amounts of Valium being taken. At all other lags, the relationship was still weaker, and--with one minor exception--positive. Thus, on average, the amount of Valium a person took seems only very weakly related to how much anxiety the person reported--either before or after the Valium-taking.

Table 5.19 presents similar results for the relationships between Valium-taking and ratings of life quality. The findings here are very similar to those just described for Valium and anxiety, except that the weak relationships tend to be negative--i.e., lower life quality is associated with higher amounts of Valium-taking. Only at lag 0 did the magnitude of the relationship exceed -.10, and even here it was only -.13. In conclusion, on average, the week-by-week variation in Valium-taking showed only a weak relationship to the week-by-week variation in life quality ratings.

---

[73]The number of observations (weeks) over which the correlation is computed varies according to the lag interval. At lag 0 the maximum number of observations is 24; at lag 9 (or -9) the maximum number is 15. These numbers were occasionally reduced by instances of missing data, but a correlation was not computed if there were more than three weeks of missing data.

Table 5.18

MEAN VALUES OF THE WITHIN-PERSON CORRELATION BETWEEN VALIUM-TAKING AND ANXIETY AT VARIOUS LAGS

	Anxiety before Valium				Concurrent	Anxiety after Valium			
Lag in weeks	-9	-6	-3	-1	0	1	3	6	9
Mean r	-.01	.02	.03	.08	.17	.05	.01	.02	.02

Table 5.19

MEAN VALUES OF THE WITHIN-PERSON CORRELATION BETWEEN VALIUM-TAKING AND QUALITY OF LIFE AT VARIOUS LAGS

	QOL before Valium				Concurrent	QOL after Valium			
Lag in weeks	-9	-6	-3	-1	0	1	3	6	9
Mean r	-.01	.02	-.03	-.07	-.13	-.05	-.00	-.01	.01

Are There Some Individuals for Whom Valium Shows "Beneficial" or "Detrimental" Results?

The averages just described do not answer this question, and instead one must consider the distribution of the within-person correlations. This distribution shows that there were some individuals who showed negative relationships between Valium-taking and later anxiety, and there were some who showed positive relationships between Valium-taking and later life quality. There were roughly the same number of individuals who showed opposite patterns. In fact, the distribution of each of the 18 within-person relationships (nine for Valium and anxiety, nine for Valium and life quality) came close to matching the statistical "normal" (bell-shaped) curve, had a standard deviation of about .3, covered most of the theoretically possible range from -1.0 to +1.0, and was centered at the mean value shown in Table 5.18 or 5.19. So, while there were some individuals who showed "beneficial" patterns, and about an equal number who showed "detrimental" patterns, most individuals showed only weak relationships at any lag.

Searching for Systematic Differences Between People Who Showed "Beneficial" and "Detrimental" Effects

An extensive search was made for systematic differences between people who showed "beneficial" effects of Valium and those who showed "detrimental" effects. This was accomplished by relating the 18 within-person relationship scores described previously to about 80 other variables from the study-- including standard demographic information (age, sex, race, education, and income) and most of the scales tapping social and psychological constructs described in Chapter 4. Results showed no strong relationships. Most were under .20 (the highest was only .35), and none of the stronger relationships seemed theoretically meaningful.

Additional analyses were done in a further attempt to find subgroups or variables which might differentiate people who showed "beneficial" or "detrimental" effects of Valium (as indicated by the direction and magnitude of the within-person scores). These analyses compared a group of 22 relatively "new" users (i.e., the first time they ever took Valium was within six weeks of the beginning of the study), a group of 41 "off-on" users (i.e., they did not take Valium for at least one 6-week period during the study, but then resumed use), and a randomly selected group of "other" Valium users (i.e., not "new" or "off-on" users).

In the first of these analyses, all 18 within-person scores were compared across these three groups. Although there were a few statistically significant (p < .05) differences across groups, these differences did not appear very meaningful. In each of these groups both "positive" and "negative" lags produced very similar results, indicating that it made very little difference whether reports of Valium use preceded or followed reports of anxiety (or quality of life). Thus it appeared unlikely that the differences observed could be causally associated with Valium use.

In a second analysis, the 18 within-person scores were compared across three different groups: (a) people who took Valium at some time during the study who also reported at least one anxiety-related reason for taking Valium, but who did not report any physical illnesses/problems including epilepsy, para- or quadriplegia, or diseases/problems involving the musculoskeletal system, (b) other Valium users who did not fall into the group described in (a), and (c) respondents who did not report taking Valium at any time during the study. These comparisons also produced very few significant (p < .05) differences, and those that occurred appeared likely to be due to chance.

A third additional analysis was done to check for curvilinearity in the relationship between the within-person scores and two other variables: (a) dosage of Valium being taken, and (b) compliance of the patient's Valium consumption with the doctor's prescription.[74] The check for curvilinearity was done by comparing Pearson correlations (which reflect only linear components of a relationship) with etas (which reflect both linear and curvilinear components of a relationship).

---

[74]This measure of compliance was actually a measure of underuse, because very few respondents were overusers.

These statistics were computed for relationships between each of the 18 within-person scores and both the "dosage" and the "compliance" variables at Waves 1 and 3. The "dosage" variable was coded to represent four categories of users based on the milligrams of Valium consumed during "the last 7 days:" (a) 0 mg, (b) 1-29 mg, (c) 30-59 mg, and (d) 60+ mg. The "compliance" variable was coded to represent five categories of users based on the difference between the amount of Valium prescribed and what the patient usually took per day: (a) 0 mg--i.e., perfect compliance, (b) 1-4 mg less than prescribed, (c) 5 mg less, (d) 6-10 mg less, and (e) 11+ mg less per day than prescribed. Comparisons of correlations and etas provided no evidence of curvilinearity in the relationships between the within-person scores and the "dosage" or "compliance" variables.

One final analysis would have examined the within-person scores as possible moderators of other relationships. It could not be carried out because there were not enough individuals with sufficiently large negative Valium-anxiety within-person scores.[75]

Summary

Methodologically, the analyses described here represent an elegant way of addressing the questions raised at the beginning of this portion of this chapter. The results indicate that use of Valium--on average, and for most respondents--has little relationship, either positive or negative, to anxiety or life quality when these are measured any time from 1-9 weeks after Valium-taking. While there were some respondents who showed "beneficial" effects and others who showed "detrimental" ef-

---

[75]The original plan was to create two subgroups: one containing "responders" (i.e., those who had relatively high negative Valium-anxiety scores) and the other containing "nonresponders" (i.e., those with near-zero Valium-anxiety scores). Correlations among selected variables would have been computed for each group and then comparisons made to see if relationships were stronger (or weaker) for "responders" versus "nonresponders." However, this analysis could not be carried out because there were only 36 people with lag 0 Valium-anxiety relationships which were less than or equal to -.20; this problem was even greater at other lags.

fects, the possible significance of these findings is offset by our inability to distinguish the two groups on any of the more than 80 characteristics and numerous subgroups that were examined. Unless more meaningful results later emerge for these two groups, their presence is probably best attributed to the operation of chance factors rather than to substantively important phenomena.

A Case Study Approach to Changes in Anxiety and Quality of Life

The effects of Valium use on anxiety and quality of life may be different for new users of Valium than they are for long-term users of Valium. For example, the effects of Valium may be more pronounced when Valium is initially used than after prolonged, consistent use. Twenty-nine respondents who were taking Valium at Time 1 reported that they first took Valium within six weeks of the interview; these respondents were classified "new users." In order to increase the number of respondents included in these analyses, a second group of respondents, who were labelled "on-off users",[76] was identified. These individuals did not take Valium for at least one 6-week period during the study and then resumed use of Valium. Thirty-six respondents were identified who displayed this pattern of Valium use. Like the new users, their Valium use might have more pronounced effects because they were not long-term, consistent users.

Calendar data (see Chapter 4 for a description of these measures) were used because they allowed examination of week-by-week changes in Valium use, anxiety, and quality of life-as-a-whole for the 24 weeks of the study. Specifically, the relationship between commencing Valium use and changes in anxiety and life quality levels was examined. It was necessary to examine the data on a case-by-case basis because respondents began Valium use at different points. Several different analyses were conducted with these respondents and two control groups; these analyses are discussed in the following sections.

---

[76]The terms "on-off" and "off-on" are used interchangeably throughout this report.

Analysis I

This analysis looked at episodes of beginning use of Valium (t) after a period of at least two weeks of non-use. For every such episode, we determined how anxiety changed from the week before the Valium use to the week of its use (t-1, t), from the week when use began to the following week (t, t+1), and from the week when use began to the second following week (t, t+2); parallel calculations were made for changes in life quality. Differences were measured such that positive values indicate an increase in anxiety or life quality over a given time period, while negative values indicate a decrease. As shown in the first row of Table 5.20, anxiety tended to increase during the week when Valium use began relative to what it had been in the preceding week, and tended to decrease in the weeks immediately after use began compared to the week use began. For example, the number in the upper left cell in Table 5.20 indicates that, on the average, the anxiety of new and on-off users increased by .5 from the week before they took Valium to the week they took Valium. Similarly, quality of life tended to decrease during the week that Valium use began relative to what it had been in the preceding week, and tended to increase in the weeks immediately after use began compared to the week when use began.

An examination of rows 9 and 10 in Table 5.20 shows that the same pattern held both for new users of Valium and for on-off users. The magnitude of change was somewhat greater for new users than for on-off users, but the patterns were the same.

A comparison of rows 11 and 12 in Table 5.20 shows that the same pattern occurred regardless of whether Valium use occurred early or late in the course of the study. A comparison of rows 1 and 3 or rows 2 and 4 shows that this pattern occurred regardless of whether respondents reported taking Valium for reasons related to anxiety.

Analysis II

The results of Analysis I appeared to indicate a beneficial effect of Valium use; after these respondents began taking

Valium, their anxiety diminished and their perceived life quality improved. Before attributing this change to Valium, it was necessary to conduct further analyses. Analysis II was designed to determine whether the changes in anxiety and quality of life found in Analysis I would also appear when Valium was not being used. In Analysis II, an "episode" consisted of four adjacent weeks (t-1, t, t+1, t+2) in which anxiety increased from t-1 to t, and in which Valium was never used.[77] These findings, for the same respondents examined in Analysis I, are presented in row 7 of Table 5.20. The same basic pattern was found as in the first set of analyses, that is, the initial increase in anxiety was followed by a decrease in anxiety. Similarly, an initial decrease in quality of life was followed by a increase in life quality.

The initial increase in anxiety from week t-1 to t was higher for "new" and "on/off" users during episodes when they did not take Valium (row 7) than during episodes when they did (row 1 of Table 5.20). Of course, in row 7 the change from t-1 to t had to be at least 1.0 because this was how episodes were defined, which was not true for the analyses summarized in row 1. Row 2 is comparable to row 1, except that the analyses included only episodes of Valium use in which there was a concomitant increase in anxiety of at least 1.0. Comparison of rows 7 and 2 (which used the same criterion for anxiety increases to define episodes, but differed in that row 2 episodes involved taking Valium and in row 7 they did not) shows similar patterns. Although the patterns are similar, episodes including Valium use showed higher mean changes than did episodes in which Valium was not used.

This last finding suggested that these new and on-off users chose to take Valium at times when changes in their anxiety levels were particularly large. To further examine this phenomenon, an additional analysis was conducted focusing on new and on-off users who reported taking Valium for reasons related to anxiety. This analysis examined only episodes in which anxiety rose at least 2.0 and Valium was not taken. When

---

[77]The increase had to be at least 1.0 because the scale points were whole units.

these figures (not shown) were compared to those in row 4, they showed comparable initial increases in anxiety and comparable later decreases in anxiety. However, the initial decrease in life quality was not quite as large nor were the subsequent increases at t+1 and t+2. Consequently, for these respondents there was no evidence that anxiety decreased more one week later when they used Valium than when they did not use Valium. The results for quality of life were less clear and may be suggestive of an area for future research.

Analysis III

Two other groups of respondents were examined to help clarify interpretation of these findings. First, a group of respondents who never used Valium during the course of the study was identified. A nonuser control group was selected by matching them to the new and on-off users on their within-person mean levels of anxiety and variability (standard deviation) using the 24 week-by-week "calendar" measures (see the section on within-person analysis in this chapter for a description of the logic of this type of analysis). For these respondents, episodes in which anxiety increased from t-1 to t were identified and compared with the episodes that followed. The results of this analysis are presented in row 8 of Table 5.20. This pattern of results was comparable to the pattern found for new and on-off users for episodes in which anxiety increased from t-1 to t and Valium either was or was not taken (rows 2 and 7, respectively--as described in the previous section).

Finally, a random subset of Valium users other than the new and on-off users was examined. Again, episodes of beginning use of Valium after a period of at least two weeks of non-use were identified. In one analysis, all such episodes were used in calculations (row 5 of Table 5.20), in a second analysis only episodes which were also associated with an increase in anxiety were included (row 6 of Table 5.20). Results showed the same pattern that all other analyses have shown: anxiety tended to increase during week t relative to week t-1, and tended to decrease in weeks t+1 and t+2 compared to week t. Quality of life showed the converse. It should be noted that

242

the findings are somewhat weaker for this group of Valium users than for the new and on-off users (row 1 versus row 5; row 2 versus row 6).

Summary and Conclusions

The results of Analysis I could be interpreted as showing either (a) a beneficial effect of Valium (note the increase in anxiety as Valium is begun and the decline after people have taken Valium, and the reversed pattern--as seems reasonable-- for quality of life) or (b) a "natural" over-time variation in anxiety and quality of life that has been synchronized with Valium-taking, but cannot be attributed to Valium-taking. Analysis I shows that the basic pattern appeared for both new and on-off users, and for both early and late episodes of Valium use during the study. Analysis II, which showed the same pattern of anxiety changes described above even when people did not take Valium, and Analysis III, which showed comparable findings for two different control groups, suggest that explanation b is more likely than a, particularly in the case of anxiety. For quality of life, the results were similar, but differences were consistent enough to suggest that this might be a fruitful area for future research. It might be noted that new and on-off users, compared to other Valium users, took Valium when they experienced larger increases in anxiety and larger decreases in life quality. The number of respondents in these analyses was quite small, so caution must be exercised in drawing conclusions from these results.

Alternative Ways of Dealing with Anxiety

A variety of potential methods of handling anxiety, other than Valium use, were examined in this study. These concepts, and hypotheses regarding their effects on strain, are described in detail in Chapter 2. A brief review of some of these hypotheses regarding anxiety will be presented here, however, as background for some analyses which will be presented later in this section.

Four specific coping-like and defense-like strategies of dealing with stress and strain were examined: religious beliefs, maintaining a positive approach, reinterpretation of

243

Table 5.20

	$Anx_{t-1,t}$	$Anx_{t,t+1}$	$Anx_{t,t+2}$	$QOL_{t-1,t}$	$QOL_{t,t+1}$	$QOL_{t,t+2}$
(1) New & on-off users of Valium: off Valium 2 weeks & then resume use (n=65)	.5	-.5	-.7	-.7	.8	.8
(2) New & on-off users of Valium: off Valium 2 weeks & then resume use with concomitant increase in anxiety (n=65)	1.9	-1.1	-1.0	-1.8	1.2	1.4
(3) New & on-off users of Valium who report taking Valium for reasons related to anxiety: off Valium 2 weeks & then resume use (n=58)	.6	-.5	-.7	-.8	.8	.9

Table 5.20
(continued)

	$Anx_{t-1,t}$	$Anx_{t,t+1}$	$Anx_{t,t+2}$	$QOL_{t-1,t}$	$QOL_{t,t+1}$	$QOL_{t,t+2}$
(4) New & on-off users of Valium who report taking Valium for reasons related to anxiety: off Valium 2 weeks & then resume use with concomitant increase in anxiety (n=58)	1.9	-1.2	-1.0	-1.7	1.2	1.4
(5) Valium users (not on-off or new users): off Valium 2 weeks & then resume use (n=61)	.4	-.4	-.3	-.2	.0	-.1
(6) Valium users (not on-off or new users): off Valium 2 weeks & then resume use with concomitant increase in anxiety (n=61)	1.5	-.7	-.7	-.8	.5	.3

245

Table 5.20
(continued)

	$Anx_{t-1,\ t}$	$Anx_{t,\ t+1}$	$Anx_{t,\ t+2}$	$QOL_{t-1,\ t}$	$QOL_{t,\ t+1}$	$QOL_{t,\ t+2}$
(7) New & on-off users of Valium: periods in which they are not taking Valium but their anxiety increases (n=65)	1.5	-.6	-.8	-.8	.2	.4
(8) Nonusers of Valium: periods in which anxiety increases (n=65)	1.6	-.7	-.8	-.8	.4	.4
(9) New users of Valium only: off Valium 2 weeks & then resume use (n=29)	.5	-.5	-.9	-1.2	.9	.9

Table 5.20
(continued)

	Anx$_{t-1,\,t}$	Anx$_{t,\,t+1}$	Anx$_{t,\,t+2}$	QOL$_{t-1,\,t}$	QOL$_{t,\,t+1}$	QOL$_{t,\,t+2}$
(10) On-off users of Valium only: off Valium 2 weeks & then resume use (n=36)	.4	-.5	-.4	-.5	.5	.7
(11) New & on-off users of Valium: off Valium & then resume use in first 12 weeks of study	.4	-.3	-.6	-.8	.5	.6
(12) New & on-off users of Valium: off Valium & then resume use in last 12 weeks of study	.6	-.8	-.6	-.9	1.0	1.1

events, and seeking help from others. The use of each of these techniques could be related to anxiety. For example, individuals capable of maintaining a positive approach may be less anxious than other individuals because of their optimistic perspective. In addition to these four strategies, several others were examined: social support, perceptions of control, and use of other affect-modifying substances (e.g., alcohol, caffeine, and other drugs).

It was hypothesized that social support exerts some of its beneficial effects by providing individuals with information about other methods of coping with stress (Abbey, 1983; Schaefer, Coyne, & Lazarus, 1981; Wortman, in press). A person may either seek out this social support or be provided with it without asking when supporters note that the person is under stress. In either case, this information might improve coping and, in turn, might lead to a reduction in anxiety (Lazarus, 1981).

Perceptions of control might also be related to anxiety. Individuals with high levels of perceived internal control may feel less anxious than do individuals with low levels of perceived internal control because they feel capable of directing events in a way that will benefit them. They may be more likely to attempt to engage in active coping because they have more confidence that they will be able to have an impact on the external environment. Conversely, individuals with high levels of perceived internal control may feel more anxious than individuals with low levels of perceived internal control because they feel personally responsible but are ambivalent about what to do or how to achieve their wishes (Janoff-Bulman & Brickman, 1982). With parallel reasoning, hypotheses can be generated regarding the potential anxiety-provoking or anxiety-reducing effects of perceived control by others.

Finally, use of other substances might influence individuals' anxiety levels or their responses to anxiety. For example, alcohol use may reduce anxiety or anxiety may increase alcohol use. Psychotherapy may also be related to anxiety in the sense that anxious people may be more likely to seek therapy.

248

Bivariate correlations between these variables and anxiety at Time 1 are presented in Table 5.21. Several coping-like or defense-like strategies were related to anxiety. For example, the more respondents used reinterpretation, which involves trying to understand why something occurred and to find meaning in its occurrence, the greater their anxiety (r = .27). This may be because the cognitive effort exerted in the attempt to find meaning is anxiety-provoking. It is also possible that the greater respondents' anxiety, the greater their use of reinterpretation. The causal direction of all the findings in this section is unclear because only cross-sectional analyses were conducted. Social support was weakly related to anxiety such that the greater the social support, the lower the anxiety (r= -.18). Social support may have anxiolytic effects. Alternatively, this finding could indicate that people with low levels of anxiety do best at establishing supportive relationships.

Perceived internal control over one's personal life was weakly related to anxiety such that the greater one's level of perceived internal control, the lower one's anxiety (r= -.15). Conversely, perceptions that others control one's personal life and emotions were positively related to anxiety (r= .25, r= .34 respectively). Anxiety was also positively correlated with the use of CNS depressant-like drugs other than Valium (r= .26), street drugs (r= .16), and cigarette-smoking (r= .24). Receiving psychotherapy within the previous year was also positively correlated with anxiety (r= .34).

The moderating effects of these same variables on the relationship between stress and anxiety are presented in Table 5.22. It was hypothesized that these various coping-like and defense-like techniques might moderate the relationship between stress and anxiety. As can be seen from Table 5.22, social support moderated the relationship between stress and anxiety. For individuals with high levels of social support there was a significantly weaker relationship between negative life events and anxiety than there was for individuals with low levels of social support. This same trend was exhibited for the relationship between anxiety and role ambiguity in the personal

249

Table 5.21

TIME 1 CORRELATIONS BETWEEN SOME ALTERNA-
TIVE WAYS OF COPING AND ANXIETY'

	Hopkins Anxiety r
Religious beliefs	.08
Positive approach	.16**
Reinterpretation	.27**
Seek help from others	.10*
Informational social support	-.11*
Esteem social support	-.18**
Perceived internal control over personal life	-.15**
Perceived internal control over emotions	-.02
Perceived control by others over personal life	.25**
Perceived control by others over emotions	.34**
Caffeine	.04
Alcohol	.10*
Street drugs	.16**
CNS depressant-like drugs	.26**
CNS stimulant-like drugs	.07
Cigarettes	.24**
Psychotherapy	.34**
Valium	.30**

* p< .05
**p< .01
'An examination of the correlations between calendar anxiety
and these variables at 12 different lags indicates that the
strongest relationships are usually at lag 0.

life, but it was not statistically significant. There were no other statistically significant moderating effects (except for the non-replicated one for Valium use shown in the last row of the table). These findings need to be examined at later waves and longitudinally before statements about the causal ordering of these variables can be made.

Effects of Valium Use on Significant Others in Personal Life and Work Life

To what extent is the well-being of significant others influenced by whether the focal respondent takes Valium? Given the uniqueness of this question in the study of a minor tranquilizer, the results of analyses that examined these effects are detailed in this section. They are reported first for the personal life significant other (personal other) and then, for employed respondents, for the significant other in work life (work other). The analyses are confined to Wave 1 except to determine if certain key results replicated. These replications used data from Wave 4. Analyses of selected variables for all four waves of data were reported in a previous section comparing two subgroups of highly anxious Valium users--daily and new users--with highly anxious nonusers.

Personal Other Results

Who were they? Forty-six percent of the personal others were spouses. Another 1/4 were friends, and just over 1/4 (27%) were relatives. The remaining 1% (six persons out of 631 at Wave 1) fell into other categories (e.g., ex-spouse or neighbor).

Was the focal respondent's formal relationship to the personal other associated with characteristics of the personal other or of the focal respondent? Any such association might suggest that the effects of Valium use on the well-being of a significant other should be examined separately for different types of significant others. Therefore, analyses of variance were run to determine if there were mean differences in the focal respondents' emotional states and in Valium-taking for focal respondents who selected a spouse versus a friend versus a relative to serve as their personal other. It should be

251

Table 5.22

RELATIONSHIPS BETWEEN TWO SOURCES OF STRESS AND ANXIETY
AS MODERATED BY SOME ALTERNATE WAYS OF COPING

	Stressors			
	Role Ambiguity in Personal Life		Negative Life Events	
	Level of Moderator		Level of Moderator	
Moderator Variables	Low	High	Low	High
Religious beliefs	.50	.42	.30	.34
Positive approach	.56	.46	.43	.29
Reinterpretation	.43	.49	.30	.38
Seek help from others	.53	.47	.36	.39
Informational social support	.47	.39	.55	.30**
Esteem social support	.51	.37	.60	.26**
Perceived internal control over personal life	.52	.35	.40	.34
Perceived internal control over emotions	.45	.46	.47	.34
Perceived control by others over personal life	.42	.47	.42	.33

Table 5.22

RELATIONSHIPS BETWEEN TWO SOURCES OF STRESS AND ANXIETY
AS MODERATED BY SOME ALTERNATE WAYS OF COPING
(continued)

	Stressors			
	Role Ambiguity in Personal Life		Negative Life Events	
	Level of Moderator		Level of Moderator	
Moderator Variables	Low	High	Low	High
Perceived control by others over emotions	.42	.44	.37	.39
Caffeine	.56	.43	.46	.31
Alcohol	.43	.47	.34	.34
CNS depressant-like drugs	.44	.47	.28	.37
CNS stimulant-like drugs	.45	.48	.36	.34
Cigarettes	.49	.42	.36	.32
Psychotherapy	.44	.44	.33	.31
Valium	.51	.33*	.27	.36

* Difference in r's significant at p< .05
**Difference in r's significant at p< .01

noted that focal respondents could nominate only one significant other in the personal life. Consequently, this study
cannot determine if comparisons of different types of significant others for the _same_ focal respondent would produce
similar results.

Those respondents whose spouse served as their personal
other were less depressed at Waves 1 and 4 than respondents who
had a relative or friend serve in this category (respective
Wave 1 and 4 etas = .19 and .10, respectively).[78] Respondents
whose personal other was a spouse, rather than a friend or
relative, were also less anxious and angry at Wave 1 (respective Wave 1 etas = .14 and .10), but these differences were
nonsignificant at Wave 4. Type of personal other was not associated with significant differences in the amount of Valium
taken by the focal respondent in the last seven days at Waves 1
and 4.

There were some differences in the social-psychological
responses of the personal others depending on whether they were
spouses, friends, or relatives. Using Wave 1 data, spouses,
compared to friends or relatives, tended to judge the quality
of life of the focal respondent as higher (eta = .17). Spouses
tended to rate both the technical and social performance of
their focal respondent higher than did significant others who
were friends, but no differently than did relatives (both overall Wave 1 etas = .10; Wave 4 etas = .12 and .10 respectively).
Spouses, compared to nonspouses, also judged their focal
respondents as providing them with less social support and more
social conflict (etas = .20 and .40 respectively). Finally,
spouses, compared to nonspouses, perceived themselves as
providing less social support and directing more social conflict toward their focal respondents (Wave 1 etas = .21 and .44
respectively; Wave 4 etas = .11 and .31 respectively).

In summary, these findings suggest that if one interviews
the spouse as the significant other, ratings of depression of

---

[78]All etas reported in this section on the personal other
are statistically significant (minimum p< .05) unless otherwise
noted. Degrees of freedom were 2 and 622 with slight variations in the latter number for missing data.

the focal respondent are likely to be lower, ratings of the focal respondent's quality of life and performance are likely to
be higher, and ratings of social support between the pair are
likely to be lower. There were no differences by type of significant other, however, in the significant others' ratings of
their own quality of life, anxiety, or depression.

The differences that did appear could be due to a variety
of influences. Differences in the well-being of the focal
respondent, as reported by the focal respondent, may have to do
with the type of significant other one can call upon in personal life. They may also have to do with attributes of the
focal respondent as well as of the personal other which led to
the relationship. Differences among types of personal others
with respect to their perceptions of the focal respondent's
well-being may be due to differences in the amount and type of
information to which each type of personal other is exposed.
For example, a spouse may see more positive and negative behaviors than a friend or relative. Such differences may also
reflect biases in perception motivated by different
relationships, or may be due to the consequences of being able
to rely on such a relationship (Caplan, Robinson, French,
Caldwell, & Shinn, 1976, pp. 132-133). These different
hypotheses cannot be tested in this data set because each
respondent was rated by only one type of individual from the
personal life.

Relationships between Valium use by the focal respondent
and the well-being of the personal other. These analyses examined how the well-being of the significant other was related
to the focal respondent's use of Valium, alcohol, caffeine,
cigarettes, and a number of nondrug modes of coping and
defense (indices of seeking help, turning to religion, taking a
positive approach to life, and reinterpreting the meaning of
things). The analyses examined the following characteristics
of the significant other as dependent variables: overall
quality of life-as-a-whole and quality of personal life, and
anxiety and depression as measured by reduced versions of the
Hopkins scales. Other dependent variables included the amount
of time the significant other spent with the focal respondent

in the last seven days, perceptions of the quality of life of the focal respondent, the focal respondent's technical and social performance in personal life, and social support and social conflict both received from and given to the focal respondent as judged by the personal other.

Valium use and the other modes of coping and defense were generally unrelated to all of these dependent variables. Most correlations did not exceed .08 in absolute value. Only one coefficient exceeded .13 -- a negative relationship between the estimated milligrams of Valium the focal respondent took per day and the personal other's estimate of the focal respondent's quality of working life (r=-.17). This finding did not replicate at Wave 4 (r=.02, ns). The near-zero relationships for the other variables did replicate at Wave 4.

As an additional check on the findings, the relationship of Valium use to indicators of the personal other's well-being was examined separately for significant others who were spouses, friends, and relatives. As noted above, there were initial differences among these three types of significant others in their reports of the well-being and social support of the focal respondents. Those differences suggested that there might be important differences in the effects of Valium depending on the type of significant other. Only a few statistically significant findings involving Valium use were found, however, and those were neither substantively interesting nor reliable.

These analyses, of course, did not make use of the sophisticated controls incorporated in the structural equation modeling used elsewhere in this study. The analyses of covariance across all four waves, reported in a prior section of this chapter, ("Changes in stress, strain, and performance among the highly anxious: A comparison of Valium users and nonusers), did make use of more sophisticated analyses, and found essentially no effects of Valium use on the well-being of the personal other. Within the limits of the analyses detailed above, there was no evidence that Valium either improved or worsened the well-being of significant others in personal life. This conclusion appeared to hold for significant others who were spouses, friends, or relatives of the focal respondents.

Validity of the personal other data. Earlier in this chapter evidence was presented indicating that the self-report data from the focal respondents were reliable and valid. Were the data from the significant others equally reliable and valid? The reliabilities of the significant other indices were all acceptable, as reported in Chapter 4, "Measures." To evaluate the concurrent construct validity of these measures, analyses were performed to examine relationships among these measures and between them and the focal respondents' self-reports of stress, strain, social support, and other phenomena. A large number of substantial relationships appeared. These findings suggest that the significant others' self-reports were reasonably valid and were useful for the purposes of this study. For example, the higher the personal other's own anxiety and depression, the lower was the personal other's quality of personal life (r's=-.50 and -.64 respectively, both p<.001). These same relationships were very similar when measured for the focal respondents (r's=-.46 and -.67 respectively; both p<.001).

As another example, the focal respondent's self-reported quality of personal life, the personal other's report of that same variable, and the personal other's own self-reported quality of personal life were all positively intercorrelated, as shown in Figure 5.34. These data suggest a model which assumes that the effect of the focal respondent's quality of life on the personal other's quality of life operates via the personal other's perception. Perception acts as a filter in this process. Although the focal respondent's subjective quality of life was somewhat related to the significant other's subjective quality of life, the partial correlation indicates that almost all of the effect of the focal respondent's reported quality of life operated via the personal other's perception.[79] A replication of this pattern of findings appears for quality of

---

[79] It is possible, in practice, to reverse the direction of the causal arrows so that they point from right to left. The model in Figure 5.34, however, seems more plausible. Without going into details, it involves fewer assumptions and is hypothesized to produce stronger effects than the suggested alternative. The reader may wish to consider this in further detail, but it will not be pursued here.

257

life in the work domain, also shown in Figure 5.34. Other findings regarding the work other are presented shortly.

Self-ratings and personal other ratings of the quality of performance of the focal respondent also tended to be related, although the correlations were weak. For example, at Wave 1, their two ratings of technical performance were correlated .16 (p<.01) and their two ratings of social performance were correlated .20 (p<.01). Despite these weak relationships, both the focal respondent's ratings and the personal other's ratings of the focal respondent's technical performance in the personal life domains related positively to their respective subjective qualities of life in the personal domain (r's=.41 and .32 respectively). As a whole, the above findings suggest that the measures of the personal other's well-being and other perceptions by the personal other show reasonable evidence of concurrent validity. Consequently, the lack of evidence that use of Valium is associated with any beneficial or harmful effects on a significant other in personal life does not appear to be due to invalid measures of the significant other's well-being.

Work Other Results

Who were they? At Wave 1, 247 focal respondents provided a work other who completed an interview. Just over 1/2 (56%) of these significant others were co-workers, about 1/4 (26%) were a boss or supervisor, and the remainder (18%) included friends, subordinates, and relatives with whom the focal respondent worked. The last category of work others was likely to occur among focal respondents who were self-employed.

Was the relationship of the work other to the focal respondent associated with any characteristics of the focal respondent or of the work other? With regard to Wave 1 data, bosses and supervisors, compared to coworkers, evaluated the quality of work life of the focal respondent and of themselves as higher (overall etas=.21 and .14 respectively).[80] Bosses and supervisors also reported less social conflict from the fo-

---

[80]All etas presented in this section on the work other are statistically significant with a minimum p< .05, unless otherwise noted. Degrees of freedom are 2 and 244 with slight variations in the latter number for missing data.

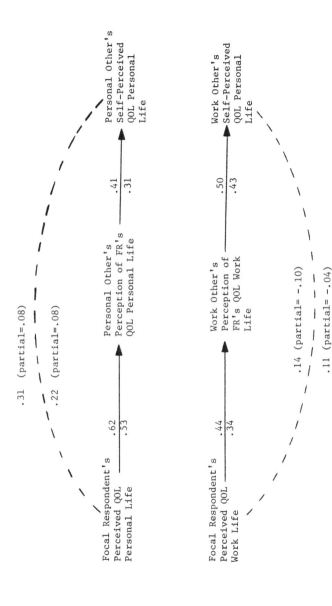

Figure 5.34 Quality of personal life as perceived by the focal respondent and significant other. Arrows represent hypothesized pathways. Zero-order and partial correlations are presented. Wave 1 data given above arrows and Wave 4 data given below arrows. All correlations except the partials are statistically significant.

cal respondent than was reported by coworkers and other categories of work others (overall eta=.18 p< .02). These findings tended to replicate at Wave 4. The reason for these effects is not clear.

There were no differences by type of work other in the work other's mean ratings of the focal respondent's technical and social performance. Care must be exercised in interpreting such findings. Each focal respondent was allowed to select a work other whom he or she knew well. Such a selection procedure could tend to reduce differences in rating perform- ance among the three categories of raters.

Bosses and supervisors on the average had higher levels of education, were older, and tended to spend less time with the focal respondent, particularly when compared to coworkers (the respective overall etas were .21, .18, and .14).

Relationships of Valium use by the focal respondent to the well-being of the work other. As was the case for the personal other, analyses of data from Waves 1 and 4 failed to show any statistically significant relationship between the amount of Valium taken by the focal respondent and the well-being of the work other. Nor were any relationships found between other modes of coping (e.g., use of alcohol, taking a positive ap- proach towards life, seeking help from others) and the well- being of the work other. These analyses were also run separately for work others who were a boss or supervisor versus a coworker of the focal respondent. The results were unchanged.

Validity of work other measures. Again one can consider whether or not the indices measuring the well-being of the work other were adequate to detect an effect if one existed. In the case of the work other, only overall quality of life-as-a- whole and of working life were measured, not anxiety or depres- sion. As was already noted with regard to Figure 5.34, the work other's perceptions of the focal respondent's quality of work life correlated positively with the focal respondent's own perceptions of quality of life at work. And the work other's perception of the focal respondent's quality of life at work related to the work other's own quality of life at work.

As other evidence of the concurrent construct validity of the work other measures, the work other's ratings of the quality of work life of the focal respondent correlated -.25 with the focal respondent's anxiety and -.20 with the focal respondent's depression as measured on the Hopkins scales (both r's p<.01). This same pattern of relationships was found in the ratings made by the personal other of the focal respondent's quality of personal life (the comparable r's were stronger, however: -.40 and -.50 respectively). The focal respondent's and work other's ratings of the focal respondent's technical performance were unrelated (for example, at Wave 1, r=.07, ns), but their ratings of the focal respondent's social performance were related (for example, at Wave 1, r=.27, p<.01).

One finding of interest has to do with who was the work other who provided the performance rating. The correlation between the focal respondent's self-ratings and the work other's ratings of the focal respondent's performance was lower when the work other was a boss or supervisor than when the work other was a coworker. For example, at Wave 1, the correlations between focal respondent and boss or supervisor ratings of technical and social performance were .01 and .15 (neither statistically significant); the respective correlations when comparing focal respondent and coworker ratings were .15 (ns) and .28 (p< .01). This result occurred despite the finding, already noted, that different types of work others did not differ significantly in the mean ratings for performance that they assigned to the focal respondent. The similarity of means for different types of raters but the difference in correlations suggests that there was no overall tendency for one group of work other raters to be more or less generous in the ratings they gave. Rather, there is a tendency for the boss and supervisor to be less concordant with the focal respondent in all directions, a potential indicator of the greater unreliability of the boss and supervisor compared to the coworker as a rater. The use of ratings by peers is of interest to administrative scientists. At least one study (in three life insurance companies) suggests that such ratings are predictive of objective employee performance (e.g., Gibson, Ivancevich, & Donnally, 1979, p. 372).

In summary, a number of work other measures were examined and found to have adequate evidence of concurrent construct validity. Consequently, any lack of effects of Valium use by the focal respondent on the well-being of the work other does not appear attributable to a lack of valid work other measures.

Summary. This section has examined the effects of Valium on the well-being of the focal respondents' significant others in personal life and in work life. No effects were found when correlational analyses were performed within Waves 1 and 4. Nor were any effects found when these analyses were repeated for different subgroups of significant others such as spouse versus friend or supervisor versus coworker. This lack of significant relationships could not be attributed to a lack of valid measures obtained from the significant other, because those measures appeared to have reasonable validity. Issues regarding the appropriate interval of causation and related design questions are a separate matter, and they are taken up in Chapter 6. Similar results occurred in analyses of covariance across all four waves of data for highly anxious daily, new, and nonusers of Valium. These results were described earlier in this chapter.

Chapter Summary

Valium users in this study tended to use medication conservatively, taking less than the prescribed amount. They also tended to drink less alcohol than nonusers, particularly during weeks in which they reported using Valium.

A variety of bivariate and multivariate analyses led to the conclusion that there was no evidence that Valium had any notable harmful or beneficial effects on the anxiety and well-being of either the user of Valium or of significant others in the personal and work lives of users. There were some exceptions to these findings, but they all occurred in analyses which either did not replicate consistently or involved small numbers of respondents. A more extensive summary follows in Chapter 6.

CHAPTER 6
SUMMARY AND DISCUSSION

This chapter summarizes a longitudinal study of the potential social effects of Valium use. The expression "social effects" refers to a wide array of variables relating to well-being and functioning in everyday life. The chapter presents a summary of the specific aims, methods, and results. Then the results are interpreted and compared to other studies of Valium use.

The study, unlike a clinical trial, was intended to examine the use of Valium as it is taken in the community at large. To gather this information, 675 persons were interviewed four times, approximately six weeks apart. Some of these respondents were selected because they had received a prescription for Valium within the past six weeks. Other respondents were selected because they had not received a prescription for any drug with psychotropic indications during that same period but had received a prescription for some other type of drug.

Summary of Purposes

Social Effects

The primary aim of the study was to determine how the use of Valium might influence a wide variety of conditions and functions characteristic of everyday life. The variables that were assessed included a variety of stressors in personal and work life, social support and social conflict, coping and defense, perceived control, quality of performance, quality of life, and the well-being of significant others. Chapter 2 describes each of these outcomes and Table 2.1 lists examples of each. The study also examined the effects of Valium use in several major life domains including the domains of work, personal life, self, physical health, and emotions.

263

The inclusion of significant others as respondents was another important facet of the study. One significant person from the focal respondent's personal life (called the "personal other") and one from work life (only for the employed; called the "work other") were interviewed about their own quality of life and their perceptions of the focal respondent's performance and well-being. In this way, the study examined how the use of Valium might influence both the person taking the medication and persons who were closely associated with the medication-taker.

Relationship of Valium Use to Use of Other Psychotropic Substances

Although this study was not explicitly designed to examine the effects of Valium use on the use of other psychotropic substances (such as other medications, alcohol, and street drugs), certain data on these substances were routinely gathered. Thus, this report is able to present some findings relating to this topic.

Anxiety

The present study included measures of anxiety so the results could be compared with those in the clinical trial literature. Furthermore, it was hypothesized that the potential social effects of taking Valium might operate via the medication's effects on anxiety. The anxiety-reducing properties of Valium have been demonstrated repeatedly in a large body of literature. The evidence appears both in early studies (see the review by Greenblatt and Shader, 1974) and in the bibliography of published studies that exists for the period between 1979 and 1983 (Bibliographic Retrieval Services, 1983).

Other Affective Strains

A number of other affective strains were also examined. They included depression, anger, and general negative and positive affects. Somatic symptoms sometimes associated with emotional upset (such as sleep disturbances, loss of appetite, and heart pounding) were also included. These states are commonly examined in clinical trials.

Summary of Methods[81]

Recruitment

It was not necessary or even desirable to obtain a random sample of the population for this study. Such a sample was not required because the main purpose was to describe relationships between Valium use and other variables rather than to produce norms or other descriptive data. On the other hand, representation of various groups was desirable. Consequently, the drawing of respondents was designed to obtain a group of respondents that represented a range of ages from 18 upwards, males and females, black and white, and a broad range of socioeconomic statuses. Chapter 3 describes how this was achieved.

Although several methods of respondent selection were considered and tried (for example, contacting patients at physicians' offices, recruiting them at pharmacies), some of these methods had serious problems. Those problems involved logistics, costs, and volunteering bias. As a result, the final method involved drawing most respondents from pharmacy records and a small number from other sources. This method and all related procedures were developed after a long series of pilot tests.

It was not possible to contact patients prior to their filling a prescription for Valium. This meant that many patients had started taking Valium prior to entering the study. Therefore, some effects of Valium use may already have begun. On the other hand, it was felt that any beneficial or harmful long-term effects could be detected if they occurred within the six-month time frame of the study.

Persons were selected from pharmacy lists either because they had received a prescription for Valium in the six weeks prior to entering the study or because they had received a prescription for any medication other than one which might be

---

[81]This fairly detailed summary of methods is intended for readers who have not read the entire report. Other readers may wish to proceed to the section of this chapter entitled "Summary of Results: Portrait of the Valium User."

indicated for treatment of emotional disorder during that same
time frame.[82]   These persons and a small number of persons from
other lists were first contacted by letter and then phoned by a
professional interviewer.[83]

Characteristics of the Respondents

Of the 675 respondents who completed all four interviews,
367 used Valium at some time during the study and 308 did not.
The pool of potential respondents was drawn to obtain approximately equal numbers of males and females. The final distributions at Wave 1 were such that there were somewhat more
females than males among Valium users (61% were females); there
were about equal numbers of females and males among the nonusers (54% were females). At Wave 1, 15% of the Valium users
and 22% of the nonusers were black.

The mean age for Valium users was about 45; for nonusers
it was about 40. Education and income were similar across
users and nonusers of Valium. Average education for all
respondents was 12 years, and average family income was about
$18,000 to $25,000 per year. As already noted, respondents
were drawn to represent a broad range on these characteristics,
rather than a random sample. For example, the distribution of
ages was approximately rectangular and the distribution for income was also rather flat. Age, education, and sex of the personal other were similar to those of the focal respondents.
About 1/2 of the work others were male (48%); 31% of the personal others were male. Personal others had known their focal
respondents for an average of 21.6 years; work others had known
their focal respondents for an average of 7.2 years.

Regarding anxiety in the past seven days, the Valium group
had a Wave 1 mean of 1.9 (SD=.6) on the Hopkins Scale and the
nonValium group had a mean of 1.5 (SD=.5; difference sig-

---

[82]Access to records was made possible under Michigan State
Law with the approval of the Michigan Board of Pharmacy and individual pharmacists.

[83]In order to preserve the confidentiality of respondents,
a small number of persons were selected from business mailing
lists. Neither the study staff nor the interviewers knew from
which list any one respondent was selected.

nificant at p <.001). The respective depression scores on the Hopkins Symptom Checklist were 1.9 (SD=.6) and 1.6 (SD=.5; difference significant at p <.001).

Initial contact with respondents. The study was described to potential respondents as an investigation of stress in the domains of work, family, and health. This description reflected the overall emphasis of the study. Only a portion of the interview dealt with medications and only the section on medications mentioned Valium, along with several other trade names, as examples of minor tranquilizers.

Respondents were informed that participation was voluntary and that the interviews were confidential and would be rendered anonymous. Respondents were told that they would be paid $5 for each of the first 3 interviews and $10 for the last. Then the respondent and interviewer signed a contract affirming these conditions, and the contract was given to the respondent to keep.

Interviews took an average of 97 minutes, and were conducted by carefully-trained interviewers from the Survey Research Center. At the end of the first interview, the focal respondent was asked to select a significant other in personal life and, if employed, one in work life. Persons so selected were contacted by the interviewer. The purposes and conditions of the study described to them were the same as those described to the focal respondent, except that no payment was involved. If they agreed to participate, they were interviewed. An attempt was made to use the same interviewer and the same significant others at each wave of data collection.

Refusal and Continuance Rates

Approximately 48% of the people contacted agreed to be interviewed. Rates of refusal and evasion were computed. They were comparable for persons chosen because they received or had not received a Valium prescription. The refusal rates were as follows: Valium group = 28.7%, Others = 25.6%; the evasion rates were: Valium = 13%, Others = 12%. For 92% of the focal respondents at Time 1, a significant other from their personal life was interviewed. Focal respondents employed 15 hours or more per week were asked for a work other, and 71% at Time 1 provided such persons who were successfully interviewed.

Continuance was high for the focal respondents throughout the study. From 91% to 98% of each preceding wave's focal respondents were reinterviewed. Approximately 90% of focal respondents continued to provide a personal other at each wave. Similarly, approximately 70% of working respondents continued to provide a work other at each wave.

The small number of persons who dropped out were somewhat more likely to be black than white, taking Valium rather than not, male, less educated, and have lower income. Age, anxiety, depression, and perceived health were unrelated to dropping out. Regardless of dropout rates, there were still sufficient numbers of respondents for analyses within and between each of the above-mentioned groups.

Quality of the Raw Data

Several steps were taken to maximize the quality of the data. They included careful monitoring of the questionnaires to ensure interviewer compliance with procedures, verification of computer card punching, and computer checks for consistency (for example, was the recorded gender of the respondent the same at successive interviews; did a person have data about role conflict at work when the person was coded as being unemployed; and so on). Several thousand such consistency checks were conducted. Checks were made on the reliability of coders in instances where open-ended questions had to be coded. Agreement among coders ranged from 77% to 96% with most agreement being above 80%. The error rate for coding closed-ended questionnaire items was about 1/10th of 1 percent.

Construction of Indices

Indices are measures made up of a set of similar items to increase the reliability of measurement. Factor analysis and other forms of item analysis were used to ensure that the measures of stress, social support, and social conflict, anxiety, quality of life, and other multi-item measures met acceptable standards for reliability. The indices generally had coefficient alphas of .60 or higher, with most coefficients

268

being in the .70s and .80s. These reliabilities held up within various subgroups, such as males, females, Valium users, non-users, and at each of the four interviews. Before constructing the indices, the items were checked to make sure they had adequate distributions and were not badly skewed. Similar checks were made on the index scores themselves.

Summary of Results: Portrait of the Valium User

In this study Valium had been prescribed most often by physicians in general practice or internal medicine. Osteopaths and psychiatrists were the next most likely to prescribe Valium. These findings are consistent with data drawn from national studies.

Most patients found their prescribing physician supportive. The small percent who made use of the services of therapists or counselors also perceived them as supportive.

The most common reasons for taking Valium mentioned by respondents were anxiety, tension, keeping calm or keeping relaxed. These reasons were mentioned by at least 64% of the Valium users. Insomnia was mentioned as a primary reason by 10% of the Valium users. The only commonly mentioned physical reason was for a pulled back or sore muscles (7%). Some of the analyses compared the social effects of Valium for persons taking the medication for anxiety-related versus other reasons (described below). There were essentially no differences.

The most commonly prescribed dosages of Valium per day ranged from 10-20 mg. As has been found elsewhere (e.g., Hulka, et al., 1976), patients prescribed specific regimens tended, on the average, to take less rather than more milligrams of Valium than were prescribed.

The large majority (83%) of persons taking Valium reported taking it within the seven days preceding each interview, and the majority of Valium users (59%) took some Valium during all four of the 6-week periods prior to each interview. Nevertheless, there were considerable ranges of dosages and patterns of use across and within the 6-week periods between interviews.

At each interview, Valium users were asked about their pattern of use during the previous six weeks. About 1/3

269

reported taking Valium "only once in a while," whereas almost half the Valium users reported taking Valium "every day or every other day the whole time" during the 6-week period prior to each interview.

Valium users tended to drink less alcohol than nonusers, particularly during weeks when they used Valium daily or every other day. Valium users also tended to smoke more cigarettes than nonusers. There was little evidence of differences with regard to caffeine or street drug use. Although Valium users tended to take more prescribed drugs of other kinds than nonusers, this difference was probably largely due to the intentional bias in recruitment procedures for the two groups.

Summary of Results: Social Effects of Valium

Cross-sectional analyses showed that use of Valium was weakly associated with indicators of distress including low quality of life, poor perceived health, and high anxiety. Such findings have been observed in other cross-sectional studies (e.g., Mellinger, et al., 1978). These relationships became near-zero when they were subsequently examined in a variety of longitudinal, multivariate analyses that examined both main effects and a number of potential moderators. The sections that follow summarize in further detail the methods used in these analyses, the results, the interpretations of the results, and the conclusions.

Main Effects: Quality of Life

The influence of Valium use on quality of life was a potential social effect of major interest. Consequently, a primary focus of the study and analysis was to determine if Valium use influenced quality of life adversely, had no effect on it, or improved it.

Several types of correlational analyses were performed to examine the relationship between weekly use of Valium and weekly levels of life quality. These analyses were performed after careful checks were made that found no marked curvilinear relationships between these variables.

The first type of analysis examined three types of relationship between weekly Valium use and weekly quality of life: (1) when both variables were measured simultaneously (i.e., both during any single 7-day period), (2) when Valium use was measured before quality of life (that is, when use of Valium was measured one to 24 weeks before quality of life), and (3) when quality of life was measured one to 24 weeks before Valium use. The logic of the analysis is that when Valium use is measured at a time prior to quality of life, then quality of life is viewed as a potential consequence of taking Valium. When Valium use is measured at a time after quality of life, then Valium use is viewed as a potential consequence of quality of life. When the use of Valium and quality of life are measured simultaneously, one cannot distinguish between outcome and antecedent.

The average zero-lag correlation was about -.12 and dropped slightly over time. There was a slight tendency for the relationship to be more strongly negative when Valium use preceded quality of life. The findings suggest that variations in Valium use and in quality of life are relatively concurrent phenomena and that Valium use and quality of life are negatively related.

A second type of analysis examined the relationship between changes in use of Valium and in quality of life. Although change scores have some psychometric disadvantages, such as greater unreliability, they have the advantage of cancelling out any systematic response error from each time point and leaving only the true change score and random error. In general, the relationships were weak regardless of whether changes in use of Valium and quality of life were lagged or examined as concurrent measures. The highest correlation using the single item measure of quality of life from the calendar was -.14, and the relationships were generally negatively-signed (that is, increases in the use of Valium were associated with decreases in the quality of life), as was the case in the first type of correlational analyses described above.

The third type of analysis made use of the multivariate procedure of structural equation modeling (LISREL IV; Joreskog

& Sorbom, 1978). This approach made use of a number of statistical controls both for measurement factors and for potentially confounding variables including perceived stress and health. These analyses showed that the predictive effect of weekly use of Valium on quality of life approximately six weeks later was near zero. Valium use neither reduced nor improved global quality of life. These results, along with those from other analyses, suggest an alternative interpretation of the modest cross-sectional association between increased use of Valium and lower quality of life. It seems likely that the modest cross-sectional association of Valium use with quality of life was probably due to the association of quality of life with anxiety, stress, and health problems. Valium users appeared to have lower life quality because of the anxiety, stress, and health problems they experienced, not because of their Valium use (see below).

Analysis of Covariance: Social Effects

The next type of analysis, like the structural equation modeling analysis, controlled for the higher levels of perceived stress and of reported poor health found among Valium users. The analysis, as detailed below, dealt with the possibility that the structural equation analyses may have shown a near-zero association between Valium use and quality of life because most users were taking Valium too infrequently to get a benefit and were less anxious than patients in typical clinical trials.

Two sets of analyses of covariance were used to examine changes in quality of life over the course of the study. The first set compared the following two subgroups of respondents: persons who took Valium daily or almost daily from six weeks prior to Wave 1 through Wave 2, and persons who took no Valium during the course of the study. Both groups were selected to have initially high levels of anxiety--levels similar to those found at the start of treatment in clinical trials. Differences between these two groups in perceived stresses and health were taken into account via the statistical controls of the analyses.

272

The daily users might have already experienced the expected anxiolytic benefits of Valium prior to the start of the study, making it difficult to detect change in their subsequent quality of life levels. Consequently, a second set of analyses of covariance were repeated focusing on a Valium-using group that consisted of a small number of respondents (n=19) who had started taking Valium for the first time within the six weeks prior to the onset of the study, and a control group selected to have a similar mean and distribution of initial levels of anxiety.

These analyses found no effects of Valium use on quality of life for daily users. For the new users, quality of life and its components showed improvement from Wave 1 to Wave 4. The fact that other analyses suggest alternative explanations, and that ratings by personal others depicted new users as having lower quality of life, suggest the need for caution in interpreting these findings.

Interaction Effects: Quality of Life and Other Outcomes

It was possible that there might be evidence of social effects of Valium for specific subgroups of respondents. If Valium reduced the quality of life of one subgroup and increased the quality of life of another subgroup, the result could be a lack of effect among the total set of respondents. Such a case is called an interaction effect because the characteristic of the subgroup interacts with Valium use to determine the medication's effect.

To search for interactions, subgroups were created that differed on variables that might influence the efficacy of Valium. These subgroups were defined on the basis of gender, whether or not Valium was taken for anxiety, amount of social support from the physician, and a large number of other variables. Then the relationship between use of Valium and several indicators of quality of life (e.g., life as a whole, personal life, work life) was examined within subgroups over at least two waves, using cross-sectional and lagged analyses.

Little evidence of such an interaction effect was found for quality of life. A few of the moderators that produced the

273

strongest effects were examined in causal models computed separately for each relevant subgroup. The effects were essentially the same regardless of the subgroup examined.

Another type of search for interactions examined the extent to which Valium use buffered (reduced) or exacerbated (increased) the relationship between stresses and quality of life and other outcomes. While there was a slight tendency for Valium use to buffer the relationship between stress and life quality, the differences were of moderate magnitude and did not always replicate. Consequently, results from interaction analyses do not alter those from the main effect analyses.

Case Study Analyses: Quality of Life

Analyses were also performed, person-by-person, comparing new, off-on, and other Valium users with nonusers with regard to how quality of life changed in the week prior to, the week during, and the two weeks after taking Valium. Off-on users were persons who did not take Valium for at least one 6-week interval between the four waves of interviews but did use Valium during a subsequent wave. Weeks during whih a clear increase in anxiety occurred were selected to determine if subsequent use of Valium improved quality of life. Quality of life decreased more for off-on and new users, compared to the other users, from the week prior to taking Valium to the week Valium use began. Quality of life also increased more after taking Valium. Similar patterns were observable in these persons when they did not take Valium and in persons who were not Valium users but who also showed an initial increase in anxiety. Specifically, quality of life returned the same amount toward its base level (an improvement) with and without the use of Valium. On the other hand, the return to baseline represented a larger absolute increase or improvement in quality of life following use of Valium than not following its use. Such a return, however, was usually accompanied by a concomitant decrease in anxiety. So the change in quality of life could have been due to a change in anxiety independent of the effect of Valium. Furthermore, quality of life decreased more prior to episodes of anxiety during which respondents took Valium than during episodes when they did not take Valium. This is an indication that people might need to experience a particularly large decrease in life quality in order to decide to take the medication. This decrease, however, could by itself have accounted for the subsequent larger improvement due to natural adjustive processes.[84] Given these alternative interpretations, it is equivocal as to whether Valium did or did not produce the greater absolute improvement in quality of life. Statistically controlling for the size of the initial decrease in life quality prior to taking Valium would not resolve this question. Instead it might control out the very conditions that could lead people to take Valium. Furthermore, the small sample size involved in these analyses makes us less confident about these findings. Consequently, these analyses did not provide clear evidence as to whether Valium affected resultant quality of life.

Within-Person Analyses: Quality of Life

Another analysis was an examination of the within-person covariation between use of Valium and quality of life analyzed separately for each respondent over the 24 weeks of the study. It was possible that some yet-unidentified Valium users might show either a negative relationship between Valium use and quality of life (that is, the more Valium, the lower the subsequent quality of life) or a positive relationship between Valium use and quality of life. If this were the case, analyses could be performed to determine if persons who showed a negative correlation between Valium use and quality of life differed from those who showed a zero correlation or from those who showed a positive correlation.

The analyses were performed in the following manner. Each person was assigned a set of scores reflecting the correlation between Valium use and quality of life based on the person's 24 weekly calendar measures. Nine such scores were computed. They reflected Valium use preceeding the assessment of life quality by one, three, six, or nine weeks; Valium use simultaneous with the assessment of life quality; and Valium use

---

[84] Such adjustive processes are sometimes referred to as "regression toward the mean."

following the assessment of life quality by one, three, six, or nine weeks. The distributions showed that such within-person scores ran nearly the full range from correlations of 1.0 to -1.0.

These scores were related to 82 variables in the study including stress, social support, coping, control, performance, use of medications and other substances, quality of life, and demographic variables. The few relationships that appeared did not exceed what would be expected by chance and were not easily explainable. Checks for curvilinearities did not produce any results which would modify the above findings. These within-person scores were also similar in the subgroups of off-on and new users. In sum, these analyses suggest that the few persons with notable negative and positive within-person correlations between Valium use and quality of life represented chance occurrences.

In considering the general absence of a relationship between use of Valium and quality of life in these findings, several points can be raised about potential artifacts of the design. These will be discussed below, following review of study findings regarding other potential social effects of Valium use.

Effects of Use of Valium on Other Variables

Sets of analyses much more limited than those described above were performed examining the strains of anger, depression, somatic complaints, and global measures of positive and negative affect. These limited analyses were also performed for measures of coping and defense, social support and social conflict, perceived control, perceived health, the well-being of personal other and work other, role performance, and use of alcohol, caffeine, and other drugs. The scope of these analyses was reduced in part because these latter variables were not measured using the calendar. Only data marking the week of each interview were available, rather than the 24 weeks of the calendar. Nevertheless, all of the just-mentioned variables were examined in multivariate as well as bivariate and univariate analyses.

Analyses were performed to determine the correlation between the amount of Valium taken in the seven days prior to each interview and about 80 major variables. Valium-taking at 14 different time points during the study was related to the other variables when they were measured at week 12, the week of the second interview. This provided lags between Valium and these variables ranging from Valium use 12 weeks before to 11 weeks after the measurement of the variable. A broad scan of over 1,000 zero-order relationships was involved. With few exceptions, all relationships were very low, and there were no sharp peaks associated with particular lags. The highest relationships were between Valium-taking and attitudes about tranquilizers ($r=.35$; that is, the more Valium taken, the more positive one's attitudes). Most relationships were under .20 and most that were significant suggested that the greater the use of Valium, the higher the stress and strain, the lower the social support, and so forth. In general, more Valium was associated with less desirable levels of outcome variables.

Multivariate analyses using structural equation modeling and covariance analysis examined quality of performance in personal life as a potential outcome. The analyses showed virtually no effect of Valium use on weekly levels of quality of performance.

Searches for interaction effects of Valium were also conducted. As noted in the previous section on quality of life, this was done by examining relationships of Valium use to the many other variables in this study for the many subgroups described in earlier text on this type of analysis. Over 6,000 analyses were conducted involving a hypothesized moderator, predictor, and dependent variable. Although 14% of the tests were significant at the $p< .05$ level, most were of weak magnitude. Furthermore, the percent of significant findings must be viewed with caution. It does not take into account the extent to which these separate effects involved predictors and dependent variables which were correlated with one another and which measured similar variables.

Another search for interactions involved examining Valium as a moderator of the stress-strain relationship. In general,

277

there appeared to be more instances in which Valium buffered the effects of stresses on strain than instances in which it exacerbated the effects of such stresses. However, the interpretation of these findings is unclear because they are largely cross-sectional and do not always replicate as expected. Even the appearance of more buffering than exacerbating effects has to be viewed with caution. To the extent that predictors were intercorrelated (as were outcomes), a single strong buffering effect could lead to several apparent replications involving correlated measures. The value of these findings at this time is largely to suggest new avenues for basic research related to such potential moderator effects. The reader is referred to Chapter 5 and Appendix T, which review both moderating analyses in more detail.

Another form of analysis, described above, was also applied to the search for effects of Valium on many other variables. This was the analysis of covariance in which users of Valium who took the medication daily from six weeks prior to Wave 1 through Wave 2, new users, and persons who did not take Valium at any of the four waves were compared across the four waves. All of the respondents selected for this analysis had relatively high anxiety scores on the Hopkins at Wave 1, levels similar to those found in typical clinical drug trials.

The only differences between the users of Valium and nonusers involved quality of life (described in the preceding section) and alcohol. Daily users consumed significantly less alcohol than nonusers. This finding is similar to one reported in Chapter 5 comparing the alcohol use of all daily users with nonusers regardless of level of anxiety. Daily users may have been complying with physician instructions not to use alcohol with Valium, or they may have been using Valium in place of alcohol, or both. No such effect was present for new users, but this does not necessarily imply that they were or were not complying with advice to avoid alcohol consumption.

Interpretations: Social Effects

In sum, the basic finding of this study is that Valium use has little effect, either beneficial or detrimental, on quality

278

of life and a number of other social effects. A number of potential interpretations of this finding are described below.

Interpretation 1. One interpretation is that there are no social effects, either harmful or beneficial, of using Valium which occur within the time frame of this study (a minimum of one week to a maximum of six months).

Interpretation 2. A related interpretation is that if there are social effects, beneficial or harmful, which occur in less than the 7-day time frame of this study (for example, an effect that lasts only a few hours or a day), this study would not necessarily be able to detect them. This would be the case particularly if these effects were weak to begin with. This would also be true for effects which take longer than the 6-month span of this study to develop. (However, it might be noted that most users had taken Valium prior to entering the study, which effectively expands this 6-month time span.)

If one interprets the data as indicating that, at most, only short-range effects are present, then the study has addressed and allayed the main concerns expressed about the potential negative social effects of Valium. Most of those concerns (e.g., Cooperstock & Hill, 1982) deal with major, relatively lasting alterations in the well-being of the person. Of course, this study cannot rule out the possibility that there are effects which take more than six months to develop or that such effects had already occurred and stabilized. Dealing with these issues would require following new users over a longer span of follow-up than was available in this study.

Interpretation 3. Another interpretation is that any social effects could have occurred prior to the start of the study because many of the Valium users in this study had been taking Valium for a number of years. If so, their levels of performance, perceived control, and other potential social effects could have stabilized before they entered the study. There is no way to answer this question without prior measurements.

Interpretation 4. It is possible, of course, that there were no social effects because patients did not take Valium in

279

the amounts that are considered clinically effective. This is an unlikely interpretation. Longitudinal analyses of highly anxious daily users as well as other analyses using daily dosage or pattern of use (e.g., daily versus intermittent) as a control failed to produce any evidence that dosage altered the effect of Valium use on potential social effects.

Interpretation 5. If one assumes that any social effects of Valium use would occur because Valium reduces anxiety, then, if Valium does not have a significant anxiolytic effect as it is generally used, it would not have any social effects either. For example, one could hypothesize that Valium use increases social support because it is easier to be supportive of a less anxious person. This is not implausible given that, even in clinical trials, the magnitude of the effects is often weak, although statistically significant. The magnitude of such findings in clinical trials is uncovered only after rigorous controls are introduced to ensure that the patients follow certain regimens and meet certain screening criteria for anxiety.

Interpretation 5 is plausible only if one assumes that any social effects of Valium must operate via the anxiolytic effects of Valium. This need not be the case, however. There might be direct effects, such as psychological dependence of the person on a medication rather than on other resources. Over 1000 correlational cross-sectional and lagged analyses, a large number of analyses of covariance of highly anxious persons, and over 6000 subgroup analyses, however, failed to uncover any notable direct social effects of Valium use.

To examine the possibility that Valium use did not have social effects because it did not produce anxiolytic effects as an intermediate step, a number of analyses were performed. Anxiety was measured in this study both to link it with clinical trials and as a way of exploring the extent to which social effects might occur via the anxiolytic pathway. The next section summarizes the analyses of Valium's relationship to anxiety.

Summary of Results: Effects of Valium on Anxiety

Detection of effects of Valium use on anxiety in this study poses some challenges. For one thing, the study was designed to search for long-term social effects rather than potentially short-lived changes in anxiety. Second, given that Valium is commonly used as an anxiolytic, there was an awareness that any cross-sectional correlational analysis of the links between Valium and anxiety might partly reflect the effects of Valium on anxiety as well as the triggering effects of anxiety on the behavior of taking Valium. These two effects could combine to obscure the drug's anxiety-reducing effects: if the effect of anxiety on taking Valium were stronger than the effect of Valium on resultant anxiety, then any cross-sectional relationship might show a weak but positive correlation between Valium use and anxiety (the more Valium, the more anxiety, and vice-versa).

With these potential complications in mind, the analyses were begun. A full range of analyses, using procedures already described, were applied to study the link between use of Valium and weekly anxiety.

Main Effects: Anxiety

After finding no evidence of marked curvilinearity, a number of linear bivariate analyses were carried out to examine the relationship of Valium use to anxiety. These analyses made use of the 24 weeks of calendar data and the lags described above in the section on Valium use and quality of life.

Regardless of whether Valium was examined as antecedent, consequent, or simultaneous to anxiety, the bivariate relationship was modest. The maximum correlation coefficient using the single-item measure of anxiety from the calendar data was about .15, and was about .30 using the Hopkins Symptom Checklist. The correlation was always positive. That is, higher Valium use was moderately associated with higher anxiety. The relationship was strongest when Valium and anxiety were measured simultaneously. There was a tendency for the relationship to be slightly stronger when anxiety followed Valium-taking rather than vice versa. These data would suggest

281

that the strongest of these relatively weak effects are simultaneous, that each causes the other, and/or that anxiety and Valium-taking are caused by some third variable, such as a health problem or a stressful event. Analyses described later provide a basis for evaluating the feasibility of each of these explanations.

The second type of analysis examined the relationship between changes in the use of Valium and changes in anxiety from wave to wave. The rationale for this relationship was summarized earlier.

The results of the change score analysis confirmed the pattern just described. All relationships were relatively weak (never exceeding the low .20s) and positive regardless of whether changes in Valium use were examined as antecedent, simultaneous with, or consequent to changes in anxiety. The strongest relationships occurred for the simultaneous measures. The lagged relationships were nearly equal regardless of whether change in Valium use was examined as antecedent or consequent to change in anxiety.

A third type of analysis examined the effects of weekly Valium use on anxiety using the multivariate procedure of structural equation modeling (Joreskog & Sorbom, 1978). This procedure provided opportunities for detailed statistical controls. These controls took into account the findings that Valium users had higher initial levels of anxiety and reported more stresses and poorer health than did the other respondents. This procedure also provided opportunities for statistical estimates of measurement error so that tests of the effects of Valium use on anxiety could take into account such error. These analyses showed that the positive relationship between Valium use and concurrent as well as later anxiety (six weeks later) was spurious. The use of these controls reduced the positive correlation of Valium use with concurrent and with later anxiety to one that was approximately zero. The near-zero relationship, of course, is different from the negative relationship between Valium use and subsequent anxiety that has been observed repeatedly in clinical trials. Partly to understand this difference between the findings from this study and from the clinical trials, the series of analyses described below was undertaken.

Analysis of Covariance: Anxiety

Two sets of analyses of covariance were also used to investigate the effects of different subgroups of Valium users on mean levels of anxiety across the four waves of the study. One analysis selected only daily or almost-daily users of Valium and the other selected only new users. Both analyses matched these respondents with nonusers who, like the users of Valium, were further selected to have initially high levels of anxiety as measured on the Hopkins Symptom Checklist. As a result of these restrictions, both analyses included small numbers of respondents (for example--36 daily users and 19 new users).

Both analyses produced the same results. Although anxiety declined from Wave 1 to Wave 2 and then levelled off somewhat for the Valium groups, the nonusers showed a similar decline. So when level of anxiety, regularity of use, or prior use experience (all new users) were controlled, there was no evidence of any association between use of Valium and subsequent level of anxiety, a finding similar to that derived from the structural equation modeling analyses.

Search for Interactions: Anxiety

Other analyses attempted to search for additional subgroups of respondents for whom use of Valium might have different effects on anxiety. Many subgroups (such as males, females, respondents high versus low on stress, and so on) were examined to determine if the type of person, the level of stress the person faced, social support, the way in which Valium was used, use of other drugs, or any of a large number of other variables might potentially moderate the effects of Valium use on anxiety.

More such effects were found than might be expected by chance alone. Most of the effects were small in magnitude, however, and tended to show low replicability. Fully satisfactory interpretations of these findings are not available. A few of the moderators which produced the strongest effects were examined in causal models computed separately for each relevant subgroup. These analyses indicated that the estimated effects of Valium on anxiety were essentially the same regardless of the subgroup examined. The interested reader is referred to Chapter 5 for further details.

Case Study Analyses: Comparing Pre- and Post-Valium Anxiety

The analysis of covariance of daily and new users, described above, examined weekly use of Valium and weekly levels of anxiety at each of the four waves of the study. Another analysis was attempted that made use of much shorter time intervals than the six-week intervals between waves. Using data from the calendar, changes in anxiety levels of new users were examined for the week prior to, during, and after Valium use began. Changes in anxiety levels were also examined in this manner among users who stopped taking Valium for at least one six-week interval between the four waves of interviews but did use Valium during a subsequent wave--"off-on" users. The anxiety changes of both groups were compared with those for nonusers.

For both new users and off-on users of Valium, increases in anxiety tended to be higher in the week when Valium use began compared to the preceding week, and decreases in anxiety tended to be greater in the weeks immediately after use began compared to the week use began. (Similarly, as reported earlier, decreases in quality of life tended to be greater in the week Valium use began compared to the preceding week, and improvements in life quality tended to be higher in the weeks immediately after use began compared to the week when use began.) Although these findings might be interpreted as evidence for beneficial effects of Valium use on anxiety and life quality, some further analyses cast doubt on this interpretation. This same pattern of findings was also found for these same individuals at times when their anxiety increased but they did not take Valium. The same pattern of findings occurred for nonusers of Valium and for regular users of Valium.

In summary, increases in anxiety were followed by decreases in anxiety and improvements in life quality regardless of whether people took Valium or not. The later improvement might have been due to something the individual did (e.g., take Valium, learn more about the situation, deny the threat) or to spontaneous improvement. The increases in anxiety before Valium use and the decreases afterwards were both greater for new and off-on users than for other users. Regardless of the mechanisms inferred, the overall improvement in anxiety did not appear to be uniquely due to Valium use.

Another analysis examined each person's correlation between weekly use of Valium and weekly anxiety over the 24 weeks of the calendar. The method of analysis has already been described in the discussion of effects of Valium on quality of life. These analyses were performed to determine if there were some persons who showed a negative relationship of Valium use with anxiety (that is, use of Valium was associated with a subsequent reduction in anxiety) and others who showed no relationship, or a positive one. The analyses, described in more detail in the previous section on the effects on quality of life, examined lagged relationships when Valium use preceded as well as followed the rating of anxiety. Simultaneous relationships were also examined.

Subsequent analyses examined 80 variables in the study to determine whether any of these variables predicted to why some persons showed negative and others showed positive or zero relationships between Valium and anxiety. The absence of findings over a very large number of analyses was striking. It suggests that the few notable negative and positive correlations for given individuals were due to chance.

Interpretations: Anxiety

Cross-sectional surveys of the general population (e.g., Mellinger, et al., 1978) have found a positive correlation between the use of minor tranquilizers and indicators of psychic distress. The simple, first-order positive correlations between use of Valium and anxiety in this study replicate those findings.

Usually such findings have been interpreted to mean that persons who are distressed seek and receive anxiolytic medication. An alternative interpretation is that the drug therapy increases anxiety. The latter conclusion is not supported by a

285

large number of clinical trials which demonstrate the anxiolytic effects of benzodiazepines (for a review, see Greenblatt and Shader, 1974). Data from this study also suggest that this is an implausible interpretation. When statistical controls for initial levels of anxiety, stress, and perceived health were made, the positive correlation between Valium and anxiety disappeared. The resulting relationship was nearly zero. That is, Valium use appeared to be unrelated to later or earlier anxiety. How might this finding be explained?

There are a number of alternative, related explanations that have to do with how people used Valium, when they entered the study, and so on.[85] Each of these explanations will now be reviewed. Although results from this study and from other studies can suggest that some explanations are less plausible than others, this study lacks sufficient data for determining unambiguously which explanation is the most plausible one. This is partly because the study was not designed in anticipation of such results.

Interpretation 1. The first explanation is that Valium, as it is typically used by people, is ineffectual in reducing anxiety. This is a plausible argument if people take the medication in doses or for periods of time which are less than those demonstrated to be effective in the many clinical trials in which diazepam has been tested as an anxiolytic. This study has produced evidence suggesting that people may tend toward undermedication. Nevertheless, such tendencies toward taking less medication than was originally prescribed have been observed in some trials in which this medication has produced significant decreases in anxiety (Rickels, et al., 1977b).

Furthermore, this argument needs to be considered in light of the study's analyses of daily users, infrequent users, and of those who took relatively high versus relatively low doses of Valium. Most of those analyses indicated the same lack of effects of Valium on anxiety as was observed for Valium users as a whole.

---

[85]Some of these explanations have already been applied to the discussion of social effects in the preceding section.

Interpretation 2. Valium is effective in reducing anxiety, but no more so than other coping methods (e.g., obtaining help from another person or simply waiting for the problem to solve itself). This interpretation is untestable in this study. Both users of Valium and nonusers showed improvements in levels of anxiety over the four waves of the study. Whether the Valium users might have done worse, had they not taken Valium, may only be answerable unequivocally in a trial in which individuals are randomly assigned to Valium or are given a placebo. Given that some people in this study are taking Valium as needed (PRN) rather than on any fixed schedule, such a trial might well offer people the drug on a PRN schedule.[86]

Interpretation 3. Another possible explanation for a general lack of evidence of anxiolytic effects has to do with the characteristics of the respondents. There is evidence from clinical trials that Valium is not equally effective for all persons (e.g., Rickels, 1978). Individuals who have high levels of depression, whose levels of anxiety are extremely low, or who have nonsupportive physicians, for example, are less responsive to the anxiolytic effects of benzodiazepines (Rickels, 1981). This study performed analyses of such subgroups and found no evidence that level of anxiety, depression, the ratio of anxiety to depression, or physician supportiveness altered the effects of Valium on anxiety.

Interpretation 4. An alternative set of explanations of these findings concerns the methodology of the study. There are three issues here. One deals with the quality of the measures, another deals with the type of people who have entered clinical trials versus entered this study, and the third deals with being able to measure respondents at appropriate time points and over appropriate intervals.

If the measures of anxiety or of Valium-taking are unreliable or are not valid, then the observed relationship might differ from the true one. This argument is implausible for two

---

[86]We are indebted to Edward Kaim and Harry Diakoff for this design suggestion.

reasons. First, anxiety was found to have adequate internal reliability and adequate evidence of validity in terms of its relationships to measures of social stress and quality of life.[87] Second, Valium itself was correlated with anxiety in a manner found in other survey studies. On these grounds, the measures seem adequate to detect Valium's effects on anxiety.[88]

Differences in the types of people who enter clinical trials compared to those who entered this study might have influenced the results. In a clinical trial, the patients usually enter the study with high levels of anxiety and take a minor tranquilizer to reduce an already manifest set of symptoms. In this study, by contrast, many of the users of Valium might have taken the medication in anticipation of an anxiety-provoking situation. If this type of use of Valium is effective, the anxiety levels of these persons might be similar both before and after taking Valium. The respondents who might be least likely to use Valium in anticipation of anxiety, and more likely to use it in response to existing anxiety, were new and off-on users.[89] Analyses of the effects of Valium on such users, however, showed no clear-cut anxiolytic effect of Valium.

The intervals of measurement may be another potential contributor to the near-zero multivariate relationship between Valium and anxiety. The measures of use of Valium and of anxiety covered a minimum period of "the last 7 days." Episodic changes in Valium use and in anxiety which covered shorter periods than this (or which covered periods greater

---

[87]The Hopkins measure of anxiety has also been used successfully in clinical trials for screening and evaluation of change in symptomatology.

[88]This point is independent of the issue of whether measurement occurred at the right point in time, a topic discussed below.

[89]The case-by-case analysis of changes in anxiety preceding, accompanying, and following Valium use indicated that new users and off-on users showed the strongest increase in anxiety accompanying start of use of Valium compared to other users. This suggests that these persons were more likely to take Valium in response to anxiety rather than in anticipation of it.

than the maximum 24 weeks spanned by the calendar) cannot be detected.

The minimum period of seven days was selected on the grounds that this time frame is typically used in assessing anxiety with the Hopkins Symptom Checklist in clinical trials. Equally important, the social effects of interest in this study were ones that would be relatively long-lasting, certainly longer than a few hours or a couple of days. Suppose, however, that some users of Valium took the medication to manage short-term anxiety which would remit or yield to some form of coping in less than a week, regardless of Valium use. Then Valium would not be responsible for levels of anxiety a week later, any more than taking an aspirin for a headache would be likely to be responsible for the presence or absence of a headache a week later. This possibility may be less likely as a factor in clinical trials if such trials tend to include primarily patients with chronic, high levels of anxiety rather than those experiencing short-lived episodes. Long-term users of Valium in this study might be comparable to persons in trials with chronic anxiety. Unlike clinical trials, however, no washout period occurred in this study, and so data on this study's long-term users are difficult to evaluate.

Another possible reason why Valium use may appear unre-lated to anxiety in this study might have to do with the presence of only a few new users of the medication. Clinical research (Rickels, 1981) has shown that near-maximum benefit from anxiolytics may be obtained as early as one week after starting treatment. Most drug trials, like this study, do not have many new users, but the trials do include a washout period prior to the start of the drug administration. A detailed analysis of a small number of relatively new users and on-off users in this study provided an opportunity to see if their anxiety levels did change from before to after their use of Valium. Although increases in anxiety preceded use of Valium, none of the analyses demonstrated that any subsequent reduc-tions in anxiety could be attributed unambiguously to the use of Valium.

Limitations in the Clinical Trials

Finally, note that even in clinical trials it is difficult to demonstrate improvement in significant proportions of the participants. For example, in one study, 44% of the patients showed no improvement at six weeks (Hesbacher, Stepansky, Stepansky, & Rickels, 1976), and in another study 63% showed little or no improvement at one week and 38% were still unimproved at six weeks (Rickels, 1981). Rickels (1981) concluded that "benzodiazepines are completely ineffective for 25% to 30% of all patients." There also is no reason to expect that there may necessarily be long-lasting effects in those who do improve. In one study by Rickels (1978), a six-month follow-up of chronically anxious patients showed an 82% relapse rate following a completed trial of four to six weeks. Another study reported by the same investigator in the same article found no such evidence of relapse nor of improvement lasting beyond one week.

Both in clinical trials and in this study investigators face a limitation in dealing with human outpatient respondents. The measurement of use of the medication must rely either on self-report or on other methods (pill counts, biochemical assays where markers are included with the medication). All of these methods have drawbacks with regard to their validity (Dunbar, 1979).

These reasons may contribute to the diversity of findings in the clinical trials noted above. As Greenblatt and Shader (1974, pg. 1240) conclude,

> It is ironic that anxiety neurosis, the most
> common indication for benzodiazepine therapy,
> is the disorder for which their [the benzodia-
> zepines] clinical efficacy is the most difficult
> to demonstrate.

This statement may also be applicable to longitudinal field surveys.

Summary

There was a near-zero multivariate relationship between the use of Valium and anxiety. This relationship occurred consistently, and with few exceptions, in a variety of analyses both within and between persons. A number of hypotheses have been suggested for why such a relationship might occur. Some of these hypotheses were partly testable with the current data, but others were not. In our view, the most reasonable conclusion is simply that Valium--as it is commonly taken--tends to have neither strong positive nor strong negative effects on anxiety (or on a large number of other outcomes) when averaged over time spans of a week or more.

Other Findings of Interest

Although this study has the potential for examining a very large number of hypotheses regarding interrelationships among variables other than use of Valium, most of the focus of this report has been on Valium itself. Presented below are a few findings not specifically relating to Valium which appeared in the course of analyses for this study.

The study was started partly because there is a broadening interest in how medical care contributes to overall quality of life as well as to the more medically-defined conditions which it aims to treat directly. One of those conditions is anxiety. Consequently, it is of interest to find that anxiety was rather substantially associated with quality of life (cross-sectional correlations in the -.50s). This suggests that the attempt to treat anxiety medically may have the potential for substantially altering the quality of the patient's life. Such an effect should be readily noticeable because the analyses of lagged relationships shows that the relationship appears strongest when these variables reference the same point in time.

Another finding of potential clinical interest is the link between the well-being of the focal respondent and that of the significant other. As is shown in Chapter 5, the well-being of these two persons was significantly correlated in personal life via the significant other's perceptions of the focal respondent's well-being. This applied particularly in the case of husbands and wives. The link between the well-being of the two persons would suggest that when the medical profession treats one person, who is defined as "the client," there may be non-clients who indirectly benefit and who may independently contribute to the well-being of the patient. This realization is, of course, instrumental to conjoint psychotherapy and family practice medicine. It confirms the observation that the physician indirectly affects the well-being of a network of individuals.

Using Wave 1 data, analyses showed that social support was weakly and negatively related to anxiety. That is, persons who reported high social support tended to have somewhat lower levels of anxiety. These findings are cross-sectional, so there may be more than one interpretation. Although social support may be the source of the low anxiety, for example, it is possible that persons with low anxiety are more likely to elicit and receive social support from others.

Social support also moderated the relationship between stress and anxiety. The relationship between negative life events and anxiety was statistically weaker for persons with high social support compared to persons with low social support. This type of moderator effect has been observed in other research as well (e.g., Cobb, 1976; LaRocco, et al., 1980).

These findings suggest that social support may have beneficial effects on anxiety and on how stress influences anxiety. Nevertheless, the results need to be examined at later waves and longitudinally before statements about the causal ordering of these variables can be made. Analyses also need to examine different sources of social support (such as family, friends, and professional sources of counseling and therapy) to determine if their effects are similar.

Relevance of the Findings for Social Issues and Questions

In addition to the above results, there were a number of other findings from the study which bear on social issues regarding the use of Valium and other such anxiolytics. The findings and the issues that they address are presented below. The issues are drawn from literature which has reviewed them (e.g., Cooperstock & Hill, 1982).

1. Does the use of Valium numb patients so that they are unaware of feelings and emotions, and cannot report them to others?

This study did not find evidence of such an effect. Several analyses compared the levels of depression, anger, and somatic complaints for users of Valium and nonusers. The analyses also compared these affective states for different types of Valium users--daily, nondaily, and new users. The levels of emotion and the pattern of change in these emotions over the course of the study were very similar across groups. The higher levels of anxiety among Valium users throughout the period of the study also casts doubt on a numbing effect.

2. Does Valium use dull one's perception of external reality?

Most analyses suggested that correlations between stress and anxiety or between other affects and quality of life are generally no different for persons taking Valium than for persons who do not take Valium. Analyses of covariance comparing initially anxious daily, new, and nonusers of Valium showed that they perceived similar levels of quality of performance, stress, and social support. These analyses showed no evidence of a change in the level of perception due to use of Valium.[10] If there was a dulling effect, one would have expected different results.

On the other hand, some analyses of the moderating effects of Valium use, cited above, suggest that use is more likely to buffer (or "dull") than to exacerbate the effects of stress on strain. That is, Valium users exhibited a weaker relationship between some stresses and strains than did nonusers. This was particularly true for nondaily users rather than for daily users. Those findings, as noted above, were only suggestive and are open to other interpretations. Whether these findings are interpreted as evidence of dulling and whether dulling is interpreted as a benefit or not of Valium use is open to question. Note that social support also produces buffering under certain circumstances (e.g., Cobb, 1976 and findings from this study). That effect is usually viewed as beneficial. A social issue raised by this observation is whether a more positive

---

[10]Nonusers, of course, could be biased in their perceptions of external reality. The findings of this study are that users of Valium do not necessarily differ from nonusers in their perceptions.

value should be associated with any hypothesized dulling produced by social support compared to that produced by a medication. The answer to such a question may involve both values and fact. With regard to the latter, future research, if it confirms a buffering effect of Valium, might wish to compare the efficacy of such an effect with one produced by social support.

3. Does use of Valium decrease one's self-esteem?

Correlational analyses examining a number of lags found no relationships of any notable magnitude relating use of Valium to self-esteem (quality of life regarding the self) except at lag 0, where the correlation was -.23. Longitudinal analyses found that changes in self-esteem over the four waves of the study were virtually no different for daily and for new users than they were for nonusers of Valium. If there were changes they could have been too short-lived to detect, could have taken more than six months to develop, or could have occurred prior to the entry of persons into the study.

4. Does the use of Valium affect patients' perceived ability to control their lives?

Patients may feel that the medication substitutes for relying on their own resources when dealing with problems of life. Such a perception could lead to the attitude that Valium decreases their sense of personal control. Alternatively, the availability of Valium could increase the user's sense of control if it is viewed as a resource that can be used when it is needed.

Two sets of data are relevant here. One is the finding that Valium users perceived that Valium increased their control over emotions and problems of living. This, of course, can be merely a self-justification for why they were using Valium. The other evidence is the lack of any notable relationship either cross-sectionally or over time between measures of the use of Valium and measures of the amount of control reported over emotions and personal lives. If there were any losses in control, they would have had to occur either before persons entered the study, be short-lived and undetectable, or take more than six months to develop. Caution is required in ac-

cepting any one conclusion because the Valium users' judgments
that Valium did enhance their subjective control is con-
tradicted by the lack of evidence that subjective control was
so enhanced. The analyses do not resolve the contradiction.

5. Is it true that people come to view Valium as essentially a social and recreational drug, not unlike alcohol? Do
those who use Valium consume more alcohol?

Detailed person-by-person analyses showed that increases
in anxiety accompanied initiation of Valium use. This suggests
that users of the medication in this study tended to use it for
anxiolytic rather than recreational purposes.

Only one person (Wave 1 data) gave recreational reasons
for the use of Valium. This study, of course, drew respondents
primarily from pharmacies and not from sites where users of
street drugs might be more prevalent. The social issue addressed here, however, deals primarily with whether the
legitimate prescribing of Valium leads to its abuse. Given
that there was a very small minority of persons who reported
using street drugs (most such persons mentioned marijuana), the
association between use of Valium and illicit drugs for users
similar to those in this study would appear to be very weak.
As already noted above, Valium use was not related to alcohol
consumption, per se, but daily users of Valium did consume less
alcohol during the periods when they used Valium.

In Conclusion

Seeking answers has the potential both for providing
answers and for raising new questions. This study has done
both. This chapter has summarized findings from this study
which suggest that persons taking Valium believe the medication
is helpful, tend not to use street drugs, and tend to take less
Valium than their physician recommends rather than the exact
amount or more. The study has shown that users and nonusers of
Valium who are experiencing anxiety react to their stresses in
a similar manner.

A variety of analyses uncovered a general lack of significant relationships between Valium use and the many potential social effects that were examined. The effects that did
appear were present for certain subgroups and were few in num-

ber and difficult to interpret. The lack of strong relationships suggests a number of new questions. Is it the case that Valium really does not have any effects on these variables? Does the use of Valium in anticipation of stress have special effects? Did any benefit or harm occur prior to the person's entry into the study? Were there effects that could not be detected within the minimum scope of seven days or the maximum scope of six months for this study? These questions and some alternative interpretations have been discussed. Based on these data there is no way of determining which of these interpretations (either singly or in combination) best explain the overall findings. We suggest strongly, however, that future clinical trials of benzodiazepines include measures of social effects as well as of anxiety. In this way, some further resolution might be gained. Clearly, some integrative approach is needed to link this study's results with the large literature that demonstrates the anxiolytic effects of benzodiazepines.

Among other future directions for research, it may be useful to conduct trials and field studies which examine changes in anxiety and social effects at intervals shorter than one week. Such studies could include weekly as well as daily measures of potential social effects and quality of life. It would then be possible to determine the relationship between the weekly measure and the aggregation of the daily measures to determine if the weekly measures miss certain clinically significant daily changes. In general, clinical trials which assess the potential social effects evaluated in this study can play an important role in the interpretation and confirmation or disconfirmation of these results.

APPENDIX A

DESIGN OF RESPONDENT SELECTION PROCEDURES

The universe for the study includes 137 pharmacies in Wayne, Oakland and Macomb counties of Michigan. The elements or units of observation are the men and women who filled a prescription at one of these pharmacies during specified reference periods in the spring and summer of 1981. Under the research design, potential respondents were subdivided into two groups: 1) persons who had purchased diazepam during the reference period, and 2) persons who had filled a prescription for a pharmaceutical but did not purchase diazepam or another medication with potential indication for treatment of an emotional disorder during the reference period.

In addition, an original design objective was to sample equal numbers of men and women for both the diazepam group and the control group, as well as a heterogeneous group with respect to race (black/white), income, and locale (urban/suburban). Thus, analyses of the data could be performed within these subgroups. The potential respondents were selected under a two-stage sample design, a primary-stage sample of pharmacies followed by a second-stage subsampling of prescription customers from sample pharmacies.

Primary stage of Sampling

Using ZIP codes of the 137 pharmacies, the municipality and general location of each was identified. Based on its approximate physical location, each pharmacy was classified according to the race and income characteristics of the population residing in the surrounding area. The complete list of 137 pharmacies was then ordered hierarchically, first by county, then by income, and finally by race. From the ordered list, a systematic sample of 50 pharmacies was chosen, each of the 137 pharmacies having an equal probability of selection. The ordered nature of the list,

combined with systematic sample method, yields a sample of pharmacies which is implicitly stratified by locale, neighborhood income, and racial composition.

Anticipating a high level of nonresponse or nonparticipation on the part of pharmacy owners and managers, a special feature was incorporated into the primary-stage sample.' Before the sample was selected, each pharmacy was paired with another which was similar with respect to location, income, and racial stratification criteria. In the event of nonresponse on the part of a sample pharmacy, the pharmacy with which it was paired was substituted.

After sampling of pharmacies was complete, sample pharmacy owners and managers were contacted by phone, and asked to provide the Survey Research Center with permission to sample from their computer-filed customer records. If pharmacy managers agreed to cooperate in the study, they were requested to sign a written statement granting the SRC access to prescription records of their customers. When the contact of sample pharmacies was complete, 39 pharmacies had granted SRC permission to access their customer records.

To facilitate the processing of the prescription files, the 39 pharmacies were assigned to eight groups or replicates; seven groups of 5 pharmacies and one group of four. Beginning on 25 May 1981, the sampling section began to obtain customer files. The files were obtained on a weekly basis at the rate of one new pharmacy group per week for the first eight weeks of the field period. Prescription customer files were obtained only for those customers that had purchased a prescription drug within the preceding 6-week period.

'Our anticipation of high non-response was based on an early pretest. See the Method Chapter section "Procedures Considered But Rejected."

Sampling Prescription Customers from the Pharmacy Files

Upon receipt of a prescription customer file for a pharmacy, SRC staff assigned each listing to one of four strata: 1) non-diazepam group-male; 2) non-diazepam-female; 3) diazepam group-male; and 4) diazepam group-female. Non-diazepam respondents had filled a prescription in the last six weeks for a medication other than diazepam, other antianxiety agents, antidepressants, antipsychotics, antihistamines, or physician-requested compounds of an unknown nature. Subsampling rates were established individually for each of these four groups. Since, prior to the study, little was known about the prescription volume--diazepam or other drugs--of each pharmacy or the overall volume of pharmacies, the initial specification of subsampling rates was tentative. Based on numbers of prescriptions recorded for the first fourteen pharmacies, subsampling rates were set for each of the four sample strata. After data for 20 sample pharmacies had been processed, the subsampling rates were reviewed and slight adjustments were made in the non-diazepam group strata. The following table provides the within pharmacy sampling rates both before and after this adjustment was made.

Within pharmacies and separately for each of the four strata, prescription customers were subsampled at the rates specified in Table A below, and this information was transmitted to the field operations staff for contact and interview.

Table A

Within Pharmacy Sampling Rates

Strata	Rate Before Adjustment	Rate After Adjustment
DIAZEPAM GROUP		
Male	1/1	1/1
Female	1/1	1/1
NON-DIAZEPAM GROUP		
Male	1/73	1/85
Female	1/136	1/120

The University of Michigan

SURVEY RESEARCH CENTER

INSTITUTE FOR SOCIAL RESEARCH
THE UNIVERSITY OF MICHIGAN
ANN ARBOR, MICHIGAN 48106

Appendix B
Initial Letter to Potential Respondents

Dear

The University of Michigan's Survey Research Center is currently conducting a study on the effects of stress on health, work, and everyday life. The University needs to interview a wide range of people, and we would like you to share your opinions on these important issues.

One of our interviewers will be calling at your home soon in connection with this survey. We want to let you know in advance about the visit so that you will not mistake our interviewer for a salesperson. Each of our interviewers carries a University of Michigan employee identification card and is happy to show it. If you wish to confirm the interviewer's assignment, please do not hesitate to call the University collect at (313) 763-5847.

The University of Michigan's Survey Research Center has been conducting national surveys for 30 years on topics of public interest and scientific concern. Most people have found that talking with the interviewer was interesting and worthwhile. Your specific answers to the survey will be kept in complete confidence. People interviewed can never be identified from any of the publications or reports based on this survey.

Our interviewer will be happy to answer any further questions you may have.

Sincerely,

Dr. Robert D. Caplan
Project Director

Your interviewer will be: _____

July, 1981

Appendix C
Persuasion Letter

Dear

One of our interviewers called you recently in connection with a study we are conducting. I understand you did not wish to participate at that time. Of course, the final decision rests with you. I thought that if you knew more about the nature of our work and the importance of the study, you might reconsider and grant an interview.

For the past 33 years the Survey Research Center of the University of Michigan has been conducting surveys to get an accurate picture of the opinions and expectations of the American people. I want to make it clear that in a study such as this there are no right or wrong answers: we are just trying to learn how people feel about things.

Your participation is very important. Our sampling procedure is scientifically designed to give us the best picture possible of issues dealing with stress and health in daily life. It is vital to the accuracy of this research to represent many views and attitudes, including those of people similar to you.

The identity of the persons with whom we talk is never disclosed to anyone. Every interview is held in strict confidence. Most people find that they very much enjoy being interviewed by a member of our staff of professional interviewers. The results of all the interviews taken are combined in a report which is statistical in nature.

The results of our surveys are used by people in universities, government, and private organizations. The surveys help people gain a better understanding of current social issues. A report on this study will be sent to you, if you wish, when it is completed.

I am enclosing a recent issue of the ISR Newsletter, which contains articles based on some of the research which is done here. If you are interested, you can subscribe to this Newsletter at no charge, simply by writing to the editor.

Our interviewer will call you again a few days after you receive this letter. We sincerely hope that you will decide to take part in this important study of stress and health in daily life. It may be that the things we learn from this research will improve the quality of all our lives.

Thank you very much for your time and consideration.

Sincerely,

Robert D. Caplan, Ph.D.
Senior Study Director

The University of Michigan

CERTIFICATE OF AGREEMENT

Appendix D

Certificate of Agreement

1. Participants in the Survey Research Center's Study of Stress: Work, Family and Health will be paid a total of $25 for four interviews-- $5 upon completion of the first, second and third interviews, and $10 upon completion of the final interview.

2. All information which would permit identification of the people being interviewed as part of this project will be held in strict confidence. No information that would allow identification will be disclosed or released to others for any purpose.

_____
Signature of Interviewer

1. I agree to participate in all four interviews.

2. I understand that the information from this interview must be very accurate in order to be useful. This means that I must do my best to give accurate and complete answers. I agree to do this.

_____
Signature of Respondent

300

SURVEY
RESEARCH
CENTER

INSTITUTE FOR
SOCIAL RESEARCH
THE UNIVERSITY
OF MICHIGAN

ANN ARBOR,
MICHIGAN 48106

Summer 1981

Dear _____:

has volunteered to take part in a survey being conducted by The University of Michigan's Survey Research Center to study the effects of stress on health, work, and everyday life.

Part of our study requires that we talk to someone who knows the participant well. Since you were named as such a person we would like to interview you briefly on the telephone.

A professional interviewer from the University will call you today or tomorrow to ask you a few questions. The interview generally lasts about 15 minutes. The interviewer will be glad to answer any questions you may have at that time.

Accompanying this letter is a booklet containing answer categories to some of the questions you will be asked. Please keep this booklet by the telephone. The interviewer will refer you to the appropriate page as she asks the questions.

All interviews are strictly confidential. No one will see your answers except the staff at The University of Michigan where your answers will be added to the answers of others for a statistical report. Names will never be used in the report.

Your participation is completely voluntary. However, I think you will enjoy the interview and knowing that you have made a valuable contribution to this research.

Sincerely,

Robert D. Caplan, Ph.D.
Senior Study Director
Institute for Social Research
The University of Michigan

RDC:PO

Project 45
(464911)

SURVEY
RESEARCH
CENTER

INSTITUTE FOR
SOCIAL RESEARCH
THE UNIVERSITY
OF MICHIGAN
ANN ARBOR,
MICHIGAN 48106

Summer 1981

ISR

Dear _____ :

_____ has volunteered to take part in a survey being conducted by The University of Michigan's Survey Research Center to study the effects of stress on health, work and everyday life.

Part of our study requires that we talk to someone familiar with the participant's work life. Since you were named as such a person we would like to interview you briefly on the telephone.

A professional interviewer from the University will call you today or tomorrow to ask you a few questions. The interview generally lasts 5 to 10 minutes. The interviewer will be able to answer any questions you may have at that time.

Accompanying this letter is a booklet containing answer categories to some of the questions you will be asked. Please keep this booklet by the telephone. The interviewer will refer you to the appropriate page as she asks the questions.

All interviews are strictly confidential. No one will see your answers except the staff at The University of Michigan where your answers will be added to the answers of others for a statistical report. Names will never be used in the report.

Your participation is completely voluntary. However, I think you will enjoy the interview and knowing that you have made a valuable contribution to this research.

Sincerely,

Robert D. Caplan, Ph.D.
Senior Study Director
Institute for Social Research
The University of Michigan

RDC:WO

Project 45
(462491)

SURVEY RESEARCH CENTER / INSTITUTE FOR SOCIAL RESEARCH / THE UNIVERSITY OF MICHIGAN / ANN ARBOR, MI

University of Michigan Study of Stress: Work, Family, and Health

Dear Participant:

I want you to know how much we value and appreciate your participation in our study. You are making an important contribution to science. Hopefully this research will give all of us a better understanding of how people cope with the demands and challenges of daily life.

Your interviewer looks forward to interviewing you again. In this way we can learn about things that stay the same and things that change in people's lives. On behalf of your interviewer and our staff, I want to thank you for your cooperation.

Sincerely,

Robert D. Caplan, Ph.D.
Senior Study Director

ISR

SURVEY RESEARCH CENTER / INSTITUTE FOR SOCIAL RESEARCH / THE UNIVERSITY OF MICHIGAN / ANN ARBOR, MI

University of Michigan Study of Stress: Work, Family, and Health

Dear Participant:

This is just a reminder that your fourth, and final, interview for our study should take place soon. Preliminary results indicate that this research endeavor will prove to be a valuable and relevant contribution to our understanding of how people deal with stress. The success of this study is due to your effort and cooperation.

If you would like to receive a report describing the results of this study, please tell your interviewer. It will probably take us approximately one year to fully analyze the information and prepare this report, but we will be happy to send it to you if you are interested.

Sincerely,

Robert D. Caplan, Ph.D.
Senior Study Director

Appendix I

Time 4 Questionnaires

Table of Contents

Time 4 Focal Respondent Questionnaire . . . I - 2

Events Calendar . . . . I - 63

Personal Other Questionnaire . . . . I - 68

Work Other Questionnaires . . . . I - 81

For Office Use Only

SRC | SURVEY RESEARCH CENTER
INSTITUTE FOR SOCIAL RESEARCH
THE UNIVERSITY OF MICHIGAN
ANN ARBOR, MICHIGAN 48106

STUDY OF STRESS: WORK, FAMILY AND HEALTH

Fall/Winter 1981
Project 45
(462491)

TIME IV

1. Interviewer's Label

8. FOCAL R ID # _____

2. Your Interview Number _____

3. Date of Interview _____

4. Length of Interview _____ Minutes

5. Length of Edit _____ Minutes

6. PERSONAL OTHER INTERVIEW?

   | 1. YES | | 5. NO |

7. WORK OTHER INTERVIEW?

   | 1. YES | | 5. NO |

INTERVIEWER: PRE-EDIT EVENTS CALENDAR AND PAGE 15

READ:

Just as before, I will be asking you about things that have changed and things that have stayed the same in your life. (To do this, I'll ask you some questions that are new. But many of the questions will be the same, only dealing with things now as compared to when you were last contacted.) Don't try to remember how you answered last time, just answer in terms of how you feel now.

Again, let me remind you that your comments are confidential. The only persons who will see them are the people at the University who tabulate them for the survey results. Also, let me remind you that you are free to skip over any questions that you do not wish to answer.

SECTION A

00. EXACT TIME NOW: _____

A1. First, I need to know again who lives with you. I don't need their names, just their ages and their relationships to you. This may not have changed since last time, but I need to check just to make sure.

MEMBERS OF THE HOUSEHOLD BY RELATIONSHIP TO RESPONDENT	SEX	AGE
1. RESPONDENT		
2.		
3.		
4.		
5.		
6.		
7.		
8.		

A2. (ASK IF UNCLEAR) Are you married, separated, divorced, widowed or have you never been married?

| 1. MARRIED AND LIVING WITH SPOUSE | 2. SEPARATED | 3. DIVORCED | 4. WIDOWED | 5. NEVER MARRIED |

A9. In the last seven days how much has your physical health kept you from doing the things you want to do? Would you say it interfered not at all, just a little, some, quite a bit, or a great deal?

1. NOT AT ALL	2. JUST A LITTLE	3. SOME	4. QUITE A BIT	5. A GREAT DEAL

A10. During the last seven days how well have you been sleeping? Would you say very poorly, poorly, all right, well, or very well?

1. VERY POORLY	2. POORLY	3. ALL RIGHT	4. WELL	5. VERY WELL

A11. (RB, P. 1) I am going to read you a list of problems or complaints that people sometimes have. Please tell me how much each has bothered or distressed you in the last seven days, including today. How much were you bothered by...

	NOT AT ALL (1)	A LITTLE BIT (2)	QUITE A BIT (3)	EXTREMELY (4)
a. nervousness or shakiness inside in the last 7 days?				
b. pains in the heart or chest in the last 7 days?				
c. trembling?				
d. suddenly scared for no reason?				
e. How much in the last seven days have you been bothered by a feeling of being trapped or caught?				
f. crying easily?				
g. blaming yourself for things?				
h. feeling lonely?				
j. worrying or stewing about things?				
k. feeling no interest in things?				
m. feeling fearful?				
n. heart pounding or racing?				
p. soreness of your muscles?				

A3. Since you were last interviewed, what have been the most pleasant events or developments that have taken place in your life? (Anything else?)

A4. Since you were last interviewed, what have been the most unpleasant events or developments that have taken place in your life? (Anything else?)

A5. Now I want to ask you some questions about your physical health. How would you rate your health at present--excellent, good, fair, or poor?

4. EXCELLENT	3. GOOD	2. FAIR	1. POOR

A6. How worried are you about your physical health these days? Would you say you are extremely worried, somewhat worried, slightly worried, or not at all worried?

4. EXTREMELY WORRIED	3. SOMEWHAT WORRIED	2. SLIGHTLY WORRIED	1. NOT AT ALL WORRIED

A7. Compared to five years ago, would you say your physical health has been getting a lot better, a little bit better, staying about the same, getting a little worse, or getting a lot worse?

5. A LOT BETTER	4. LITTLE BIT BETTER	3. ABOUT THE SAME	2. LITTLE WORSE	1. A LOT WORSE

A8. What kinds of physical health problems have you been dealing with these days? (PROBE FOR PHYSICAL SYMPTOMS)

(RB, P. 1) In the last 7 days, how much were you bothered by...

	NOT AT ALL (1)	A LITTLE BIT (2)	QUITE A BIT (3)	EXTREMELY (4)
q. feeling blue?				
r. thoughts of ending your life?				
s. trouble getting your breath?				
t. hot or cold spells?				
u. numbness or tingling in parts of your body?				
v. having to avoid certain places or activities because they frighten you?				
w. feeling hopeless about the future?				
x. weakness in parts of your body?				
y. feeling tense or keyed up?				
z. heavy feelings in your arms or legs?				
aa. difficulty in falling asleep or staying asleep?				
bb. pains in the lower part of your back?				
cc. loss of sexual interest or pleasure?				
dd. feeling low in energy or slowed down?				
ee. poor appetite?				

A12. In the last seven days, how upset have you been emotionally—very upset, quite upset, somewhat upset, or not at all upset?

| 4. VERY UPSET | 3. QUITE UPSET | 2. SOMEWHAT UPSET | 1. NOT AT ALL UPSET |

A13. What do you usually do to make yourself feel better when you're upset emotionally? (RESPONSE WILL BE USED IN B1, kk, P. 9)

_____

_____

_____

_____

IF MORE THAN ONE MENTION

A13a. Which do you do the most? (CIRCLE ANSWER ABOVE; RESPONSE WILL BE USED IN B1, kk, P. 9)

A14. (RB, P. 1) In the last seven days, how much have you felt...

	NOT AT ALL (1)	A LITTLE BIT (2)	QUITE A BIT (3)	EXTREMELY (4)
a. irritated or annoyed?				
b. furiously angry?				
c. mad at someone?				
d. so angry that you felt like hitting someone?				

A15. I want to ask you some questions about what the last several weeks have been like for you; that is, from the week you were last interviewed to now.

If you have the pocket calendar (I/the other interviewer) gave you or one of your own, you could look at it. It may help you remember some of the things that happened.

Again I'm going to write down what you tell me on this calendar and then ask you some questions about how you felt. So I want you to think carefully and try to recall events that happened that will help you remember how you felt each week.

Let's start with this week, beginning with Sunday, _____ (DATE). (NOTE: "THIS WEEK" STARTS WITH PREVIOUS SUNDAY.)

(ENTER DATES AND ABBREVIATION OF EVENTS ON CALENDAR.)

(IF R CAN'T THINK OF ANY EVENTS, PROBE: "Anything at work; Anything at home; Anything pleasant; Anything about your health?")

6

A16. R REFERRED TO A CALENDAR FOR THIS INFORMATION.

1. YES	5. NO

A17. First I want to ask you about feeling anxious, uptight, nervous, or worried. Some people feel anxious or worried almost all the time. Others rarely feel anxious at all. Still others may feel anxious some weeks and not others.

(TURN TO ANXIETY CHART.)

Just as you did before I want you to describe how much anxiety you have felt over the last several weeks using this chart.

[IF NECESSARY: Each one of these rows (POINT TO ROW) represents a week, going back to the week you were last interviewed. The squares, from the left to right, represent the amount of anxiety you felt beginning with extreme anxiety or nervousness...

...(and ending with no anxiety or nervousness./

...followed by quite a bit of anxiety or nervousness, some anxiety or nervous- ness, a little anxiety or nervousness, or no anxiety or nervousness.)

For each week, put an "X" in the box that best represents how anxious you felt. (Let's start with this week, from Sunday, _____ (DATE) to today.) How anxious have you felt this week?

Now think about the week before.]

(FOR WEEK OF LAST INTERVIEW:) This last week refers to the week that you were interviewed, and I want you to recall that week up to the time of the interview. That would be from Sunday _____ to _____ . (Just those
                                            (DAY, DATE OF LAST INTERVIEW)
days.) You mentioned _____ for that week so I have already written (this/these) event(s) down. You don't need to try and remember what you marked last time. Simply check the box that best describes how much anxiety you felt those days.

A18. (R3, P. 2) When you were filling in the chart, how much did you remember exactly and how much did you have to guess how you felt?

1. REMEMBERED EXACTLY	2. REMEMBERED MOSTLY	3. REMEMBERED PARTLY AND GUESSED PARTLY	4. GUESSED MOSTLY	5. GUESSED ALMOST ALL

7

A19. Now let's talk about how you've been feeling about your life as a whole during that same period.

(TURN TO LIFE AS A WHOLE CHART.)

[On this chart, the squares from the left to the right represent how you feel about your life as a whole, with the first square meaning delighted, the next one pleased,...

...(and so on to terrible./

...the next mostly satisfied, then mixed, about equally satisfied and dissatis- fied, the next mostly dissatisfied, the next unhappy, and finally at the end terrible.)]

Please fill in this chart too.

A20. (R3, P. 2) When you were filling in the chart, how much did you remember exactly and how much did you have to guess how you felt?

1. REMEMBERED EXACTLY	2. REMEMBERED MOSTLY	3. REMEMBERED PARTLY AND GUESSED PARTLY	4. GUESSED MOSTLY	5. GUESSED ALMOST ALL

B1. (RB, P. 3) I want you to tell me how much you've done each of the following things in the last seven days.

	NOT AT ALL (1)	JUST A LITTLE (2)	SOME (3)	QUITE A BIT (4)	A GREAT DEAL (5)
a. How much did you daydream about a better world or think ahead to a better time in the last seven days?					
b. How much did you talk to someone about your feelings in the last seven days?					
c. How much did you make decisions about what can and cannot be done?					
d. How much did you blame yourself for anything?					
e. How much did you pray?					
f. ...get people to change the demands being made on you?					
g. ...turn to some other activity to take your mind off things?					
h. ...try not to expect too much of yourself?					
j. ...learn as much as possible about any problems you might have?					
k. ...tell yourself that something is someone else's reponsibility?					
m. ...make compromises or trade-offs to make the best of things?					
n. ...take things out on other people?					
p. ...prepare for the worst that could happen?					
q. ...keep your feelings to yourself?					
r. ...try to improve yourself so you could handle things better?					
s. ...drink coffee, tea, or cola to keep yourself going?					
t. ...try to find meaning in something that happened?					

(In the last seven days, how much did you...)

	NOT AT ALL (1)	JUST A LITTLE (2)	SOME (3)	QUITE A BIT (4)	A GREAT DEAL (5)
u. ...ask someone you respect for advice?					
v. ...try to understand why something happened?					
w. ...rely on your religious beliefs?					
x. ...tell yourself you won't let things get to you?					
y. ... stand your ground and fight for what you wanted?					
z. ...find new faith or some new truth about life?					
aa. ...look on the bright side of things?					
bb. ...get someone to help out with something?					
cc. ...take responsibility for something that happened?					
dd. ...rediscover what is important in life?					
ee. ...let all your feelings out?					
ff. ...carry on your life as usual?					
gg. ...decide that you've changed or grown as a person as a result of something that might have happened?					
hh. ...accept whatever happened since nothing could be done about it?					
jj. ...view something that happened as a challenge?					
kk. You told me before that when you are emotionally upset, you usually _____. (FROM A13, P. 5) How much have you been doing this in the last seven days?					

10

B2. (RB, P. 4) We're interested in knowing how sure or unsure you have been in the last seven days about certain things in your personal life. By personal life I mean your relationships with people you feel close to.

	VERY SURE (1)	FAIRLY SURE (2)	NEITHER SURE NOR UNSURE (3)	FAIRLY UNSURE (4)	VERY UNSURE (5)
a. In the last seven days, how sure or unsure have you been about whether the people in your personal life would approve of the way you you were doing things?					
b. How sure or unsure have you been about whether you were doing the right things in your personal life?					
c. (How sure or unsure have you been) about whether you could keep up with all the responsibilities and demands in your personal life?					
d. (How sure or unsure have you been) about whether you were making the right decisions in your personal life?					
e. (How sure or unsure have you been) about what others expected of you in your personal life?					
f. (How sure or unsure have you been) about what your personal life will be like in the near future?					

B3. (RB, P. 5) In the last seven days how well have you been doing the following things in your personal life?

	VERY POORLY (1)	NOT VERY WELL (2)	ALL RIGHT (3)	VERY WELL (4)	EXCEPTIONALLY WELL (5)
a. Getting along with others in your personal life?					
b. Handling responsibilities and daily demands in your personal life?					
c. Making the right decisions?					
d. Avoiding arguing with others?					
e. Handling disagreements by compromising and meeting other people halfway?					

B4. (RB, P. 6) These next questions ask you to think about how well you've been doing in various areas of your life in the last seven days -- how successful you've been in having your life be what you wanted.

	NOT AT ALL (1)	JUST A LITTLE (2)	SOME (3)	MOST (4)	ALL (5)
a. In the last seven days to what extent has your personal life been what you wanted it to be?					
b. What about yourself-- in the last seven days how much have you been the kind of person you wanted to be?					
c. To what extent have your health and physical condition been what you wanted them to be?					
d. (ASK EVERYONE) In the last seven days to what extent have you achieved what you wanted in your work? ☐ R SAYS NOT EMPLOYED					
e. To what extent has your life as a whole been what you wanted it to be?					

309

B5. (RB, P. 7) In the last seven days...

	NOT AT ALL (1)	JUST A LITTLE (2)	SOME (3)	QUITE A BIT (4)	A GREAT DEAL (5)
a. How much has what happened in your personal life depended on what other people said and did?					
b. How much has it depended on what you said and did?					
c. How much has it depended on luck, either good or bad?					
d. How much would you like what happens in your personal life to depend on what other people say and do?					
e. How much would you like it to depend on what you say and do?					
f. How much would you like it to depend on luck?					

13

B6. (RB, P. 7) Now, I'm going to read you a set of similar but slightly different questions. We're doing this for statistical reasons.

	NOT AT ALL (1)	JUST A LITTLE (2)	SOME (3)	QUITE A BIT (4)	A GREAT DEAL (5)
a. In the last seven days how much have things in your personal life been influenced or determined by other people?					
b. How much have they been influenced or determined by you?					
c. How much by chance?					
d. Now think ahead to the future. In the near future how much do you expect other people to influence or determine things in your personal life?					
e. In the near future how much do you expect to be the one who influences or determines things in your personal life?					
f. How much do you expect them to be influenced or determined by chance?					
g. How much would you like things in your personal life to be influenced or determined by other people?					
h. How much would you personally like to be the one who influences or determines things?					
j. How much would you like them to be influenced or determined by chance?					

I - 16

B7. (RB, P. 7) Now I want to ask you some questions about how much real enjoyment you have gotten from different parts of your life in the last seven days.

	NOT AT ALL (1)	JUST A LITTLE (2)	SOME (3)	QUITE A BIT (4)	A GREAT DEAL (5)
a. How much have you really enjoyed your personal life?					
b. What about yourself, in the last seven days, how much have you really enjoyed being the kind of person you've been--the way you've acted and felt?					
c. How much have you really enjoyed your health and physical condition?					
d. (IF R ANSWERED B4d) In the last seven days how much have you really enjoyed your work? [ ] R SAID NOT EMPLOYED					
e. How much have you really enjoyed your life as a whole?					

B8. What were you thinking about when you answered these last few questions about enjoying your life?

_____

_____

_____

PROBE AS APPROPRIATE: (1) Can you give me some examples?
(2) How about things at home?
(3) What about your relationships with your friends?

I - 17

SECTION C

C1. INTERVIEWER CHECKPOINT: CHECK WORK STATUS FROM ITEM 13 ON COVER SHEET

[ ] R WAS EMPLOYED

Last time you were interviewed you said you were working as _____, JOB TITLE.

Are you still working at this job with the same employer?

1. YES   5. NO → GO TO C2
TURN TO P. 18, C19

[ ] R WAS NOT EMPLOYED

Last time you were interviewed you said you were _____ STATUS
are you still _____ or has this changed?

1. STILL THE SAME   5. CHANGED → GO TO C3
TURN TO P. 16, C8

[ ] R WAS DISABLED ──→ TURN TO P. 24, SECTION D

C2. Are you now working at a different job, temporarily laid off, unemployed, retired, disabled, a student, a homemaker or what?

WORKING
1. DIFFERENT JOB
TURN TO P.16, C4

2. TEMPORARILY LAID OFF
TURN TO P.16, C7

3. UNEMPLOYED
TURN TO P.16, C6

4. RETIRED   5. DISABLED
TURN TO P. 16, C7

6. STUDENT   7. HOMEMAKER
TURN TO P. 16, C6

8. OTHER (SPECIFY): _____

C3. Are you now working, temporarily laid off, unemployed, retired, disabled, a student, a homemaker or what?

1. WORKING
TURN TO P.18, C16

2. LAID OFF
TURN TO P.16, C9

3. UNEMPLOYED
TURN TO P.16, C9

4. RETIRED   5. DISABLED
TURN TO P.24, SECTION D

6. STUDENT   7. HOMEMAKER
TURN TO P.16, C9

8. OTHER (SPECIFY): _____

R WORKING DIFFERENT JOB

C4. Did you quit your last job voluntarily or were you laid off or fired?

| 1. QUIT | 5. LAID OFF, FIRED |

C5. When did you stop working on your last job , what date?

MONTH _____   DAY _____

TURN TO P. 18, C16

R WAS WORKING, NOW NOT WORKING

C6. Did you quit your last job voluntarily or were you laid off or fired?

| 1. QUIT | 5. LAID OFF, FIRED |

C7. When did you stop working (on your last job), what date?

MONTH _____   DAY _____

C8. INTERVIEWER CHECKPOINT

☐ 1. R IS RETIRED OR DISABLED ──→ TURN TO P. 24, SECTION D

☐ 2. OTHER NONWORKING

C9. Are you looking for (a/another) job?

1. YES

5. NO ──→ TURN TO P. 24 , SECTION D

R NOT WORKING NOW

C10. How emotionally upsetting is it for you these days to go out looking for a job? Would you say it is not at all upsetting, somewhat upsetting, quite upsetting, or very upsetting?

| 1. NOT AT ALL UPSETTING | 2. SOMEWHAT UPSETTING | 3. QUITE UPSETTING | 4. VERY UPSETTING |

C11. (RB, P. 8) How difficult is it these days to find a job within commuting distance for a person with your skills, training, and experience?

| 1. NOT AT ALL DIFFICULT | 2. SLIGHTLY DIFFICULT | 3. SOMEWHAT DIFFICULT | 4. VERY DIFFICULT | 5. EXTREMELY DIFFICULT OR IMPOSSIBLE |

C12. (RB, P. 9) How likely is it that in the near future you will be able to find a job with enough income and fringe benefits?

| 1. VERY UNLIKELY | 2. NOT VERY LIKELY | 3. EQUALLY LIKELY AND UNLIKELY | 4. SOMEWHAT LIKELY | 5. VERY LIKELY OR CERTAIN |

C13. (RB, P. 9) How likely is it that in the near future you will be able to find a job you'd be willing to do?

| 1. VERY UNLIKELY | 2. NOT VERY LIKELY | 3. EQUALLY LIKELY AND UNLIKELY | 4. SOMEWHAT LIKELY | 5. VERY LIKELY OR CERTAIN |

C14. How long ago was it that you looked for a job?

_____ DAYS / WEEKS / MONTHS / YEARS   AGO   (CIRCLE ONE)

C15. When was the last time you actually applied for a job?

_____ DAYS / WEEKS / MONTHS / YEARS   AGO   (CIRCLE ONE)

TURN TO P. 24, D1

R WORKING NOW

1 - 20

C16. When did you start your new job, what date?

MONTH _____ DAY _____

C17. What is your job title, or what sort of work do you do on your job?

C17a. Tell me a little more about what you do.

C17b. What kind of business or industry is that?

C17c. What do they make or do at the place where you work?

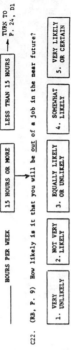

C18. About how many days do you usually work on your (main) job in an average week, including any overtime?

_____ DAYS PER WEEK

00. NONE   01. ONE
TURN TO P. 19, C20

8. IRREGULAR OR SEASONAL

C18a. How many is it during the weeks you do work?

_____ DAYS PER WEEK

C19. Think back to when you were last interviewed. Aside from any vacations, layoffs, or strikes (or any time you were unemployed), approximately how many days of work have you missed since you were last interviewed?

_____ DAYS MISSED   MORE THAN ONE

C19a. Were these all in a row or on separate occasions?

1. ALL IN A ROW   2. SEPARATE OCCASIONS
TURN TO P. 19, C20

_____ SEPARATE OCCASIONS

C19b. How many separate occasions were there? By that I mean one or more days at a time?

1 - 21

C20. During the last two weeks that you worked, approximately how many times did you arrive at work late?

_____ TIMES   98. WORKS OWN HOURS

C21. About how many hours do you usually work on your (main) job in an average week, including any overtime (during the weeks you work)?

_____ HOURS PER WEEK   15 HOURS OR MORE   LESS THAN 15 HOURS ──→ TURN TO P. 24, D1

C22. (RB, P. 9) How likely is it that you will be out of a job in the near future?

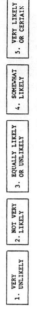

| 1. VERY UNLIKELY | 2. NOT VERY LIKELY | 3. EQUALLY LIKELY OR UNLIKELY | 4. SOMEWHAT LIKELY | 5. VERY LIKELY OR CERTAIN |

C23. (RB, P. 9) How likely is it that (an employer/your clients or customers) will still value your job skills six months from now?

| 1. VERY UNLIKELY | 2. NOT VERY LIKELY | 3. EQUALLY LIKELY OR UNLIKELY | 4. SOMEWHAT LIKELY | 5. VERY LIKELY OR CERTAIN |

C24. (RB, P. 9) How likely is it that you will remain employed for the next year (at any job)?

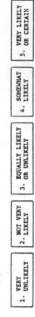

| 1. VERY UNLIKELY | 2. NOT VERY LIKELY | 3. EQUALLY LIKELY OR UNLIKELY | 4. SOMEWHAT LIKELY | 5. VERY LIKELY OR CERTAIN |

C25. Have you worked at your job in the last seven days?

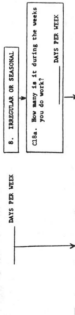

1. YES   5. NO
TURN TO P. 20, C26

C25a. How long ago did you last work? _____ WEEKS AGO

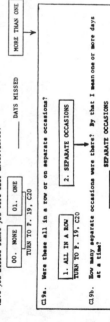

READ: Since you haven't worked in the last week, I want you to answer the following questions about your job in terms of the last week you worked.

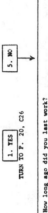

20

C26. We're interested in knowing how **sure** or **unsure** you were **in** the last (seven days/week you worked) about certain things on your job.

	VERY SURE (1)	FAIRLY SURE (2)	NEITHER SURE NOR UNSURE (3)	FAIRLY UNSURE (4)	VERY UNSURE (5)
a. (RB, P. 10) In the last (seven days/week you worked) how sure or unsure were you about whether others would approve of the way you were doing your work?					
b. How sure or unsure were you about whether you were doing the right things on your job?					
c. In the last (seven days/week you worked) how sure or unsure were you about whether you could keep up with all the responsibilities and demands of your job?					
d. (How sure or unsure were you) about whether you were making the right decisions on your job?					
e. ...about what others expected of you at work?					

C27. (RB, P. 11) In the last (seven days/week you worked) how **well** were you doing the following things on your job?

	VERY POORLY (1)	NOT VERY WELL (2)	ALL RIGHT (3)	VERY WELL (4)	EXCEPTIONALLY WELL (5)
a. Getting along with others at work?					
b. Handling the responsibilities and daily demands of your work?					
c. Making the right decisions?					
d. Avoiding arguing with others?					
e. Handling disagreements by compromising and meeting other people half-way?					
f. Performing without mistakes?					
g. Getting things done on time?					

I - 24

I - 25

C28. (RB, P. 12) Conflicts can occur in any job. I'm going to read you a list of problems and for each one I'd like you to tell me how much you have been faced with something similar on your job in the last (seven days/week you worked).

	NOT AT ALL (1)	JUST A LITTLE (2)	SOME (3)	QUITE A BIT (4)	A GREAT DEAL (5)
a. In the last (seven days/week you worked), how much did key people you work with ask you to do things that conflicted with your own sense of what should be done?					
b. How much did key people you work with give you things to do which conflicted with one another?					
c. In the last (seven days/week you worked), how much did key people you work with see things about your job differently from the way you do?					
d. How much did key people you work with give you things to do which conflicted with other work you had to do?					

C29. In the last (seven days/week you worked), were you faced with any other problems on your job? (Tell me about them).

_____

_____

_____

314

24

I - 26

SECTION D

315

ASK EVERYONE

D1. (RB, P. 12) I want to ask you several questions about your relationships with people (at work and) in your personal life during the last seven days. As I ask each question, I'd like you to think of someone in particular, but it doesn't have to be the same person for each question.

	NOT AT ALL (1)	JUST A LITTLE (2)	SOME (3)	QUITE A BIT (4)	A GREAT DEAL (5)
a. In the last seven days, how much could you count on some one person to give you useful information and advice if you wanted it?					
b. How much could you count on some one person to be a source of encouragement and reassurance if you wanted it?					
c. How much did some one person misunderstand the way you think and feel about things?					
d. ...listen if you wanted to confide about things that were important to you?					
e. ...criticize you unjustly?					
f. ...act in ways that showed he or she appreciated you?					
g. ...argue with you about something?					
h. ...treat you with respect?					
j. In the last seven days, how much did some one person get on your nerves?					
k. How much did some one person act in an unpleasant or angry manner toward you?					
m. ...show that he or she cared about you as a person?					
n. ...ignore you or not include you in important aspects of his or her life?					
p. ...show that he or she disliked you?					

25

I - 27

```
1. IF R MENTIONS MORE THAN
   ONE PERSON FOR A QUES-
   TION, ASK: "Were you
   thinking of one person
   more than the other(s)?"
   CIRCLE CHOICE IF ANY.

2. IF A RELATIONSHIP LIKE
   SON OR FRIEND IS MEN-
   TIONED MORE THAN ONCE,
   PROBE: "Is that the same
   (son/friend)?" AND USE
   INITIALS OR FIRST NAME
   TO DISTINGUISH THEM.

3. IF R RESISTS BECAUSE
   "NOT AT ALL" IN D1:
   "Sometimes people are
   thinking of someone in
   in particular. Did
   you have anyone in mind
   when I asked how much
   someone..., if so, who?"
```

D2. Now let me go back over these questions and ask you who you were thinking about for each one. I don't need their names, just their relationship to you. Who is the person you were thinking about when I asked...

a. ...who you could count on to give you useful information and advice?

b. ...who could be a source of encouragement and reassurance?

c. ...who misunderstood the way you think and feel about things?

d. ...who listened when you wanted to confide about things?

e. ...who criticized you unjustly?

f. ...who acted in ways that showed he or she appreciated you?

g. ...who argued with you?

h. ...who treated you with respect?

j. ...who got on your nerves?

k. ...who acted in an unpleasant or angry manner toward you?

m. ...who showed he or she cared about you as a person?

n. ...who ignored you or didn't include you in important aspects of his or her life?

p. ...who showed that he or she disliked you?

SECTION E: QUALITY OF LIFE

E1. (RB, P. 13) We want to find out how you feel about various aspects of your life. I'm going to read you a list of things. On page 13 of your Respondent Booklet is a scale with the number 7 for delighted, 6 for pleased, and so forth on to 1 for terrible.

As I read each one please tell me what number best describes the feelings you have now—taking into account what has happened in the last seven days. If you have no feelings at all, or never thought about it, or if the question doesn't apply to you, just tell me.

7	6	5	4	3	2	1
DELIGHTED	PLEASED	MOSTLY SATISFIED	MIXED (ABOUT EQUALLY SATISFIED & DISSATISFIED)	MOSTLY DISSAT- ISFIED	UNHAPPY	TERRIBLE

O= NO FEELINGS, NEVER THOUGHT ABOUT IT, OR DOESN'T APPLY

(Here's the first one:)

_____ E1a. How do you feel about the way you handle problems that come up in your life?

_____ E1b. How do you feel about your work?

_____ E1c. How do you feel about your children?

_____ E1d. ...your (wife/husband), your marriage?

_____ E1e. ...your romantic life?

_____ E1f. (How do you feel about) your friends and acquaintances?

_____ E1g. ...the people you work with—your co-workers?

_____ E1h. ...what you are accomplishing in your life?

_____ E1j. ... your physical appearance, the way you look to others?

_____ E1k. ...your own health and physical condition?

_____ E1m. ...your (family) income?

_____ E1n. (How do you feel about) yourself?

_____ E1o. ...the sleep you get?

_____ E1p. ...how secure you are financially?

_____ E1q. (How do you feel about) the extent to which you can adjust to changes in your life?

_____ E1r. ...how tense or nervous you've been?

_____ E1s. ...the work you do on the job—the work itself?

_____ E1t. ...your personal life?

_____ E1u. And now the last one: How do you feel about your life as a whole?

E2. Taking all things together, how would you say things are these days—would you say you're very happy, pretty happy, or not too happy these days?

3. VERY HAPPY	2. PRETTY HAPPY	1. NOT TOO HAPPY

E3. Most people worry more or less about some things. Would you say you never worry, worry a little, worry sometimes, worry a lot, or worry all the time?

1. NEVER	2. A LITTLE	3. SOMETIMES	4. A LOT	5. ALL THE TIME

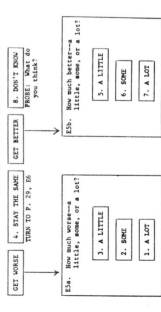

E4. Since you were last interviewed, do you think things in your life got worse, stayed the same, or got better?

GOT WORSE	4. STAYED THE SAME	GOT BETTER	8. DON'T KNOW
	GO TO E5		PROBE: What do you think?

E4a. How much worse--a little, some, or a lot?

3. A LITTLE
2. SOME
1. A LOT

E4b. How much better--a little, some, or a lot?

5. A LITTLE
6. SOME
7. A LOT

E5. Now, think ahead to the future. Over the coming six weeks do you think things in your life will get worse, stay the same, or get better?

GET WORSE	4. STAY THE SAME	GET BETTER	8. DON'T KNOW
	TURN TO P. 29, E6		PROBE: What do you think?

E5a. How much worse--a little, some, or a lot?

3. A LITTLE
2. SOME
1. A LOT

E5b. How much better--a little, some, or a lot?

5. A LITTLE
6. SOME
7. A LOT

E6. (RB, P. 14) Next, I have some questions about how emotionally upset various parts of your life have made you feel in the last seven days.

	NOT AT ALL (1)	JUST A LITTLE (2)	SOME (3)	QUITE A BIT (4)	A GREAT DEAL (5)
a. How much has your personal life made you feel emotionally upset?					
b. What about yourself, in the last seven days how much has the kind of person you've been made you feel emotionally upset?					
c. How much has your health and physical condition made you feel emotionally upset?					
d. (IF R ANSWERED B4d) In the last seven days how much has your work made you feel emotionally upset? [ ] R SAID NOT EMPLOYED					
e. How much has your life as a whole made you feel emotionally upset?					

E7. (RB, P. 14) The next few questions have to do with your feelings and emotions in general.

I - 32

	NOT AT ALL (1)	JUST A LITTLE (2)	SOME (3)	QUITE A BIT (4)	A GREAT DEAL (5)
a. In the last seven days how much have your feelings and emotions depended on what other people said and did?					
b. How much have they depended on what you said and did?					
c. How much have your feelings and emotions depended on luck, either good or bad?					
d. How much would you like your feelings and emotions to depend on what other people say and do?					
e. How much would you like them to depend on what you say and do?					
f. How much would you like your feelings and emotions to depend on luck?					

E8. Again I'm going to read you some similar but slightly different questions for statistical reasons.

	NOT AT ALL (1)	JUST A LITTLE (2)	SOME (3)	QUITE A BIT (4)	A GREAT DEAL (5)
a. (RB, P.14) In the last seven days how much have your feelings and emotions been influenced or determined by other people?					
b. How much have they been influenced or determined by you yourself?					
c. How much by chance?					

31

I - 33

	NOT AT ALL (1)	JUST A LITTLE (2)	SOME (3)	QUITE A BIT (4)	A GREAT DEAL (5)
d. Now think ahead to the future. In the near future how much do you expect other people to influence or determine what your feelings and emotions will be?					
e. In the near future how much do you expect to be the one who influences or determines what they will be?					
f. How much do you expect them to be influenced or determined by chance?					
g. How much would you like your feelings and emotions to be influenced or determined by other people?					
h. How much would you personally like to be the one who influences or determines them?					
j. How much would you like them to be influenced or determined by chance?					

COMPARE EACH MEDICATION IN MEDICATION CHART TO SELECTED PRESCRIPTION DRUG LIST BELOW

F4. FOR EACH MEDICATION IN CHART WHICH APPEARS ON LIST, ENTER A CHECK (✓) AT F4

F5. FOR EACH MEDICATION IN CHART WHICH IS ASTERISKED (*) ON LIST, ENTER A CHECK (✓) AT F5

SELECTED PRESCRIPTION DRUG LIST

Aldoril
Aldomet
Ambenyl Expectorant
Antivert
*Atarax
*Ativan

Benadryl Elixer
Benadryl
Bendectin
Benylin
*Butisol

*Centrax
*Chlordiazepoxide
*Combid
*Compazine

*Dalmane
Darvocet
Darvon
Darvon Compound
Dilantin
Dimetane Expectorant
Dimetane Expectorant VC
Donnagel
Donnatal
Drixoral

*Elavil
Empirin with Codeine
Equagesic
*Equanil

Fastin
Flexeril
Fiorinal
Fiorinal with Codeine

*Haldol

Inderal
Ionamin

*Librax
*Librium
*Limbitrol
Lomotil
*Luminal

*Mellaril
*Meprobamate
*Miltown

Naldecon
*Nembutal
Novahistine DH

Ornade

Paregoric
Percodan
Perlactin
Phenaphen with Codeine
*Phenergen Expectorant
*Phenergen VC Expectorant
*Phenobarbital

Ritalin
Robaxin-750
Robaxisal
Robitussin AC
Rondec DM

Ser-Ap-Es
*Serax
*Sinequan
*Stelazine
Sudafed

Talwin
Tenuate
*Thorazine
Tigan
*Tofranil
*Tranxene
Tussionex
Tuss-ornade
Tylenol with Codeine
Tylenol #1, #2, #3, and #4

*Valium
*Vistaril

F6. INTERVIEWER CHECKPOINT (SEE COLUMNS F4 AND F5 IN MEDICATION CHART)

☐ 1. THERE ARE NO ✓S IN EITHER F4 OR F5 FOR ANY MEDICATION → TURN TO P. 41, F50

☐ 2. NO MEDICATION HAS 2 ✓S, BUT ONE OR MORE HAS ONE → TURN TO P. 38, F28

☐ 3. ONLY ONE MEDICATION HAS 2 ✓S → CIRCLE IN CHART AND ENTER NAME AT (P.34, F7)

☐ 4. MORE THAN ONE MEDICATION HAS 2 ✓S, ONE IS VALIUM → CIRCLE VALIUM IN CHART AND ENTER (AT P. 34, F7)

☐ 5. MORE THAN ONE MEDICATION HAS 2 ✓S, NONE IS VALIUM → CIRCLE FIRST MEDICATION IN CHART WITH 2 ✓S & ENTER (AT P. 34, F7)

SECTION F: MEDICATIONS I-34

F1. Now I'd like to ask you some more questions about your health, especially about any medications you've been taking. Please think carefully. People sometimes forget to mention medications they take regularly such as insulin or Inderal or tranquilizers. Have you taken any prescription medicines in the last seven days?

☐ 1. YES ↓
☐ 5. NO → GO TO F2

F1a. What is the name of the medication you took? (Anything else?) (ENTER BELOW AND ASK F2)

F2. How about since you were last interviewed. Can you remember taking any (other) prescription medicines in the last six weeks?

☐ 1. YES ↓
☐ 5. NO → GO TO F2b, CHECKPOINT

F2a. What is the name of the medication you took? (Anything else?) (ENTER BELOW)

F2b. INTERVIEWER CHECKPOINT: (SEE COVER SHEET ITEM 14)

☐ 1. R MENTIONED (ALL) MEDICATION(S) LISTED ON COVER SHEET OR NO MEDICATIONS LISTED ON COVER SHEET → GO TO F2d

☐ 2. R FAILED TO MENTION ONE OR MORE MEDICATIONS LISTED ON COVER SHEET

F2c. (FOR EACH MEDICATION ON COVER SHEET R DID NOT MENTION:) Last time you were interviewed you mentioned taking (NAME OF MEDICATION). Have you taken any of this medication in the last six weeks?

IF YES
ENTER IN CHART BELOW

IF NO
ENTER AT P. 41, F51, F53, F55 AND RETURN TO F2d

F2d. INTERVIEWER CHECKPOINT

☐ 1. AT LEAST ONE MEDICATION IS ENTERED IN CHART BELOW

☐ 2. NO MEDICATION IS ENTERED IN CHART BELOW → TURN TO P. 41, F50

F3. May I see the bottle(s) so I can copy some information off the label? (IF NO BOTTLE, ASK A THROUGH E REGARDING HOW IT WAS PRESCRIBED.)

F4. ✓ ON LIST	F5. ✓ ON LIST	A. NAME OF MEDICATION	A. DATE FILLED	B. STRENGTH (mg., etc.)	C. # TIMES PER DAY	D. # PILLS EA TIME	E. # IN BOTTLE WHEN FULL	F. # PILLS IN BOTTLE (1)	G. FROM MEMORY (2)
		1.							
		2.							
		3.							
		4.							
		5.							
		6.							
		7.							
		8.							

F7. Now I want to ask you some additional questions about (some of) the medication(s) you mentioned.

Are you still taking _____ or have you stopped taking it?
ENTER NAME OF MEDICATION

| 1. STILL TAKING GO TO F8 | 5. STOPPED TAKING → |

F7a. Why did you stop taking it?
_____
_____

F8. For what reason (are/were) you taking it?
_____
_____

F9. How long ago did you first take (MEDICATION)?
_____ DAYS / WEEKS / MONTHS / YEARS AGO (CIRCLE ONE)

F10. How long ago did you last take it?
_____ DAYS/ WEEKS / MONTHS AGO (CIRCLE ONE)
□ TODAY
□ YESTERDAY

F11. On the days you (take/took) it, how many times a day (do/did) you usually take it?
_____ TIMES A DAY

F12. How many pills or capsules (or teaspoons) (do/did) you usually take each time?
_____ EACH TIME

F13. (RB, P. 15) During the period you took (MEDICATION) over the last year, which of these statements best describes how often you took it?

| 1. ONLY ONCE IN A WHILE | 2. SOME WEEKS ALMOST EVERY DAY, OTHER WEEKS NOT AT ALL | 3. AT LEAST ONCE A WEEK THE WHOLE TIME | 4. EVERY DAY OR EVERY OTHER DAY THE WHOLE TIME |

F13a. (RB, P. 15) Since you were last interviewed which of these statements best describes how often you took it?

| 1. ONLY ONCE IN A WHILE | 2. SOME WEEKS ALMOST EVERY DAY, OTHER WEEKS NOT AT ALL | 3. AT LEAST ONCE A WEEK THE WHOLE TIME | 4. EVERY DAY OR EVERY OTHER DAY THE WHOLE TIME |

F14. What kind of doctor prescribed this (MEDICATION) (a general practitioner, a surgeon, a psychiatrist, or what)?

KIND OF DOCTOR _____

F15. (RB, P. 16) When you visit your (KIND OF DOCTOR), how much time is there to discuss with him or her all the things you want to talk about?

| 1. NONE | 2. A LITTLE | 3. SOME | 4. A LOT | 5. A GREAT DEAL |

F16. (RB, P. 17) Would you say your (KIND OF DOCTOR) is very cold towards people, somewhat cold towards people, neither cold nor warm, somewhat warm, or very warm towards people?

| 1. VERY COLD | 2. SOMEWHAT COLD | 3. NEITHER COLD NOR WARM | 4. SOMEWHAT WARM | 5. VERY WARM |

F17. Has your (KIND OF DOCTOR) ever recommended that you see (a/another) psychologist, (a/another) psychiatrist, or any other kind of counselor?

| 1. YES | 5. NO |

F18. Now I want you to describe how often you took (MEDICATION) over the last several weeks, using this chart.

(TURN TO PATTERN OF MEDICINE USE CHART IN EVENTS CALENDAR. ENTER NAME OF MEDICATION AT TOP, REMIND R OF EVENTS.)

If you took it every single day during the week you would put an "X" in this box, if you took it every day except one, you would mark this box....
...(and so on/
...if you took it a few days you would mark this box, just one day this box.
or no days that week you'd mark this box.)
Please mark it for each week, just as you did before.

F19. (RB, P. 18) When you were filling in the chart, how much did you remember exactly and how much did you have to guess how often you took (MEDICATION)?

| 1. REMEMBERED EXACTLY | 2. REMEMBERED MOSTLY | 3. REMEMBERED PARTLY AND GUESSED PARTLY | 4. GUESSED MOSTLY | 5. GUESSED ALMOST ALL |

F20. Now let's do another chart describing the number of (MEDICATION) pills (or capsules/teaspoons) you took each week.

(TURN TO DOSAGE CHART, ENTER NAME OF MEDICATION, CIRCLE TYPE OF DOSAGE.)

For each week, put an "X" in the box that represents the number of (pills/capsules, teaspoons) you took that whole week—(15 or more, 10-14, 5-9, 1-4, or none).

(You can look at the chart you just filled out if that will help you remember.)

F21. When you were filling in the chart, how much did you remember exactly and how much did you have to guess how many you took?

| 1. REMEMBERED EXACTLY | 2. REMEMBERED MOSTLY | 3. REMEMBERED PARTLY AND GUESSED PARTLY | 4. GUESSED MOSTLY | 5. GUESSED ALMOST ALL |

F22. How (do/did) you decide when to take (MEDICATION)?

☐ TAKE IT AS PRESCRIBED

F23. (RB, P. 19) To what extent (does/did) (MEDICATION) make you feel better?

| 1. NOT AT ALL | 2. JUST A LITTLE | 3. SOMEWHAT | 4. QUITE A LOT | 5. A GREAT DEAL |

F24. (RB, P. 20) How helpful (do/did) you find (MEDICATION)?

| 1. NOT AT ALL | 2. JUST A LITTLE | 3. SOMEWHAT | 4. VERY | 5. EXTREMELY |

F25. (RB, P. 21) And if you (don't didn't) take your (MEDICATION) how much discomfort (do/did) you feel?

| 1. NONE OR VERY LITTLE | 2. A SMALL AMOUNT | 3. SOME | 4. A LOT | 5. AN EXTREME AMOUNT | 8. DON'T KNOW; ALWAYS TAKE IT |

F26. Think about how (MEDICATION) affects your control over your emotions. Does it increase your control, decrease it, or not really affect it at all?

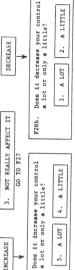

| INCREASE | 3. NOT REALLY AFFECT IT
GO TO F27 | DECREASE |

F26a. Does it increase your control a lot or only a little?

| 5. A LOT | 4. A LITTLE |

F26b. Does it decrease your control a lot or only a little?

| 1. A LOT | 2. A LITTLE |

F27. Think about how it affects your ability to deal with the problems in your life. Does it increase your ability to deal with them, decrease it, or not really affect it at all?

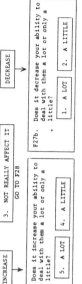

| INCREASE | 3. NOT REALLY AFFECT IT
GO TO F28 | DECREASE |

F27a. Does it increase your ability to deal with them a lot or only a little?

| 5. A LOT | 4. A LITTLE |

F27b. Does it decrease your ability to deal with them a lot or only a little?

| 1. A LOT | 2. A LITTLE |

F28a. Think back to the first time you were interviewed this summer. Between then and now, did you at any point stop taking (MEDICATION) for a while and then start taking it again?

| 1. YES | 5. NO → GO TO F28c |

F28b. When you started taking (MEDICATION) again, had you discussed it with your doctor or did you just decide to take it?

| 1. DISCUSSED WITH DOCTOR | 5. JUST DECIDED TO TAKE IT |

F28c. INTERVIEWER CHECKPOINT (SEE MEDICATION CHART, P. 32)

1. ☐ THERE IS ONE OR MORE UNCIRCLED MEDICATION WITH ONE OR MORE CHECKMARK(S) → ENTER EACH CHECKMARKED, UNCIRCLED MEDICATION AT F29, F36, F43, AND GOLD SUPPLEMENTAL MEDICATION FORM AND TURN TO P. 38, F29

2. ☐ THERE ARE NO UNCIRCLED MEDICATIONS WITH ANY CHECKMARKS → TURN TO P. 41, F50

F35. INTERVIEWER CHECKPOINT, SEE F36 BELOW

[ ] 1. THERE IS NO MEDICATION ENTERED BELOW ──→ TURN TO P. 41, F50
[ ] 2. THERE IS A MEDICATION ENTERED BELOW

F36. And now I want to ask you the same questions about ___ENTER NAME OF MEDICATION.
How long ago did you first take (MEDICATION)?
___ DAYS / WEEKS / MONTHS / YEARS AGO (CIRCLE ONE)

F37. How long ago did you last take it?
___ DAYS / WEEKS / MONTHS AGO (CIRCLE ONE) [ ] TODAY [ ] YESTERDAY

F38. On the days you take it, how many times a day do you usually take it? (How many times a day when you used to take it?)
___ TIMES A DAY

F39. How many pills or capsules (or teaspoons) (do/did) you usually take each time?
___ EACH TIME

F40. (RB, P. 15) During the period you took (MEDICATION) over the last year, which of these statements best describes how often you took (MEDICATION)?

| 1. ONLY ONCE IN A WHILE | 2. SOME WEEKS ALMOST EVERY DAY, OTHER WEEKS NOT AT ALL | 3. AT LEAST ONCE A WEEK THE WHOLE TIME | 4. EVERY DAY OR EVERY OTHER DAY THE WHOLE TIME |

F41. (RB, P. 15) Since you were last interviewed which of these statements best describes how often you took it?

| 1. ONLY ONCE IN A WHILE | 2. SOME WEEKS ALMOST EVERY DAY, OTHER WEEKS NOT AT ALL | 3. AT LEAST ONCE A WEEK THE WHOLE TIME | 4. EVERY DAY OR EVERY OTHER DAY THE WHOLE TIME |

F28d. INTERVIEWER INSTRUCTION (SEE P. 33, F6)   NO MEDICATION HAS 2 CHECKMARKS BUT ONE OR MORE HAS 1 CHECKMARK.

FOR EACH MEDICATION WITH A CHECKMARK AT F4, ENTER NAME OF MEDICATION AT F29, F36, F43 AND GOLD SUPPLEMENTAL MEDICATION FORM (FROM BACK OF INSTRUCTION BOOK) AND CONTINUE BELOW.

F29. Now I'm going to ask you a few questions about ___ENTER NAME OF MEDICATION.
How long ago did you first take (MEDICATION)?
___ DAYS / WEEKS / MONTHS / YEARS AGO (CIRCLE ONE)

F30. How long ago did you last take it?
___ DAYS / WEEKS / MONTHS AGO (CIRCLE ONE) [ ] TODAY [ ] YESTERDAY

F31. On the days you take it, how many times a day do you usually take it? (How many times a day when you used to take it?)
___ TIMES A DAY

F32. How many pills or capsules (or teaspoons) (do/did) you usually take each time?
___ EACH TIME

F33. (RB, P. 15) During the period you took (MEDICATION) over the last year, which of these statements best describes how often you took (MEDICATION)?

| 1. ONLY ONCE IN A WHILE | 2. SOME WEEKS ALMOST EVERY DAY, OTHER WEEKS NOT AT ALL | 3. AT LEAST ONCE A WEEK THE WHOLE TIME | 4. EVERY DAY OR EVERY OTHER DAY THE WHOLE TIME |

F34. (RB, P. 15) Since you were last interviewed, which of these statements best describes how often you took it?

| 1. ONLY ONCE IN A WHILE | 2. SOME WEEKS ALMOST EVERY DAY, OTHER WEEKS NOT AT ALL | 3. AT LEAST ONCE A WEEK THE WHOLE TIME | 4. EVERY DAY OR EVERY OTHER DAY THE WHOLE TIME |

I - 42

F42. INTERVIEWER CHECKPOINT, SEE F43 BELOW

☐ 1. THERE IS NO MEDICATION ENTERED BELOW ——→ TURN TO P. 41, F50
☐ 2. THERE IS A MEDICATION ENTERED BELOW

F43. And now I want to ask you the same questions about _____ENTER NAME OF MEDICATION_____.
How long ago did you first take (MEDICATION)?

_____ DAYS / WEEKS / MONTHS / YEARS AGO (CIRCLE ONE)

F44. How long ago did you last take it?

_____ DAYS / WEEKS / MONTHS AGO (CIRCLE ONE)   ☐ TODAY   ☐ YESTERDAY

F45. On the days you take it, how many times a day do you usually take it? (How many times a day when you used to take it?)

_____ TIMES A DAY

F46. How many pills or capsules (or teaspoons) (do/did) you usually take each time?

_____ EACH TIME

F47. (RB, P. 15) During the period you took (MEDICATION) over the last year, which of these statements best describes how often you took (MEDICATION)?

| 1. ONLY ONCE IN A WHILE | 2. SOME WEEKS ALMOST EVERY DAY, OTHER WEEKS NOT AT ALL | 3. AT LEAST ONCE A WEEK THE WHOLE TIME | 4. EVERY DAY OR EVERY OTHER DAY THE WHOLE TIME |

F48. (RB, P. 15) Since you were last interviewed which of these statements best describes how often you took it?

| 1. ONLY ONCE IN A WHILE | 2. SOME WEEKS ALMOST EVERY DAY, OTHER WEEKS NOT AT ALL | 3. AT LEAST ONCE A WEEK THE WHOLE TIME | 4. EVERY DAY OR EVERY OTHER DAY THE WHOLE TIME |

F49. INTERVIEWER CHECKPOINT

☐ 1. NO MEDICATIONS ARE ENTERED ON GOLD SUPPLEMENTAL MEDICATION FORM ——→ TURN TO P. 41, F50
☐ 2. MEDICATION IS ENTERED ON GOLD SUPPLEMENTAL MEDICATION FORM ——→ TURN TO GOLD SUPPLEMENTAL MEDICATION FORM(S)

323

I - 43

F50. INTERVIEWER CHECKPOINT (FROM F2c, P. 32)

☐ 1. THERE IS NO MEDICATION ENTERED BELOW ——→ TURN TO P. 42, SECTION G
☐ 2. THERE IS A MEDICATION ENTERED BELOW

F51. (You said you haven't taken any _____(ENTER NAME OF MEDICATION)_____ since you were last interviewed.) Why haven't you been taking it?

_____

F52. INTERVIEWER CHECKPOINT

☐ 1. THERE IS NO MEDICATION ENTERED BELOW ——→ TURN TO P. 42, SECTION G
☐ 2. THERE IS A MEDICATION ENTERED BELOW

F53. You also haven't taken any _____(ENTER NAME OF MEDICATION)_____ since you were last interviewed. Why haven't you been taking it?

_____

F54. INTERVIEWER CHECKPOINT

☐ 1. THERE IS NO MEDICATION ENTERED BELOW ——→ TURN TO P. 42, SECTION G
☐ 2. THERE IS A MEDICATION ENTERED BELOW

F55. You also haven't taken any _____(ENTER NAME OF MEDICATION)_____ since you were last interviewed. Why haven't you been taking it?

_____

NOTE: IF R NO LONGER TAKING ADDITIONAL MEDICATIONS, ASK F55 ABOUT THEM AS WELL AND RECORD ON BACK OF QUESTIONNAIRE.

SECTION G
I - 44

ASK EVERYONE

G1. Have you been hospitalized since your last interview?

1. YES   5. NO ──→ GO TO G2

G1a. How many nights have you spent in the hospital (altogether)? _____ NIGHTS

G2. Since you were last interviewed have you received any kind of therapy or counseling from a minister, a psychologist, a psychiatrist, a marriage counselor, or any other kind of therapist?

1. YES   5. NO ──→ TURN TO P. 43, G8

G3. What type of professional did you see?

a.

b.

G4. When was the last time you saw or talked with your (KIND OF PROFESSIONAL)?

a.

b.

G5. Do you plan on seeing this person again?

a. 1. YES   5. NO   b. 1. YES   5. NO

G6. (RB, P. 16) When you visit your (KIND OF PROFESSIONAL) how much time is there to discuss with him or her all the things you want to talk about?

1. NONE	2. A LITTLE	3. SOME	4. A LOT	5. A GREAT DEAL
a				
b				

G7. (RB, P. 17) Would you say your (KIND OF PROFESSIONAL) is very cold toward people, somewhat cold towards people, neither cold nor warm, somewhat warm, or very warm towards people?

1. VERY COLD	2. SOMEWHAT COLD	3. NEITHER COLD NOR WARM	4. SOMEWHAT WARM	5. VERY WARM
a				
b				

G8. I would like to ask you about alcoholic beverages—that is, wine, beer, and liquor. Again, think back over the last seven days. On how many of the last seven days did you drink any alcoholic beverages?

_____ DAYS   0. NONE

GO TO G9

G8a. How about in the last month, (on how many days did you have any alcoholic beverages)?

_____ DAYS IN LAST MONTH   00. NONE ──→ TURN TO P. 44, G11

G8b. When you drink alcoholic beverages, how many drinks do you usually have per day? By drink I mean a shot or a glass.

_____ # DRINKS PER DRINKING DAY

_____ PINTS

_____ FIFTHS

G8c. In the last month, what's the largest number of drinks you have had at one time?

_____ # DRINKS

_____ PINTS

_____ FIFTHS

TURN TO P. 44, G11

G9. In the last seven days, on the days that you drank alcoholic beverages, how many drinks did you usually have? By drink I mean a shot or a glass.

_____ # DRINKS PER DRINKING DAY

_____ PINTS

_____ FIFTHS

G10. In the last seven days, what's the largest number of drinks you have had at one time?

_____ # DRINKS

_____ PINTS

_____ FIFTHS

G11. Since you were last interviewed have you taken any street drugs such as PCP, Uppers, Downers, Speed, Quaaludes, Mescaline, Marijuana, Heroin, or Methadone?

1. YES
GO TO G12

5. NO →

G11a. Since you were last interviewed have you taken any drugs which you haven't already mentioned, just to get high or to get in a good mood?

1. YES → (ENTER IN CHART BELOW AND ASK G13 and G14 FOR EACH.)

5. NO → TURN TO P. 45, G15

G12. What drugs have you taken? (ENTER IN CHART BELOW AND ASK G13 and G14 FOR EACH.)

G13. How many times have you taken (DRUG) since you were last interviewed? (ENTER BELOW)

ASK IF NOT EVERY DAY IN G13

G14. How many times in the last seven days? (ENTER BELOW)

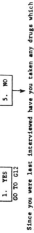
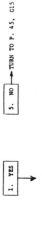

NAME OF DRUG	G13 TIMES TAKEN SINCE LAST INTERVIEWED	G14 TIMES TAKEN IN LAST 7 DAYS
1.	☐ EVERY DAY	
2.	☐ EVERY DAY	
3.	☐ EVERY DAY	
4.	☐ EVERY DAY	

G15. Do you smoke cigarettes, cigars, or a pipe? (Which?)

1. YES, CIGARETTES | 2. YES, CIGARS | 3. YES, PIPE

5. NO → GO TO G16

G15a. Thinking back over the last seven days, about how many (cigarettes/ cigars, pipefulls) have you smoked per day over the last seven days?

CIGARETTES OR PACKS _____ PER DAY

CIGARS _____ PER DAY

PIPEFULLS _____ PER DAY

G16. On the average, how many cups of regular coffee, by that I mean caffeinated coffee, did you drink each day during the past seven days?

_____ CUPS PER DAY

G17. On the average, how many cups of tea did you drink each day during the past seven days?

_____ CUPS PER DAY

G18. On the average, about how many cola drinks did you have each day during the past seven days?

_____ DRINKS PER DAY

(INCLUDE COCA COLA, COKE, TAB, PEPSI, RC, DR. PEPPER, ANY DRINKS CALLED "COLA", OR ANY "DIET" FORM OF THESE DRINKS.)

(IF R ASKS: A "DRINK" MEANS 12 OUNCES.)

G19. In the last seven days, how long has it been taking you to fall asleep at night?

_____ MINUTES _____ HOURS

SECTION H

H1. How tall are you?

_____ FEET   _____ INCHES

H2. About how much do you weigh?

_____ POUNDS

H3. **Think about how much money you (and your family) usually have coming in each month. Last month, did you have more money than usual, less than usual, or about the same amount as usual?**

| 3. MORE MONEY | 1. LESS MONEY | 2. ABOUT THE SAME AMOUNT |

H4. **Now think about the expenses you (and your family) have in the average month. Last month did you have more expenses than usual, less than usual, or were your expenses about the same as usual?**

| 3. MORE EXPENSES | 1. LESS EXPENSES | 2. ABOUT THE SAME EXPENSES |

H5. I'd like to ask you some more questions about medications. What is your general impression of the medications doctors prescribe for their patients? Do you think they usually do more good than harm, usually do more harm than good, or usually don't have much of an effect one way or the other?

| 3. USUALLY MORE GOOD THAN HARM | 1. USUALLY MORE HARM THAN GOOD | 2. USUALLY NO EFFECT ONE WAY OR THE OTHER | 8. NO OPINION |

H6. Now I want you to think back. Has a doctor __ever__ given you a prescription for a medication that you did __not__ have filled?

| 1. YES | 5. NO | 8. CAN'T RECALL |

TURN TO P. 50, H7

H6a. What kind of medication was it?

a. _____

b. _____

c. _____

d. _____

e. _____

f. _____

H6b. Do you remember the name of the medication?

a. _____

b. _____

c. _____

d. _____

e. _____

f. _____

H6c. About when was that? (MONTH AND YEAR)

a. _____ MONTH _____ YEAR

b. _____ MONTH _____ YEAR

c. _____ MONTH _____ YEAR

d. _____ MONTH _____ YEAR

e. _____ MONTH _____ YEAR

f. _____ MONTH _____ YEAR

H6d. Why didn't you have the prescription filled for (MEDICATION)?

a. _____

b. _____

c. _____

d. _____

e. _____

f. _____

I - 52

H7. How much have you read or heard from any source or anybody about tranquilizers—a great deal, a fair amount, very little, or nothing at all?

| GREAT DEAL 4. | FAIR AMOUNT 3. | VERY LITTLE 2. | NOTHING AT ALL 1. | NO OPINION 8. |

GO TO H8

H7a. Where, specifically, did you hear or read this information? (CHECK ALL THAT APPLY.)

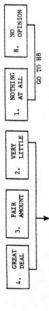

☐ DOCTOR 10.
☐ FRIEND/ACQUAINTANCE/NEIGHBOR 20.
☐ MAGAZINE 30.
☐ NEWSPAPER 31.
☐ PASTOR/RABBI/RELIGIOUS PERSON 50.
☐ RADIO 60.
☐ TELEVISION 61.
☐ OTHER (SPECIFY): _____ 97.
☐ DON'T KNOW 98.

H8. Based on what you know about tranquilizers, do you generally approve or generally disapprove of the present use of them, or are you undecided?

| 3. GENERALLY APPROVE | 1. GENERALLY DISAPPROVE | 2. UNDECIDED |

I - 53

H9. (RB, P. 22) I'm going to read you some statements about tranquilizers. After I read each one, I want you to tell me how much you agree or disagree with the statement.

	STRONGLY DISAGREE (1)	DISAGREE (2)	NEITHER AGREE NOR DISAGREE (3)	AGREE (4)	STRONGLY AGREE (5)
a. Tranquilizers work very well to make a person more calm and relaxed.					
b. Using tranquilizers just prevents people from working out their problems for themselves.					
c. Tranquilizers help people get through the day.					
d. Tranquilizers help people regain control over the stresses in their lives.					
e. It is better to use willpower to solve problems than it is to use tranquilizers.					
f. Tranquilizers cause people to lose some control over what they do.					
g. Tranquilizers are safe to take.					

H10. Some health authorities say Americans do not always get or take medication when they need it. Others say medication is used too much in this country. Thinking only about tranquilizers, which of these opinions do you agree with more? Americans do not always get the tranquilizers they need; or Tranquilizers are used too much in this country; or About the right amount of tranquilizers are used in this country?

| 3. DO NOT ALWAYS GET WHAT NEED | 1. USED TOO MUCH | 2. ABOUT RIGHT AMOUNT | 8. NO OPINION |

TURN TO P.52, H11

TURN TO P.52, H11

H10a. Why do you say that?

_____
_____
_____

H14. Have you done anything different in your life as a result of these interviews?

| 1. YES | 5. NO ──▶ GO TO H15 |

H14a. Can you describe what you did that was different?

_____

_____

_____

_____

H15. (RB, P. 24) How much have you learned about yourself by participating in these interviews?

| 1. DIDN'T LEARN ANYTHING | 2. LEARNED A LITTLE | 3. LEARNED SOME | 4. LEARNED QUITE A LOT | 5. LEARNED A GREAT DEAL |

H16. (RB, P. 25) How much have you been disturbed or upset by these interviews?

| 1. NOT AT ALL | 2. A LITTLE | 3. SOME | 4. QUITE A LOT | 5. A GREAT DEAL |

H11. I am going to ask you a *few* questions now about your use of tranquilizers. You may already have answered similar questions before but I need to get the information here.

Have you ever taken a tranquilizer _every day_ or almost every day for a week at a time or more?

| 1. YES | 5. NO | 8. DON'T KNOW/UNSURE |

GO TO H12

H11a. What was the longest period of time during which you took a tranquilizer every day or almost every day--was it less than a month, between one and three months, or longer than three months?

| 1. LESS THAN A MONTH | 2. BETWEEN ONE AND THREE MONTHS | 3. LONGER THAN THREE MONTHS | 8. DON'T KNOW |

GO TO H13

H12. Have you _ever_ taken a tranquilizer?

| 1. YES | 5. NO | 8. DON'T KNOW |

[ASK EVERYONE]

H13. (RB, P. 23) And now, just a few final questions. We are very interested in your opinion about what it has been like to be interviewed. We're interested in knowing both positive and negative things.

To what extent has being interviewed affected your life?

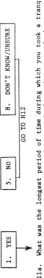

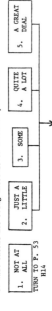

| 1. NOT AT ALL | 2. JUST A LITTLE | 3. SOME | 4. QUITE A LOT | 5. A GREAT DEAL |

TURN TO P. 53
H14

H13a. In _what ways_ has being interviewed affected your life?

_____

_____

_____

(PROBE AS NECESSARY: Anything good? Anything bad?)

(IF NOT CLEAR, ASK: Is this something you would consider good or bad?)

H17. How do you feel overall about the interviews you have had?

_____

_____

_____

_____

CONTACTING SIGNIFICANT OTHERS (16 OR OLDER)

J1. INTERVIEWER CHECKPOINT (SEE COVER SHEET SUMMARY FORM)

☐ 1. THERE WAS A PERSONAL OTHER INTERVIEWED FOR R AT ANY PREVIOUS INTERVIEW

☐ 2. NO PERSONAL OTHER WAS INTERVIEWED AT ANY PREVIOUS INTERVIEW → TURN TO P. 56, J7

J2. We would like to reinterview the (person/people) in your personal (and work) life that we talked with before. (He/She/They) already told us that it would be alright for us to contact them again, but I want to check with you to make sure that you are still in touch with (him/her/them).

Have you seen or talked with (NAME OF PERSONAL OTHER) in the last week?

1. YES
ENTER INFORMATION ON YELLOW
PERSONAL OTHER COVER SHEET
TURN TO P.57, J12

5. NO →

J3. If possible, I would prefer to interview someone else who first of all knows you well, who second of all you have talked with in the last seven days, and finally who you usually talk with at least once a week. Is there someone else we could interview?

5. NO →

USE PERSONAL OTHER FROM
BEFORE IF STILL APPROPRIATE

(_____)
(RELATIONSHIP)

1. YES

J4. About how many hours do you see or talk with (OTHER) in the average week?
(_____)
_____ HOURS

J5. How much time have you spent together or talked on the phone with (OTHER) in the last seven days?
_____ HOURS

J6. CRITERIA TO BE USED IF A DIFFERENT PERSONAL OTHER IS TO BE SELECTED:

1. KNOWS R WELL
2. SPENT SOME TIME WITH R IN THE LAST SEVEN DAYS
3. TYPICALLY SPENDS TIME WITH R
4. AVAILABLE TO BE INTERVIEWED DURING THE NEXT 72 HOURS

NOTE: OTHER MUST KNOW R WELL, BUT DOESN'T HAVE TO BE THE PERSON WHO KNOWS HIM/HER BEST. ANYONE WHO KNOWS R WELL IS ELIGIBLE. SELECT ONE WHO KNOWS HIM/HER WELL AND HAS SEEN OR TALKED WITH R IN THE LAST SEVEN DAYS IF POSSIBLE. ACCEPT SOMEONE WHO HAS NOT TALKED WITH R IN THE LAST SEVEN DAYS IF NECESSARY.

* ENTER INFORMATION ON YELLOW PERSONAL OTHER COVER SHEET, TURN TO P. 57, J12

NO PERSONAL OTHER WAS INTERVIEWED AT PREVIOUS INTERVIEW TIME

J7. As you may remember, we are interested in how one person's life affects the lives of people close to them and so we would like to interview one person who comes in close contact with you. The interview will be by phone and last only 10 or 15 minutes. Sometimes we find people are too critical of themselves and in order to get a more balanced picture we will be asking some questions about their views of you and the things you have to do. We'll also ask them some questions about their satisfaction with their own lives. Let me show you a copy of the questionnaire so that you can look it over and see what we will be asking. (SHOW R B5 IN PERSONAL QUESTIONNAIRE)

(IF R IS HESITANT) Let me assure you that your answers would never be revealed to this individual nor would we ever discuss his or her answers with you.

I would like to interview someone who first of all knows you well, who second of all you have talked with in the last seven days, and finally who you usually talk with at least once a week.

J8. Who would that be? (RELATIONSHIP)

_____

J9. About how many hours do you see or talk with (OTHER) in the average week?

_____ HOURS

J10. How much time have you spent together or talked on the phone with (OTHER) in the last seven days?

_____ HOURS

J11. CRITERIA TO BE USED IF MORE THAN ONE PERSON COULD BE SELECTED:

1. KNOWS R WELL
2. SPENT SOME TIME WITH R IN THE LAST SEVEN DAYS
3. TYPICALLY SPENDS TIME WITH R
4. AVAILABLE TO BE INTERVIEWED DURING THE NEXT 72 HOURS

NOTE: OTHER MUST KNOW R WELL, BUT DOESN'T HAVE TO BE THE PERSON WHO KNOWS HIM/ HER BEST. ANYONE WHO KNOWS R WELL IS ELIGIBLE. SELECT ONE WHO KNOWS HIM/HER WELL AND HAS SEEN OR TALKED WITH R IN THE LAST SEVEN DAYS IF POSSIBLE.

ACCEPT SOMEONE WHO HAS NOT TALKED WITH R IN THE LAST SEVEN DAYS IF NECESSARY.

* ENTER INFORMATION ON YELLOW PERSONAL OTHER COVER SHEET, TURN TO P. 57, J12

331

J12. INTERVIEWER CHECKPOINT

☐ 1. R DOES NOT WORK 15 OR MORE HOURS A WEEK ───▶ TURN TO P. 58, J18

☐ 2. R WORKS 15 OR MORE HOURS A WEEK AND WORK OTHER WAS INTERVIEWED BEFORE

☐ 3. R WORKS 15 OR MORE HOURS A WEEK AND WORK OTHER WAS NOT INTERVIEWED BEFORE ───▶ GO TO J14

J13. I (also) want to interview the person you work with that we interviewed before. Do you still see (WORK OTHER) regularly?

☐ 1. YES   ☐ 5. NO

ENTER INFORMATION ON GREEN COVER SHEET AND GO TO P. 58, J18

J14. I would like to interview someone you work with who first of all knows your work well, secondly, that you have talked with in the last seven days (or the last week you worked), and third who you usually talk with often.

Who would that be? (RELATIONSHIP)

_____

J15. About how many hours do you see or talk with (OTHER) in the average week?

_____ HOURS

J16. How much time have you spent together or talked on the phone with (OTHER) in the last seven days?

_____ HOURS

J17. CRITERIA TO BE USED IF MORE THAN ONE PERSON COULD BE SELECTED:

1. KNOWS R'S WORK WELL
2. SPENT SOME TIME WITH R IN THE LAST SEVEN DAYS (OR LAST WEEK R WORKED)
3. TYPICALLY SEES OR TALKS TO R EVERY WEEK
4. AVAILABLE TO BE INTERVIEWED DURING THE NEXT 72 HOURS

IF FOCAL R REFUSES TO GIVE NAME WITHOUT ASKING THE PERSON FIRST, ARRANGE TO CALL R AFTER (HE/SHE) HAS ASKED PERMISSION (OR LOOKED UP NUMBER, ETC.)

* ENTER INFORMATION ON GREEN COVER SHEET, GO TO P. 58, J18

I – 60

J18. It is important that I talk with (both of these/this) person(s) soon. If you think you will be seeing (him/her/them) within the next day, I would like you to give (him/her/them) this Respondent Booklet.

IF ONE OR BOTH "OTHERS" ARE NEW: I have (a) letter(s) to go with the Respondent Booklet(s).

HAND R RESPONDENT BOOKLET(S) AND LETTER(S) AS APPROPRIATE.

IF "OTHER" IS NEW: I would appreciate it if you would call (NAME OF PERSONAL AND/OR WORK OTHERS) to let (him/her/them) know I will be calling, so that they will know it's all right to talk to me.

CONFIRM FOCAL R'S ADDRESS ON COVER SHEET.

J19. This was your last interview. On behalf of the entire research staff I want to thank you for your cooperation and assistance. Your answers have been very helpful. Do you have any comments you would like to add?

_____

_____

_____

(PAY R $10.00 AND GET RECEIPT.)

EXACT TIME NOW: _____

I – 61

SECTION K: BY OBSERVATION

K1. R'S SEX: | 1. MALE | | 2. FEMALE |

K2. R'S RACE: | 1. BLACK | | 2. WHITE | | 7. OTHER (SPECIFY): _____ |

K3. RATE THE RESPONDENT ON EACH OF THE FOLLOWING:

	NOT AT ALL (1)	SLIGHTLY (2)	SOME-WHAT (3)	FAIRLY (4)	VERY (5)	CAN'T RATE (8)
a. During the interview, how much did R appear to be frank in (his/her) answers?						
b. How much did R appear to be tense, nervous, or jittery?						
c. How much did R appear to be sad, blue, or depressed?						
d. How much did R appear to be warm and friendly?						
e. How much did R appear to be interested in providing useful answers?						
f. How much did R appear to understand the questions?						

K4. IF ANYONE WAS PRESENT DURING THE INTERVIEW OTHER THAN R AND INTERVIEWER GIVE THE FOLLOWING DETAILS FOR EACH:

	PERSON 1	PERSON 2	PERSON 3
a. Relationship to R			
b. Present for how much of the interview?			
c. How closely was (s)he listening?	1. CLOSELY 2. CASUALLY 3. HARDLY AT ALL	1. CLOSELY 2. CASUALLY 3. HARDLY AT ALL	1. CLOSELY 2. CASUALLY 3. HARDLY AT ALL
d. Did (s)he make any comments on R's answers?			

[ ] NO ONE PRESENT

K5. THUMBNAIL SKETCH

EVENTS CALENDAR

THIS WEEK: SUN. _____ TO TODAY

LAST WEEK: SUN. _____ TO SAT.

2 WEEKS AGO: SUN. _____ TO SAT.

3 WEEKS AGO: SUN. _____ TO SAT.

4 WEEKS AGO: SUN. _____ TO SAT.

5 WEEKS AGO: SUN. _____ TO SAT.

WEEK OF IW: SUN. _____ TO _____ (DAY AND DATE OF LAST IW)

TIME   2   3   4   (CIRCLE ONE)

FOCAL R ID NUMBER _____

YOUR INTERVIEW NUMBER _____

DATE OF INTERVIEW _____

Interviewer's Label

PROJECT 45
(462491)

333

LIFE AS A WHOLE

1 - 65

	THIS WEEK: SUN. ___ TO TODAY	LAST WEEK: SUN. ___ TO SAT.	2 WEEKS AGO: SUN. ___ TO SAT.	3 WEEKS AGO: SUN. ___ TO SAT.	4 WEEKS AGO: SUN. ___ TO SAT.	5 WEEKS AGO: SUN. ___ TO SAT.	WEEK OF IW: SUN. ___ TO (DAY AND DATE OF LAST IW)
TERRIBLE (1)							
UNHAPPY (2)							
MOSTLY DISSATISFIED (3)							
MIXED (ABOUT EQUALLY SATISFIED & DISSATISFIED) (4)							
MOSTLY SATISFIED (5)							
PLEASED (6)							
DELIGHTED (7)							

ANXIETY CHART

1 - 44

	THIS WEEK: SUN. ___ TO TODAY	LAST WEEK: SUN. ___ TO SAT.	2 WEEKS AGO: SUN. ___ TO SAT.	3 WEEKS AGO: SUN. ___ TO SAT.	4 WEEKS AGO: SUN. ___ TO SAT.	5 WEEKS AGO: SUN. ___ TO SAT.	WEEK OF IW: SUN. ___ TO (DAY AND DATE OF LAST IW)
NO ANXIETY OR NERVOUSNESS (1)							
A LITTLE ANXIETY OR NERVOUSNESS (2)							
SOME ANXIETY OR NERVOUSNESS (3)							
QUITE A BIT OF ANXIETY OR NERVOUSNESS (4)							
EXTREME ANXIETY OR NERVOUSNESS (5)							

NUMBER OF MEDICATION _____ I - 67

PILLS CAPSULES TEASPOONS (CIRCLE ONE) EACH WEEK

	NONE (1)	1 TO 4 (2)	5 TO 9 (3)	10 TO 14 (4)	15 TO 24 (5)	25 OR MORE (6)
THIS WEEK: SUN. _____ TO TODAY						
LAST WEEK: SUN. _____ TO SAT.						
2 WEEKS AGO: SUN. _____ TO SAT.						
3 WEEKS AGO: SUN. _____ TO SAT.						
4 WEEKS AGO: SUN. _____ TO SAT.						
5 WEEKS AGO: SUN. _____ TO SAT.						
WEEK OF IW: SUN. _____ TO _____ (DAY AND DATE OF LAST IW)						

PATTERN OF MEDICATION USE _____ I - 66

NAME OF MEDICATION _____

	NONE AT ALL (1)	JUST ONE DAY THE WHOLE WEEK (2)	A FEW DAYS (3)	EVERY DAY EXCEPT ONE (4)	EVERY DAY THE WHOLE WEEK (5)
THIS WEEK: SUN. _____ TO TODAY					
LAST WEEK: SUN. _____ TO SAT.					
2 WEEKS AGO: SUN. _____ TO SAT.					
3 WEEKS AGO: SUN. _____ TO SAT.					
4 WEEKS AGO: SUN. _____ TO SAT.					
5 WEEKS AGO: SUN. _____ TO SAT.					
WEEK OF IW: SUN. _____ TO _____ (DAY AND DATE OF LAST IW)					

335

TIME IV

Fall/Winter 198_
Project 45
(462491)

STUDY OF STRESS: WORK, FAMILY AND HEALTH

For Office Use Only

SRC SURVEY RESEARCH CENTER
INSTITUTE FOR SOCIAL RESEARCH
THE UNIVERSITY OF MICHIGAN
ANN ARBOR, MICHIGAN 48106

1. Interviewer's Label

6. FOCAL R ID # _____

2. Your Interview Number: _____

3. Date of Interview: _____

4. Length of Interview: _____ (Minutes)

5. Length of Edit: _____ (Minutes)

PERSONAL LIFE QUESTIONNAIRE

(IF PERSONAL OTHER HAS BEEN INTERVIEWED BEFORE:
Just as before, I will be asking you about
things that have changed and things that have
stayed the same in your and (FOCAL R'S) lives.
To do this I'll be asking many of the same questions you were asked last time. Don't try to
remember how you answered last time, just answer
in terms of how you feel now.)

READ TO ALL RESPONDENTS:

Before we begin I would like to (assure/remind) you that the information you
provide us with will be kept in complete confidence. The interview is voluntary; if we should come to any question which you don't want to answer, just
let me know and we'll go on to the next question.

SECTION A

A0. EXACT TIME NOW: _____

A1. INTERVIEWER CHECKPOINT

☐ 1. PERSONAL OTHER IS SAME AS TIME I ☐ TIME II ☐ TIME III ☐ → GO TO A5
(CHECK ALL THAT APPLY)

☐ 2. NEW PERSONAL OTHER

A2. About how long have you known (NAME OF FOCAL R)?

_____ MONTHS / YEARS (CIRCLE ONE)

A3. How old are you? _____ YEARS

A4. What is the highest grade of school or year of college you have completed?

GRADES OF SCHOOL

| 00 | 01 | 02 | 03 | 04 | 05 | 06 | 07 | 08 | 09 | 10 | 11 | 12 |

COLLEGE

| 13 | 14 | 15 | 16 | 17+ |

A5. What is your relationship to (FOCAL R)?

☐ 1. SPOUSE
☐ 2. EX-SPOUSE
☐ 3. ROMANTICALLY ATTACHED FRIEND
☐ 4. FRIEND
☐ 5. RELATIVE (SPECIFY): _____
☐ 7. OTHER (SPECIFY): _____

A6. (ASK IF NECESSARY) Do you live in the same household with (FOCAL R)?

☐ 1. YES   ☐ 5. NO

A7. In the average week, approximately how many hours do you spend with (FOCAL R), either in person or on the phone? (IF R ASKS, DON'T INCLUDE TIME EITHER IS SLEEPING.)

_____ HOURS

A8. Now think back over the last 7 days. Approximately how many hours have you spent with (FOCAL R), either in person or on the phone, in the last 7 days?

_____ HOURS

A9. INTERVIEWER CHECKPOINT (SEE A8)

☐ 1. PERSONAL OTHER HAS SPENT 0 HOURS WITH (FOCAL R) IN LAST 7 DAYS

☐ 2. PERSONAL OTHER HAS SPENT SOME TIME WITH (FOCAL R) IN THE LAST 7 DAYS → TURN TO P. 3, SECTION B

A9a. How long has it been since you last saw or talked with (FOCAL R)?

_____ WEEKS AGO

A9b. When I ask you the following questions about (FOCAL R'S) life, please answer in terms of the last week in which you talked to (him/her).

SECTION B

B1. (RB, P. 1) We would like your opinion about how (FOCAL R) felt about (his/her) life during the last (7 days/week you talked to [him/her]).

(IF R DOES NOT HAVE RESPONDENT BOOKLET: I want you to think of a scale going from 7 to 1 with 7 meaning delighted, 6 meaning pleased, 5 mostly satisfied, 4 mixed, that is, equally satisfied and dissatisfied, 3 mostly dissatisfied, 2 unhappy, and 1 terrible.)

As I read each statement please tell me how you think (FOCAL R) felt--taking into account what happened in the previous seven days. If the question doesn't really apply or if you have no opinion please tell me.

7	6	5	4	3	2	1
DELIGHTED	PLEASED	MOSTLY SATISFIED	MIXED (ABOUT EQUALLY SATISFIED AND DISSATISFIED)	MOSTLY DISSAT- ISFIED	UNHAPPY	TERRIBLE

0 = NO OPINION; NEVER THOUGHT ABOUT IT OR DOESN'T APPLY

_____ B1a. How do you think (he/she) felt about (his/her) personal life? By personal life I mean (his/her) relationships with people (he/she) feels close to. (What number on the scale?)

_____ B1b. How do you think (he/she) felt about (his/her) (wife/husband), (his/her) marriage?

_____ B1c. (How do you think [he/she] felt about) (his/her) romantic life?

_____ B1d. (How do you think [he/she] felt about) (his/her) friends and acquaintances?

_____ B1e. (How do you think [he/she] felt about) (his/her) work?

_____ B1f. (How do you think [he/she] felt about) the people (he/she) works with--(his/her) co-workers?

_____ B1g. (How do you think [he/she] felt about) the work (he/she) does on the job--the work itself?

_____ B1h. (How do you think [he/she] felt about) (his/her) life as a whole?

B2. (RB, P. 2) In the last (7 days/week you saw or talked to [FOCAL R]), how much do you think (he/she) really enjoyed (his/her) personal life? (Would you say not at all, just a little, some, quite a bit, or a great deal?)

| 1. NOT AT ALL | 2. JUST A LITTLE | 3. SOME | 4. QUITE A BIT | 5. A GREAT DEAL |

4

B3. (RB, P. 2) In the last (7 days/week you talked to [FOCAL R]), how much do you think (his/her) personal life made (him/her) feel emotionally upset? (Would you say not at all, just a little, some, quite a bit, or a great deal?)

| 1. NOT AT ALL | 2. JUST A LITTLE | 3. SOME | 4. QUITE A BIT | 5. A GREAT DEAL |

B4. (RB, P. 3) Now think about how well (FOCAL R) feels (he/she) has been doing in (his/her) personal life--how successful (he/she) has been in having (his/her) personal life be what (he/she) wanted. In the last (7 days/week you talked to [him/her]) would you say it was not at all what (he/she) wanted, just a little of what (he/she) wanted, some of what (he/she) wanted, most of what (he/she) wanted, or all of what (he/she) wanted?

| 1. NOT AT ALL | 2. JUST A LITTLE | 3. SOME | 4. MOST | 5. ALL |

B5. (RB, P. 4) People vary a good deal on how well they do different things. Please tell me how well you think (FOCAL R) did each of the following things in (his/her) personal and home life in the last (7 days/week you talked to [him/her]).

	VERY POORLY (1)	NOT VERY WELL (2)	ALL RIGHT (3)	VERY WELL (4)	EXCEPTIONALLY WELL (5)
a. In the last (7 days/week you talked to [him/her]) how well did (he/she) do in working around the house or apartment? (Would you say very poorly, not very well, all right, very well, or exceptionally well?)					
b. handling children? [FOCAL R DOES NOT HAVE CONTACT WITH CHILDREN]					
c. being affectionate?					
d. getting along with others in (his/her) personal life?					
e. handling responsibilities and daily demands?					
(In the last [7 days/week you talked to (FOCAL R)]) how well did (he/she) do in...					
f. making the right decisions?					
g. avoiding arguing with others?					
h. handling disagreements by compromising and meeting other people half-way?					
j. being calm in (his/her) personal life?					

5

(In the last [7 days/week you talked to (him/her)]) how well did (he/she) do in...

	VERY POORLY (1)	NOT VERY WELL (2)	ALL RIGHT (3)	VERY WELL (4)	EXCEPTIONALLY WELL (5)
k. accepting responsibilities for (his/her) own actions and behaviors?					
m. staying level-headed?					
n. giving people the time and attention they need?					
p. being pleasant?					
q. doing a good job of handling all of the things required of (him/her) in (his/her) personal life?					
r. acting in a relaxed manner?					

B6. (RB, P. 5) Now I'm going to ask you several questions about (FOCAL R'S) relationships with people in (his/her) personal life. As I read each question I want you to think of someone in particular but it doesn't have to be the same person for each question. In the last (7 days/week you talked to [him/her]) ...

	NOT AT ALL (1)	JUST A LITTLE (2)	SOME (3)	QUITE A BIT (4)	A GREAT DEAL (5)
a. How much could (FOCAL R) count on some one person in (his/her) personal life to treat (him/her) with respect? (Would you say not at all, just a little, some, quite a bit, or a great deal?)					
b. How much could (FOCAL R) count on some one person in (his/her) personal life to give (him/her) useful information and advice if (he/she) wanted it?					
c. How much could (he/she) count on someone in (his/her) personal life to act in ways that show he or she appreciates what (he/she) does?					
d. ...to show that he or she cared about (him/her) as a person?					
e. In the last (7 days/week you talked to [him/her]), how much did some one get on (FOCAL R'S) nerves?					
f. How much did some one person misunderstand the way (he/she) thinks and feels about things?					

(In the last 7 days)

	NOT AT ALL (1)	JUST A LITTLE (2)	SOME (3)	QUITE A LOT (4)	A GREAT DEAL (5)
g. How much did someone in (his/her) personal life act in an unpleasant or angry manner toward (him/her)?					
h. ...show that he or she disliked (him/her)?					

B7. (RB, P. 5) In the last (7 days/week you saw or talked to [FOCAL R])...

	NOT AT ALL (1)	JUST A LITTLE (2)	SOME (3)	QUITE A BIT (4)	A GREAT DEAL (5)
a. How much could you count on (FOCAL R) to treat you with respect? (Would you say not at all, just a little, some, quite a bit, or a great deal?)					
b. In the last (7 days/week you talked to [him/her]), how much could (FOCAL R) count on you to treat (him/her) with respect?					
c. How much could you count on (FOCAL R) to give you useful information and advice if you wanted it?					
d. In the last (7 days/week you talked to [him/her], how much could (FOCAL R) count on you to give (him/her) useful information and advice if (he/she) wanted it?					
e. How much could you count on (FOCAL R) to show that (he/she) cared about you as a person?					
f. How much could (FOCAL R) count on you to show that you cared about (him/her) as a person?					
g. How much did (FOCAL R) get on your nerves?					
h. How much did you get on (FOCAL R'S) nerves?					
j. How much did (FOCAL R) act in an unpleasant or angry manner towards you?					
k. How much did you act in an unpleasant or angry manner towards (him/her)?					
m. How much did (FOCAL R) show that (he/she) disliked you?					
n. How much did you show (FOCAL R) that you disliked (him/her)?					

B8. All things considered, how do you think (FOCAL R) feels about (his/her) life these days?

_____

_____

_____

SECTION C

C1. (RB, P. 6) We are interested in how the well-being of one person like (FOCAL R) affects the well-being of another person, like you. So now we want to find out how you feel about your own life.

(IF R DOES NOT HAVE RESPONDENT BOOKLET: Again, think of a scale from 7 to one with 7 meaning delighted, 6 pleased, 5 mostly satisfied, 4 mixed, equally satisfied and dissatisfied, 3 mostly dissatisfied, 2 unhappy and 1 terrible.)

As I read each statement please tell me how you feel now--taking into account what has happened during the last 7 days. If the question doesn't really apply or if you have no opinion please tell me.

7 DELIGHTED	6 PLEASED	5 MOSTLY SATISFIED	4 MIXED (ABOUT EQUALLY SATISFIED AND DISSATISFIED)	3 MOSTLY DISSAT-ISFIED	2 UNHAPPY	1 TERRIBLE

0 = NO OPINION; NEVER THOUGHT ABOUT IT OR DOESN'T APPLY

____ C1a. How do you feel about your own personal life?

____ C1b. How do you feel about your (wife/husband), your marriage?

____ C1c. Your romantic life?

____ C1d. How do you feel about your friends and acquaintances?

____ C1e. How do you feel about your life as a whole?

C2. (RB, P. 7) In the last 7 days how much have you really enjoyed your personal life? (Would you say not at all, just a little, some, quite a bit, or a great deal?)

1. NOT AT ALL	2. JUST A LITTLE	3. SOME	4. QUITE A BIT	5. A GREAT DEAL

C3. (RB, P. 7) In the last 7 days how much has your personal life made you feel emotionally upset? (Would you say not at all, just a little, some, quite a bit, or a great deal?)

1. NOT AT ALL	2. JUST A LITTLE	3. SOME	4. QUITE A BIT	5. A GREAT DEAL

C4. (RB, P. 8) Now think about how well you've been doing in your personal life-- how successful you've been in having it be what you wanted. In the last 7 days would you say your personal life was not at all what you wanted, just a little of what you wanted, some of what you wanted, most of what you wanted, or all of what you wanted?

1. NOT AT ALL	2. JUST A LITTLE	3. SOME	4. MOST	5. ALL

C5. (RB, P. 9) I'm going to read you a list of symptoms. Please tell me how much each one has bothered or distressed you in the last 7 days. The first one is...

	NOT AT ALL (1)	A LITTLE BIT (2)	QUITE A BIT (3)	EXTREMELY (4)
a. nervousness or shakiness inside. (Has this bothered you not at all, a little bit, quite a bit, or extremely?)				
b. Suddenly scared for no reason?				
c. A feeling of being trapped or caught?				
d. Crying easily?				
e. Trembling?				
f. Blaming yourself for things?				
g. Feeling lonely?				
h. Feeling no interest in things?				
j. Feeling fearful?				
k. Feeling tense or keyed up?				

C6. Are you working now, unemployed, retired, a student, (a homemaker), or what?

| 1. WORKING NOW | 2. UNEMPLOYED | 3. RETIRED | 4. STUDENT | 5. HOME-MAKER | 7. OTHER (SPECIFY) |

GO TO C7

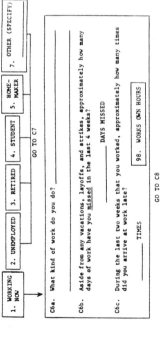

C6a. What kind of work do you do? _____

C6b. Aside from any vacations, layoffs, and strikes, approximately how many days of work have you missed in the last 4 weeks?
_____ DAYS MISSED

C6c. During the last two weeks that you worked, approximately how many times did you arrive at work late?
_____ TIMES | 98. WORKS OWN HOURS

GO TO C8

C7. Are you looking for work?

1. YES | 5. NO → GO TO C8

C7a. Just how likely is it that in the not too distant future you will be able to find a job you'd be willing to do? Would you say it is very unlikely, somewhat unlikely, equally likely and unlikely, somewhat likely, or very likely?

1. VERY UNLIKELY | 2. SOMEWHAT UNLIKELY | 3. EQUALLY LIKELY AND UNLIKELY | 4. SOMEWHAT LIKELY | 5. VERY LIKELY

C8. These are all the questions I have for you. Do you have any comments you would like to add?
_____
_____
_____

C9. I want to thank you very much for helping us.

IF INTERVIEWED BEFORE: We won't be calling you for any more interviews. The information you have given us will be very useful.

C10. EXACT TIME NOW: _____

341

SECTION D: BY OBSERVATION

D1. R'S SEX: | 1. MALE | | 2. FEMALE |

D2. RATE THE RESPONDENT ON EACH OF THE FOLLOWING:

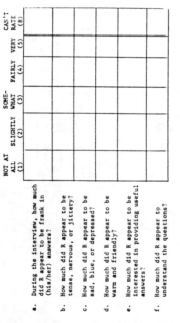

	NOT AT ALL (1)	SLIGHTLY (2)	SOME-WHAT (3)	FAIRLY (4)	VERY (5)	CAN'T RATE (8)
a. During the interview, how much did R appear to be frank in (his/her) answers?						
b. How much did R appear to be tense, nervous, or jittery?						
c. How much did R appear to be sad, blue, or depressed?						
d. How much did R appear to be warm and friendly?						
e. How much did R appear to be interested in providing useful answers?						
f. How much did R appear to understand the questions?						

D3. INTERVIEW DONE: | 1. IN PERSON | | 2. OVER PHONE |

D3a. FOCAL R PRESENT?

| 1. YES | 5. NO |

D3b. WITH RESPONDENT BOOK?

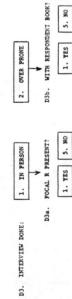

| 1. YES | 5. NO |

D4. THUMBNAIL SKETCH:

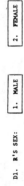

For Office Use Only

TIME IV

Fall/Winter 1981
Project 45
(462491)

STUDY OF STRESS: WORK, FAMILY AND HEALTH

1. Interviewer's Label

SURVEY RESEARCH CENTER
INSTITUTE FOR SOCIAL RESEARCH
THE UNIVERSITY OF MICHIGAN
ANN ARBOR, MICHIGAN 48106

2. Your Interview Number: _____

3. Date of Interview: _____

4. Length of Interview: _____ (Minutes)

5. Length of Edit: _____ (Minutes)

6. FOCAL R ID # _____

WORK RELATED QUESTIONNAIRE

INTERVIEWER: REMEMBER TO PRE-EDIT P. 2, A8a

(IF WORK OTHER HAS BEEN INTERVIEWED BEFORE:
Just as before, I will be asking you about
things that have changed and things that have
stayed the same in your and (FOCAL R'S) lives.
To do this I'll be asking many of the same questions you were asked last time. Don't try to
remember how you answered last time, just answer
in terms of how you feel now.)

READ TO ALL RESPONDENTS:

Before we begin I would like to assure/remind) you that the information you
provide us with will be kept in complete confidence. The interview is voluntary; if we should come to any question which you don't want to answer, just
let me know and we'll go on to the next question.

A0. EXACT TIME NOW: _____

A1. INTERVIEWER CHECKPOINT

1. WORK OTHER IS SAME AS [ ] TIME I [ ] TIME II [ ] TIME III ———→ GO TO A6
   (CHECK ALL THAT APPLY)

2. [ ] NEW WORK OTHER

A2. **What is your relationship to (NAME OF FOCAL R)?**

| 1. BOSS OR SUPERVISOR | 2. CO-WORKER | 7. OTHER (SPECIFY): _____ |

A3. About how long have you known (him/her)?

_____ MONTHS/YEARS
(CIRCLE ONE)

A4. How old are you?

_____ YEARS OLD

A5. What is the highest grade of school or year of college you have completed?

GRADES OF SCHOOL

| 00 | 01 | 02 | 03 | 04 | 05 | 06 | 07 | 08 | 09 | 10 | 11 | 12 |

COLLEGE

| 13 | 14 | 15 | 16 | 17+ |

A6. In the average week, approximately how many hours do you spend with (FOCAL R),
either in person or on the phone?

_____ HOURS

A7. Now think back over the last 7 days. Approximately how many hours have you spent
with (FOCAL R), either in person or on the phone, in the last 7 days?

_____ HOURS

I - 84

SECTION B

B1. (RB, P. 1) We would like your opinion about how (FOCAL R) felt about (his/her) life (during the last 7 days/ _____ weeks ago).

(IF R DOES NOT HAVE RESPONDENT BOOKLET: I want you to think of a scale going from 7 to one with 7 meaning delighted, 6 meaning pleased, 5 mostly satisfied, 4 mixed, that is, equally satisfied and dissatisfied, 3 mostly dissatisfied, 2 unhappy, and 1 terrible.)

As I read each statement please tell me how you think (FOCAL R) felt--taking into account what happened in the previous 7 days. If the question doesn't really apply or if you have no opinion please tell me.

7	6	5	4	3	2	1
DELIGHTED	PLEASED	MOSTLY SATISFIED	MIXED (ABOUT EQUALLY SATISFIED AND DISSATISFIED)	MOSTLY DISSAT- ISFIED	UNHAPPY	TERRIBLE

0 = NO OPINION; NEVER THOUGHT ABOUT IT OR DOESN'T APPLY

_____ Bla. How do you think (he/she) felt about (his/her) work? (What number on the scale?)

_____ Blb. How do you think (he/she) felt about the people (he/she) worked with-- (his/her) co-workers?

_____ Blc. (How do you think [he/she] felt about) the work (he/she) does on the job--the work itself?

_____ Bld. (How do you think [he/she] felt about) (his/her) life as a whole?

B2. (RB, P. 2) (In the last 7 days/ _____ weeks ago) how much do you think (he/she) really enjoyed (his/her) work? (Would you say not at all, just a little, some, quite a bit, or a great deal?)

| 1. NOT AT ALL | 2. JUST A LITTLE | 3. SOME | 4. QUITE A BIT | 5. A GREAT DEAL |

B3. (RB, P. 2) How much do you think (his/her) work has made (him/her) feel emotionally upset (in the last 7 days/ _____ weeks ago)? (Would you say not at all, just a little, some, quite a bit, or a great deal?)

| 1. NOT AT ALL | 2. JUST A LITTLE | 3. SOME | 4. QUITE A BIT | 5. A GREAT DEAL |

I - 83

A8. INTERVIEWER CHECKPOINT (SEE COVER SHEET, ITEM 5a)

☐ 1. FOCAL R HAS WORKED IN LAST WEEK ───→ TURN TO P. 3, SECTION B

☐ 2. FOCAL R HAS NOT WORKED IN LAST WEEK

A8a. When we talked with (FOCAL R), (he/she) had not worked in the last _____ weeks. So when I ask the following questions, please answer in terms of the same week (he/she) told us about. The week of _____ DATE which was _____ weeks ago.

B6. (RB, P. 5) Now I'm going to ask you several questions about (FOCAL R'S) relationships with people at work. As I read each question I want you to think of someone in particular but it doesn't have to be the same person for each question.

	NOT AT ALL (1)	JUST A LITTLE (2)	SOME (3)	QUITE A BIT (4)	A GREAT DEAL (5)
(In the last 7 days/____ weeks ago)...					
a. how much could (FOCAL R) count on some one person at work to treat (him/her) with respect? (Would you say not at all, just a little, some, quite a lot, or a great deal?)					
b. how much could (FOCAL R) count on some one person at work to give (him/her) useful information and advice if (he/she) wanted it?					
c. how much could (he/she) count on someone at work to act in ways that show he or she appreciates what (he/she) does?					
d. ...show that he or she cared about (him/her) as a person?					
e. (In the last 7 days/____ weeks ago), how much did some one person get on (FOCAL R'S) nerves?					
f. How much did some one person misunderstand the way (he/she) thinks and feels about things?					
g. How much did someone at work act in an unpleasant or angry manner toward (him/her)?					
h. ...show that he or she disliked (him/her)?					

B4. (RB, P. 3) Now think about how well (FOCAL R) feels (he/she) has been doing in (his/her) work--how successful (he/she) has been in having (his/her) work life be what (he/she) wanted. (In the last 7 days/____ weeks ago), would you say it was not at all what (he/she) wanted, just a little of what (he/she) wanted, some of what (he/she) wanted, most of what (he/she) wanted, or all of what (he/she) wanted?

1. NOT AT ALL	2. JUST A LITTLE	3. SOME	4. MOST	5. ALL

B5. (RB, P. 4) People vary a good deal on how well they do different things. Please tell me how well you think (FOCAL R) did each of the following things at work (in the last 7 days/____ weeks ago).

	VERY POORLY (1)	NOT VERY WELL (2)	ALL RIGHT WELL (3)	VERY WELL (4)	VERY EXCEPTIONALLY WELL (5)
(In the last 7 days/____ weeks ago) how well did (he/she) do in...					
a. working without unnecessary supervision? (Would you say very poorly, not very well, all right, very well or exceptionally well?)					
b. performing without mistakes?					
c. getting things done on time?					
d. getting along with others?					
e. handling responsibilities and daily demands?					
(In the last 7 days/____ weeks ago) how well did (he/she) do in...					
f. making the right decisions?					
g. avoiding arguing with others at work?					
h. handling disagreements by compromising and meeting other people half-way?					
j. being calm at work?					
(In the last 7 days/____ weeks ago) how well did (he/she) do in...					
k. accepting responsibility for (his/her) actions and behaviors?					
m. staying level headed?					
n. giving people the time and attention they need?					
p. being pleasant?					
q. doing a good job or handling all the things required of (him/her) at work?					
r. acting in a relaxed manner?					

SECTION C

C1. (RB, P. 6) We are interested in how the well-being of one person like (FOCAL R) affects the well-being of another person, like you. So now we want to find out how you feel about your own life.

(IF R DOES NOT HAVE RESPONDENT BOOKLET: Again, think of a scale from 7 to one with 7 meaning delighted, 6 pleased, 5 mostly satisfied, 4 mixed, equally satisfied and dissatisfied, 3 mostly dissatisfied, 2 unhappy and 1 terrible.)

As I read each statement please tell me how you feel now—taking into account what has happened during the last 7 days. If the question doesn't really apply or if you have no opinion please tell me.

DELIGHTED	PLEASED	MOSTLY SATISFIED	MIXED (ABOUT EQUALLY SATISFIED AND DISSATISFIED)	MOSTLY DISSAT-ISFIED	UNHAPPY	TERRIBLE
7	6	5	4	3	2	1

0 = NO OPINION; NEVER THOUGHT ABOUT IT OR DOESN'T APPLY

___ C1a. How do you feel about your work?

___ C1b. How do you feel about the people you work with—your co-workers?

___ C1c. (How do you feel about) the work you do on your job—the work itself?

___ C1d. (How do you feel about) your life as a whole?

C2. (RB, P. 7) In the last 7 days how much have you really enjoyed your work? (Would you say not at all, just a little, some, quite a bit or a great deal?)

1. NOT AT ALL	2. JUST A LITTLE	3. SOME	4. QUITE A BIT	5. A GREAT DEAL

C3. (RB, P. 7) In the last 7 days how much has your work made you feel emotionally upset? (Would you say not at all, just a little, some, quite a bit, or a great deal?)

1. NOT AT ALL	2. JUST A LITTLE	3. SOME	4. QUITE A BIT	5. A GREAT DEAL

B7. (RB, P. 5) (In the last 7 days/_____ weeks ago)....

	NOT AT ALL (1)	JUST A LITTLE (2)	SOME (3)	QUITE A BIT (4)	A GREAT DEAL (5)
a. how much could you count on (FOCAL R) to treat you with respect? (Would you say not at all, just a little, some, quite a lot, or a great deal?)					
b. (In the last 7 days/_____ weeks ago), how much could (FOCAL R) count on you to treat (him/her) with respect?					
c. how much could you count on (FOCAL R) to give you useful information and advice if you wanted it?					
d. how much could (FOCAL R) count on you to give (him/her) useful information and advice if (he/she) wanted it					
e. (In the last 7 days/_____ weeks ago), how much could you count on (FOCAL R) to show that (he/she) cared about you as a person?					
f. how much could (FOCAL R) count on you to show that you cared about (him/her) as a person?					
g. how much did (FOCAL R) get on your nerves?					
h. how much did you get on (FOCAL R'S) nerves?					
j. how much did (FOCAL R) act in an unpleasant or angry manner towards you?					
k. how much did you act in an unpleasant or angry manner towards (him/her)?					
m. how much did (FOCAL R) show that (he/she) disliked you?					
n. how much did you show (FOCAL R) that you disliked (him/her)?					

B8. All things considered, how do you think (FOCAL R) feels about (his/her) job these days?

_____

_____

C4. (RB, P. 8) Now think about how well you've been doing in your work--how successful you've been in having your work life be what you wanted. In the last 7 days would you say your work life was not at all what you wanted, just a little of what you wanted, some of what you wanted, most of what you wanted, or all of what you wanted?

| 1. NOT AT ALL | 2. JUST A LITTLE | 3. SOME | 4. MOST | 5. ALL |

C5. These are all the questions I have for you. Do you have any comments you would like to add?

_____

_____

_____

C6. I want to thank you very much for helping us.

(IF INTERVIEWED BEFORE): We won't be calling you for any more interviews. The information you have given us will be very useful.

C7. EXACT TIME NOW: _____

SECTION D: BY OBSERVATION

D1. R'S SEX: | 1. MALE | | 2. FEMALE |

D2. RATE THE RESPONDENT ON EACH OF THE FOLLOWING:

	NOT AT ALL (1)	SLIGHTLY (2)	SOME-WHAT (3)	FAIRLY (4)	VERY (5)	CAN'T RATE (8)
a. During the interview, how much did R appear to be frank in (his/her) answers?						
b. How much did R appear to be tense, nervous, or jittery?						
c. How much did R appear to be sad, blue, or depressed?						
d. How much did R appear to be warm and friendly?						
e. How much did R appear to be interested in providing useful answers?						
f. How much did R appear to understand the questions?						

D3. INTERVIEW DONE WITH RESPONDENT BOOK? | 1. YES | | 5. NO |

D4. THUMBNAIL SKETCH:

SECTION D: BY OBSERVATION

D1. R'S SEX: | 1. MALE | | 2. FEMALE |

D2. RATE THE RESPONDENT ON EACH OF THE FOLLOWING:

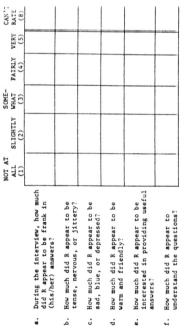

	NOT AT ALL (1)	SLIGHTLY (2)	SOME-WHAT (3)	FAIRLY (4)	VERY (5)	CAN'T RATE (8)
a. During the interview, how much did R appear to be frank in (his/her) answers?						
b. How much did R appear to be tense, nervous, or jittery?						
c. How much did R appear to be sad, blue, or depressed?						
d. How much did R appear to be warm and friendly?						
e. How much did R appear to be interested in providing useful answers?						
f. How much did R appear to understand the questions?						

D3. INTERVIEW DONE: | 1. IN PERSON | | 2. OVER PHONE |

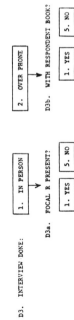

D3a. FOCAL R PRESENT? | 1. YES | | 5. NO |

D3b. WITH RESPONDENT BOOK? | 1. YES | | 5. NO |

D4. THUMBNAIL SKETCH:

APPENDIX J

DEFINITIONS OF INDICES, DERIVED
MEASURES, AND SELECTED ITEMS'

AFFECT

Y277 FXIDX AFF HOP ANX
FRs' ratings of their anxiety-like symptoms in the last 7
days (from Hopkin's Symptom Checklist).

Y278 FXIDX AFF HOP DEP
FRs' ratings of their depression-like symptoms in the last 7
days (from Hopkin's Symptom Checklist).

Y279 FXIDX AFF HOP SOMAT
FRs' ratings of their somatic symptoms in the last 7 days
(from Hopkin's Symptom Checklist).

Y274 FXIDX AFF UM ANX-DEP
FRs' ratings of a combination of their symptoms associated
with anxiety and with depression in the last 7 days.

Y276 FXIDX AFF UM CARDVAS
FRs' ratings of their symptoms which deal with the
cardiovascular system (e.g., heart beating hard) in the last
7 days.

Y271 FXIDX AFF ANGER
FRs' ratings of their anger in the last 7 days.

Y280 P1IDX AFF PO ANXIETY
POs' ratings of their anxiety-like symptoms in the last 7
days.

'Variable numbers and names are those actually used on the
computer file. The following is a key to symbols and
abbreviations:

Y = Wave number, ranging from 5 to 8, where 5 = Wave 1,
6 = Wave 2, 7 = Wave 3, and 8 = Wave 4

F or FR = Focal respondent

P or PO = Personal other

W or WO = Work other

X = Wave number, ranging from 1 to 4, where 1 = Wave 1,
2 = Wave 2, 3 = Wave 3, and 4 = Wave 4

IDX = Index

350

Y281 P1IDX AFF PO DEPRESS
POs' ratings of their depression-like symptoms in the last 7
days.

QUALITY OF LIFE

Y202 FXIDX QOL SELF DT + AC
FRs' general feelings about themselves (i.e., their own
functioning) over the last 7 days.

Y204 FXIDX QOL PL DT + AC
FRs' general feelings about their own personal lives
(including own marriage, spouse, and/or romantic lives) over
the last 7 days.

Y206 P1IDX QOL FR PL DT + AC
POs' perceptions of how FRs feel about their own personal
lives over the last 7 days.

Y208 P1IDX QOL PO PL DT + AC
POs' general feelings about their own personal lives
(including own marriage, spouse, and/or romantic lives) over
the last 7 days.

Y209 FXIDX QOL PEOPLE DT
FRs' general feelings about their friends and/or coworkers
over the last 7 days.

Y210 FXIDX QOL MAT W-B DT
FRs' general feelings about their income and financial
security over the last 7 days.

Y212 FXIDX QOL WL DT + AC
FRs' general feelings about their work life over the last 7
days.

Y214 W1IDX QOL FR DT + AC
WOs' perceptions of how FRs feel about their own work lives
over the last 7 days.

Y216 W1IDX QOL WO WL DT + AC
WOs' general feelings about their work over the last 7 days.

Y217 P1IDX QOL FR WL DT
POs' perceptions of how FRs feel about their own work lives
over the last 7 days.

Y219 FXIDX QOL HLTH 3I + AC
FRs' general feelings about their health over the last 7
days.

Y220 FXIDX QOL SLEEP DT
FRs' general feelings about their sleep over the last 7 days.

Y222 FXIDX QOL LAW 2I + AC
FRs' general feelings about their life as a whole over the last 7 days.

Y223 FXIDX QOL + A
FRs' feelings of real enjoyment over the last 7 days.

Y224 FXIDX QOL - A
FRs' feelings of emotional upset over the last 7 days.

Y225 FXIDX QOL COG
FRs' feelings of things having gone well or as wanted over the last 7 days.

SOCIAL SUPPORT

Y311 FXIDX SS ACTIVE
FRs' perceptions of how much they could count on others in the last 7 days to provide informational support, e.g., listen, encourage, provide useful advice.

Y312 FXIDX SS ESTEEM
FRs' perceptions of how much they could count on others in the last 7 days to provide esteem support, e.g., to show respect, care, and appreciation.

Y314 FXIDX SS THERAPIST
FRs' perceptions of how much social support they received from their therapist, e.g., the therapist's willingness to spend time with FR and the therapist's warmth.

Y315 FXIDX SS VAL MD
FRs' perceptions of how much social support they received from the physician who prescribed Valium, e.g., the physician's willingness to spend time with FR and the physician's warmth.

Y317 P1IDX SS FR ESTEEM
POs' perceptions of how much esteem support FR could have counted on receiving from others in the last 7 days.

Y318 P1IDX SS FR TOTAL
POs' perceptions of the total amount of active and esteem support exchanged between them and FR. A combination of Y319 and Y320.

Y319 P1IDX SS PO TO FR
POs' perceptions of the amount of active and esteem support they provided to FR in the last 7 days.

Y320 P1IDX SS FR TO PO
POs' perceptions of the amount of active and esteem support FR provided to them in the last 7 days.

Y322 W1IDX SS ESTEEM
WOs' perceptions of how much esteem support FR could have counted on receiving from others in the last 7 days.

Y323 W1IDX SS FR TOTAL
WOs' perceptions of the total amount of active and esteem support exchanged between them and FR. A combination of Y324 and Y325.

Y324 W1IDX SS WO TO FR
WOs' perceptions of the amount of active and esteem support they provided to FR in the last 7 days.

Y325 FXIDX SS FR TO WO
WOs' perceptions of the amount of active and esteem support FR provided to them in the last 7 days.

SOCIAL CONFLICT

Y352 FXIDX IC
FRs' perceptions of how much they could count on others in the last 7 days to provide negative affect and disconfirmation (social conflict) e.g., to misunderstand, ignore, act angry, and show dislike.

Y353 P1IDX FR IC
POs' perceptions of how much social conflict FR could have counted on receiving from others in the last 7 days.

Y354 P1IDX IC FR TOTAL
POs' perceptions of the total amount of social conflict occurring between him/her and FR. A combination of Y355 and Y356.

Y355 P1IDX IC PO TO FR
POs' perceptions of the amount of social conflict they created for FR in the last 7 days.

Y356 P1IDX IC FR TO PO
POs' perceptions of the amount of social conflict FR created for him/her in the last 7 days.

Y357 W1IDX FR IC
WOs' perceptions of how much social conflict FR could have counted on receiving from others in the last 7 days.

Y359 W1IDX IC FR TOTAL
WOs' perceptions of the total amount of social conflict occurring between him/her and FR.

COPING AND DEFENSE

Y301 FXIDX C&D RELIGION
How much the FR used religious means to deal with stress in the last 7 days.

Y302 FXIDX C&D POS APPROACH
How much the FR thought about ways to improve self, looked at life positively and viewed stress as an opportunity in the last 7 days.

Y303 FXIDX C&D REINTERPRET
How much the FR sought some higher meaning from an adverse event in the last 7 days.

Y304 FXIDX C&D OTHERS HELP
How much the FR contacted or sought help from others in the last 7 days.

CONTROL²

Y371 FXIDX CON HAVE INT PL
How much FRs' personal lives depended on or were influenced by what FRs did or said in the last 7 days.

Y372 FXIDX CON HAVE INT EMOTI
How much FRs' feelings and emotions depended on or were influenced by what FRs said or did in the last 7 days.

Y373 FXIDX CON WANT INT PL
How much FRs wanted their personal lives to depend on or be influenced by what they said or did in the last 7 days.

Y374 FXIDX CON WANT INT EMOTI
How much FRs wanted their feelings and emotions to depend on or be influenced by what they did or said in the last 7 days.

Y375 FXIDX CON HAVE OTH PL
How much FRs' personal lives depended on or were influenced by other people in the last 7 days.

²Three dimensions of control were measured: internal control, control by others, and control by chance. Two types of control were measured for each dimension: how much control respondents had and how much they wanted. Furthermore, misfit scores were computed for each dimension (amount of control FRs wanted subtracted from the amount of control FRs had). Each control index was formed for two domains of life: personal life and emotions.

Y376 FXIDX CON HAVE OTH EMOT
How much FRs' feelings and emotions depended on or were influenced by other people in the last 7 days.

Y377 FXIDX CON WANT OTH PL
How much FRs wanted their personal lives to depend on or be influenced by other people in the last 7 days.

Y378 FXIDX CON WANT OTH EMOT
How much FRs wanted their feelings and emotions to depend on or be influenced by other people in the last 7 days.

Y379 FXIDX CON HAVE CHC PL
How much FRs' personal lives depended on or were influenced by chance or luck, either good or bad, in the last 7 days.

Y380 FXIDX CON HAVE CHC EMOT
How much FRs' feelings and emotions depended on or were influenced by chance or luck in the last 7 days.

Y381 FXIDX CON WANT CHC PL
How much FRs wanted their personal lives to depend on or be influenced by chance or luck in the last 7 days.

Y382 FXIDX CON WANT CHC EMOT
How much FRs wanted their feelings and emotions to depend on or be influenced by chance or luck in the last 7 days.

Y541 'FX INT PL S|EI-PI|'
Misfit between the amount of internal control FRs had versus wanted in their personal lives during the last 7 days. Two pairs of commensurate "have" (Ei) and "want" (Pi) items were subtracted, then their absolute values were summed.

Y542 'FX INT EF S|EI-PI|'
Misfit between the amount of internal control FRs had versus wanted over emotions and feelings during the last 7 days. Two pairs of commensurate "have" (Ei) and "want" (Pi) items were subtracted, then their absolute values were summed.

Y547 'FX OTH PL S|EI-PI|'
Misfit between the amount of control others had versus what FRs wanted them to have over FRs' personal lives during the last 7 days. Two pairs of commensurate "have" (Ei) and "want" (Pi) items were subtracted, then their absolute values were summed.

Y548 'FX OTH EF S|EI-PI|'
Misfit between the amount of control others had versus what FRs wanted them to have over FRs' emotions and feelings during the last 7 days. Two pairs of commensurate "have" (Ei) and "want" (Pi) items were subtracted, then their absolute values were summed.

Y553 'FX CHA PL S|EI-PI|'
Misfit between the amount chance controlled FRs' personal lives versus how much FRs wanted chance to control the personal lives during the last 7 days. Two pairs of commensurate "have"(Ei) and "want"(Pi) items were subtracted, then their absolute values were summed.

Y554 'FX CHA EF S|EI-PI|'
Misfit between the amount chance controlled FRs' emotions and feelings versus how much FRs wanted chance to control emotions and feelings during the last 7 days. Two pairs of commensurate "have"(Ei) and "want"(Pi) items were subtracted, then their absolute values were summed.

ROLE CONFLICT

Y241 FXIDX ROL CONFLICT WL
How much FRs felt conflicting demands from others and demands from others which conflict with FRs' views in the last 7 days.

ROLE AMBIGUITY

Y242 FXIDX ROL AMB PL
How much FRs felt ambiguity about their performance on the job with respect to others' expectations, meeting demands, and doing things right in the last 7 days.

Y243 FXIDX ROL AMB PL
How much ambiguity FRs' felt about their performance in their personal lives with respect to others' expectations, meeting demands, and doing things right in the last 7 days.

PERFORMANCE

Y245 FXIDX TCH PERF WL
FRs' assessments of the degree to which they performed accurately and met job demands in the last 7 days.

Y246 FXIDX SOC PERF WL
FRs' assessments of the degree to which they got along well and compromised with others on the job in the last 7 days.

Y249 W1IDX TCH PERF (ALL) FR WL
WOs' assessments of the degree to which FRs' performed accurately and met job demands in the last 7 days.

Y251 W1IDX SOC PRF (ALL) FR WL
WOs' assessments of the degree to which FRs' got along well with others and acted relaxed on the job in the last 7 days.

Y253 FXIDX TCH PERF PL
FR's assessments of the degree to which they handled responsibilities and made the right decisions in their personal lives in the last 7 days.

Y254 FXIDX SOC PERF PL
FRs' assessments of the degree to which they got along well and compromised with people in their personal lives in the last 7 days.

Y257 P1IDX TCH PRF (ALL) FR PL
PO's assessments of the degree to which FRs' handled responsibilities and demands and made the right decisions in their personal lives in the last 7 days.

Y259 P1IDX SOC PERF (ALL) FR PL
POs'assessments of the degree to which FRs' got along with others and acted relaxed in their personal lives in the last 7 days.

Y260 PXIDX HOME PERF FR PL
POs' assessments of the degree to which FRs took care of housework and people at home in the last 7 days.

INTERVIEWER RATINGS

Y291 FXIDX INTWR FR SINCERE
Interviewers' rating of the sincerity of FR.

Y292 FXIDX INTWR FR AFFECT
Interviewer's rating of FRs' overall symptoms of anxiety and depression.

Y293 P1IDX INTWR PO SINCERE
Interviewer's rating of POs sincerity.

Y294 W1IDX INTWR WO SINCERE
Interviewer's rating of WOs sincerity.

ATTITUDES TOWARD VALIUM

Y401 FXIDX VALIUM HELPFUL 2I
FRs' ratings of the extent to which Valium is helpful and makes them feel better.

Y402 FXIDX VALIUM HELPFUL 5I
FRs' ratings of the extent to which Valium is helpful, makes them feel better and avoid discomfort, and increases their control over their emotions and their ability to deal with problems. (First two items same as Y401.)

Y403' F4IDX ATTITUDE RE TRNQ
FRs' ratings of the extent to which they generally approve of tranquilizers, think that they are safe and help people regain control rather than lose it, that tranquilizers do not prevent people from solving problems, and that it is not better to use willpower to solve problems.

INTERVIEW IMPACT

Y404' F4IDX INTERVIEW IMPACT
FRs' ratings of the extent to which being interviewed affected their lives or caused them to live differently or learn about themselves.

CAFFEINE

Y411 FXIDX MG CAFENE/DAY L7D
Estimated total amount of milligrams of caffeine ingested by FRs' in the last 7 days based on reported cups of coffee, tea, and cola drinks.

ALCOHOL

Y412 FXIDX # ALC DRNKS L7D
Derived estimate of number of alcoholic drinks FRs consumed in the last 7 days, based on number of days on which alcohol was consumed and the usual number of drinks consumed per day.

Y413 FXIDX # ALC DRNKS LST MO
Derived estimate of number of alcoholic drinks FRs consumed in the last 30 days, based on number of days on which alcohol was consumed and the usual number of drinks consumed per day.

TOBACCO

X641 FXG48AA NUMBER CIGARETTES
The number of cigarettes smoked per day over the last 7 days.

SELECTED OPEN-ENDED VARIABLES

'Measured at T4 only.

'Measured at T4 only.

Y007 FX OPEN: POSITIVE EVENTS
FRs' current levels of happiness due to positive life events or conditions.

Y008 FX OPEN: NEGATIVE EVENTS
FRs' current levels of distress due to negative life events or conditions.

Y006 FX OPEN: PEOPLE-POS CNT
Number of other people for whom FRs have some affection and/ or respect whom FRs mention in a positive context.

Y008 FX OPEN: PEOPLE-NEG CNT
Number of other people for whom FRs have some affection and/ or respect whom FRs mention in a negative context.

VALIUM USE MEASURES

X444 FXF11 *MED TIMES A DAY
The number of times per day the respondent reports having usually taken the first asterisked medication (usually Valium) on days when the respondent took it.

X445 FXF12 *MED NO A TIME
The number of pills of the medication referred to in X444 which the respondents report usually taking each time they consume the medication.

Y501 FX DYS SINCE FIRST RX #Z
The number of days since respondents' first use of the first medication (usually Valium). Based on F9 in the interview (X440 and X441).

Y502 FX DYS SINCE LAST RX #Z
The number of days since respondents' last use of the first medication (usually Valium). Based on F10 in the interview (X442 and X443).

Y521 FX BRAC ADJUSTED VAL L7D
An estimate of the number of Valium pills consumed in the last 7 days, based on the recoding scheme described in Appendix XX. Number of pills is bracketed following the brackets inherent in the retrospective calendar such that: 0=code 1, .1-4.5=code 2, 4.6-9.5=code 3, 9.6-14.5=code 4, 14.6-24.5=code 5, and 24.6-80.0=code 6.

Y601 FX BRAC ADJ VAL*MG L7D
This variable is Y521 times the associated number of milligrams in each Valium pill. Thus, it is a bracketed, adjusted measure of the number of milligrams of Valium consumed in the last 7 days.

Y523 'FX EST.#VAL PILLS L7D'
This variable estimates the number of Valium pills taken during the last 7 days based on the usual number of pills consumed per day (X444 * X445), taking into account when the respondent last took Valium (Y502): Y523 = (7-Y502) * X444 * X445).

Y621 FX EST#VAL P*MG L7D: B1-5
This variable is Y523 times the associated number of milligrams in each Valium pill. This variable is an estimate (based on "usual" consumption) of the actual number of milligrams of Valium consumed during the last 7 days prior to the interview. Number of milligrams is bracketed to reduce skew as follows: 0=code 1, 1-25=code 2, 26-30=code 3, 31-60=code 4, 61 or more=code 6.

Y618 FX MG VALIUM PRESCRB/DAY
The number of milligrams of Valium prescribed per day. "Number of mg" (X324) times "number of times per day" (X326) times "Number of pills per time" (X327).

Y619 FX EST MG VAL TAKEN/DAY
An estimate of the number of milligrams of Valium respondents actually consumed per day. It is the "number of milligrams" (X324) times the "number of times per day usually taken" (X444) times the "number of pills per time usually taken" (X445).

Y620 FX VALIUM COMPLIANCE
A measure of compliance to the prescription regimen. It is Y618 minus Y619. A score of zero means perfect compliance, positive scores mean under-use, and negative scores mean over-use. Note: Non-Valium users are treated as missing data.

OTHER MEDICATIONS AND SUBSTANCES

Y610 FX # + & +/- DRUGS 6 WKS
This variable is a simple count of the number of different medications having a potential effect similar to Valium which the respondent took in the last six weeks (excluding Valium but including medications which could potentially produce both similar and opposite effects, i.e., "+/-" medications).

Y611 FX # - & +/- DRUGS 6 WKS
This variable is a simple count of the number of different medications having a potential effect opposite to that of Valium which the respondent took in the last 6 weeks (including medications which could potentially produce effects both similar and opposite to that of Valium, i.e., "+/-" medications).

Y617 FX # USES STREET DRG L6W
A count of the total number of times all mentioned street drugs were used in the last 6 weeks.

COMBINED STRESS MEASURES

Y261 FX COMBINED STRSS BIG 11 (Also called "Highest Stress.")
This measure of stress assigns respondents their highest score of 11 different measures of stress. Thus, respondents who were high on any one type of stress, were coded as having high stress on this measure. (See Measures Chapter for more details)

Y262 FX COMBINED STRESS BIG 3 (Also called "Multiple Stress.")
This measure of stress assigns respondents having high scores on all of three different stress measures a high score, low on all three a low score, and medium on all three a medium score. The three stress measures are role ambiguity in the personal life, social conflict, and negative life events and conditions. Individuals simultaneously experiencing high levels of all 3 stressors are scored high on this measure. (See Measures Chapter and Table XX for more details.)

MEANS AND STANDARD DEVIATIONS
OF INDICES AND SELECTED ITEMS[1] [2]

INDEX	T_1 (N=784) $\bar{X}$(SD)	T_2 (N=716) $\bar{X}$(SD)	T_3 (N=686) $\bar{X}$(SD)	T_4 (N=675) $\bar{X}$(SD)
Affect				
Y277 FXIDX AFF HOP ANX	1.6(0.6)	1.6(0.5)	1.5(0.5)	1.5(0.5)
Y278 FXIDX AFF HOP DEP	1.7(0.6)	1.6(0.5)	1.6(0.5)	1.6(0.5)
Y279 FXIDX AFF HOP SOMAT	1.7(0.6)	1.6(0.5)	1.6(0.5)	1.6(0.5)
Y274 FXIDX AFF UM ANX-DEP	2.0(0.7)	1.8(0.6)	1.8(0.6)	1.7(0.6)
Y276 FXIDX AFF UM CARDVAS	1.4(0.5)	1.4(0.5)	1.4(0.5)	1.4(0.5)
Y271 FXIDX AFF ANGER	1.7(0.8)	1.6(0.7)	1.5(0.7)	1.5(0.6)
Y280 P1IDX AFF PO ANXIETY	1.6(0.5)	1.5(0.5)	1.5(0.5)	1.5(0.5)
Y281 P1IDX AFF PO DEPRESS	1.6(0.5)	1.6(0.5)	1.5(0.5)	1.5(0.5)
Quality of Life (QOL)				
Y202 FXIDX QOL SELF DT & AC	4.3(.83)	4.4(.78)	4.4(.80)	4.4(.76)
Y204 FXIDX QOL PL DT & AC	4.1(1.1)	4.2(1.0)	4.3(.97)	4.3(.95)
Y206 FXIDX QOL FR PL DT & AC	4.0(.94)	4.1(.90)	4.1(.89)	4.2(.84)
Y208 FXIDX QOL PO PL DT & AC	4.4(.90)	4.4(.85)	4.4(.88)	4.5(.80)
Y209 FXIDX QOL PEOPLE DT	5.4(.94)	5.3(.91)	5.3(.89)	5.3(.83)
Y210 FXIDX QOL MAT W-B DT	4.3(1.6)	4.4(1.5)	4.4(1.5)	4.4(1.5)
Y212 FXIDX QOL WL DT & AC	4.0(1.0)	4.1(.93)	4.1(.90)	4.1(.94)
Y214 W1IDX QOL FR DT & AC	4.0(.78)	4.0(.83)	4.0(.74)	4.1(.77)
Y216 W1IDX QOL WO WL DT & AC	4.3(.81)	4.3(.84)	4.2(.79)	4.2(.79)

Appendix K

MEANS AND STANDARD DEVIATIONS
OF INDICES

(continued)

INDEX	T_1 (N=784) $\bar{X}$(SD)	T_2 (N=716) $\bar{X}$(SD)	T_3 (N=686) $\bar{X}$(SD)	T_4 (N=675) $\bar{X}$(SD)
Quality of Life (QOL), continued				
Y217 P1IDX QOL FR WL DT	4.7(1.3)	4.9(1.1)	4.9(1.2)	4.9(1.1)
Y219 FXIDX QOL HLTH 3I + AC	3.3(1.1)	3.5(1.0)	3.4(1.0)	3.5(1.0)
Y220 FXIDX QOL SLEEP DT	3.7(1.1)	3.7(1.1)	3.8(1.1)	3.8(1.0)
Y222 FXIDX QOL LAW 2I + AC	3.6(.66)	3.6(.63)	3.6(.64)	3.6(.62)
Y223 FXIDX QOL + A	3.3(.91)	3.4(.84)	3.3(.87)	3.4(.82)
Y224 FXIDX QOL - A	2.4(.93)	2.3(.86)	2.2(.83)	2.2(.85)
Y225 FXIDX QOL COG	3.1(.90)	3.2(.83)	3.2(.85)	3.2(.81)
Social Support (SS)				
Y311 FXIDX SS ACTIVE	4.0(.86)	3.9(.87)	3.9(.80)	3.8(.80)
Y312 FXIDX SS ESTEEM	3.9(.82)	3.9(.78)	3.9(.80)	3.9(.75)
Y314 FXIDX SS THERAPIST	3.9(.86)	4.1(.75)	4.0(.64)	4.2(.67)
Y315 FXIDX SS VAL MD	3.9(.90)	4.0(.89)	4.0(.88)	4.0(.82)
Y317 FXIDX SS FR ESTEEM	4.2(.70)	4.2(.74)	4.2(.70)	4.2(.68)
Y318 P1IDX SS FR TOTAL	4.4(.58)	4.4(.61)	4.4(.62)	4.3(.61)
Y319 P1IDX SS PO TO FR	4.5(.56)	4.4(.60)	4.4(.60)	4.4(.61)
Y320 P1IDX SS FR TO PO	4.4(.67)	4.3(.70)	4.3(.71)	4.3(.67)

Appendix K

MEANS AND STANDARD DEVIATIONS
OF INDICES

(continued)

INDEX	T_1 (N=784) $\bar{X}$(SD)	T_2 (N=716) $\bar{X}$(SD)	T_3 (N=686) $\bar{X}$(SD)	T_4 (N=675) $\bar{X}$(SD)
Social Support (SS), continued				
Y322 W1IDX SS ESTEEM	4.0(.71)	4.0(.73)	4.0(.78)	4.1(.72)
Y323 W1IDX SS FR TOTAL	4.6(.49)	4.5(.54)	4.4(.58)	4.4(.58)
Y324 W1IDX SS WO TO FR	4.6(.50)	4.5(.54)	4.4(.56)	4.4(.58)
Y325 FXIDX SS FR TO WO	4.6(.53)	4.5(.60)	4.4(.64)	4.4(.61)
Interpersonal Conflict (IC)				
Y352 FXIDX X IC (PO/WO ITEMS)	2.4(.95)	2.2(.86)	2.1(.87)	2.1(.90)
Y353 P1IDX FR IC	2.6(.95)	2.4(.87)	2.3(.87)	2.3(.85)
Y354 P1IDX IC FR TOTAL	1.7(.71)	1.7(.73)	1.6(.68)	1.6(.66)
Y355 P1IDX IC PO TO FR	1.8(.75)	1.7(.76)	1.7(.71)	1.5(.70)
Y356 P1IDX IC FR TO PO	1.6(.73)	1.7(.76)	1.6(.69)	1.6(.66)
Y357 W1IDX FR IC	2.3(.97)	2.3(.98)	2.2(.91)	2.1(.88)
Y359 W1IDX IC FR TOTAL	1.6(.79)	1.6(.79)	1.7(.89)	1.6(.80)

Appendix K

MEANS AND STANDARD DEVIATIONS
OF INDICES

(continued)

INDEX	T_1 (N=784) $\bar{X}$(SD)	T_2 (N=716) $\bar{X}$(SD)	T_3 (N=686) $\bar{X}$(SD)	T_4 (N=675) $\bar{X}$(SD)
Coping and Defense (C & D)				
Y301 FXIDX C&D RELIGION	3.2(1.4)	3.0(1.3)	3.0(1.3)	3.0(1.3)
Y302 FXIDX C&D POS APPROACH	3.0(.89)	3.0(.87)	2.9(.85)	2.8(.86)
Y303 FXIDX C&D REINTERPRET	3.1(1.1)	3.0(1.1)	2.9(1.0)	2.9(1.0)
Y304 FXIDX C&D OTHERS HELP	2.7(.92)	2.7(.87)	2.7(.83)	2.6(.86)
Control (CON)				
Y371 FXIDX CON HAVE INT PL	3.4(.91)	3.4(.88)	3.4(.87)	3.5(.89)
Y372 FXIDX CON HAVE INT EMOT	3.2(.95)	3.3(.92)	3.3(.92)	3.3(.91)
Y373 FXIDX CON WANT INT PL	4.0(.85)	4.0(.80)	4.0(.78)	4.0(.80)
Y374 FXIDX CON WANT INT EMOT	3.8(.93)	4.0(.85)	3.9(.85)	3.9(.87)
Y375 FXIDX CON HAVE OTH PL	2.7(1.1)	2.6(1.1)	2.5(1.0)	2.6(1.0)
Y376 FXIDX CON HAVE OTH EMOT	2.6(1.1)	2.5(1.1)	2.5(1.0)	2.5(1.0)
Y377 FXIDX CON WANT OTH PL	2.0(.91)	1.9(.86)	2.0(.90)	2.0(.84)
Y378 FXIDX CON WANT OTH EMOT	2.0(.94)	1.9(.89)	2.0(.86)	2.0(.84)
Y379 FXIDX CON HAVE CHC PL	2.1(.91)	1.9(.86)	1.8(.86)	1.8(.89)
Y380 FXIDX CON HAVE CHC EMOT	1.8(.82)	1.7(.79)	1.7(.83)	1.7(.83)
Y381 FXIDX CON WANT CHC PL	1.9(1.0)	1.8(.94)	1.8(1.0)	1.7(.92)

MEANS AND STANDARD DEVIATIONS
OF INDICES

(continued)

INDEX	T_1 (N=784) $\bar{X}$(SD)	T_2 (N=716) $\bar{X}$(SD)	T_3 (N=686) $\bar{X}$(SD)	T_4 (N=675) $\bar{X}$(SD)
Control (CON), continued				
Y382 FXIDX CON WANT CHC EMOT	1.7(.90)	1.6(.83)	1.7(.91)	1.7(.89)
Y541 FXIDX INT PL S|EI-PI	2.0(1.6)	1.8(1.5)	1.6(1.5)	1.5(1.4)
Y542 FXIDX INT EF S|EI-PI	2.0(1.7)	1.7(1.6)	1.6(1.5)	1.6(1.5)
Y547 FXIDX OTH PL S|EI-PI	2.5(1.8)	2.2(1.8)	1.9(1.7)	1.9(1.7)
Y548 FXIDX OTH EF S|EI-PI	2.2(1.8)	1.9(1.8)	1.8(1.7)	1.8(1.7)
Y553 FXIDX CHA PL S|EI-PI	1.7(1.5)	1.2(1.4)	1.0(1.3)	.95(1.4)
Y554 FXIDX CHA EF S|EI-PI	1.1(1.4)	.82(1.2)	.79(1.3)	.79(1.3)
Role Conflict (ROLCON)				
Y241 FXIDX ROLCON WL	2.2(1.0)	2.1(.89)	2.0(.90)	2.0(.90)
Role Ambiguity (ROLAMB)				
Y242 FXIDX ROL AMB WL	1.6(.60)	1.7(.60)	1.7(.60)	1.7(.59)
Y243 FXIDX ROL AMB PL	2.3(7.3)	2.2(.70)	2.2(.62)	2.2(.63)

Appendix K

MEANS AND STANDARD DEVIATIONS
OF INDICES

(continued)

INDEX	T_1 (N=784) $\bar{X}$(SD)	T_2 (N=716) $\bar{X}$(SD)	T_3 (N=686) $\bar{X}$(SD)	T_4 (N=675) $\bar{X}$(SD)
Performance (PERF)				
Y245 FXIDX TCH PERF WL	4.0(.53)	4.0(.60)	3.9(.52)	3.9(.51)
Y246 FXIDX SOC PERF WL	4.0(.66)	3.9(.63)	3.8(.60)	3.8(.54)
Y249 FXIDX TCH PERF(ALL) FR WL	4.2(.59)	4.0(.58)	4.0(.59)	4.0(.61)
Y251 W1IDX SOC PERF(ALL) FR WL	4.0(.70)	3.9(.63)	3.9(.66)	3.9(.67)
Y253 FXIDX TCH PERF PL	3.5(.70)	3.5(.63)	3.5(.65)	3.5(.61)
Y254 FXIDX SOC PERF PL	3.5(.73)	3.5(.75)	3.6(.76)	3.5(.67)
Y257 P1IDX TCH PERF(ALL) FR PL	3.8(.74)	3.8(.72)	3.8(.70)	3.8(.69)
Y259 P1IDX SOC PERF(ALL) FR PL	3.6(.77)	3.6(.75)	3.6(.73)	3.6(.70)
Y260 HOME PERF FR PL	3.7(.74)	3.6(.71)	3.6(.72)	3.7(.70)
Interviewer Ratings (INTWR)				
Y291 FXIDX INTWR FR SINCERE	4.8(.60)	4.7(.59)	4.8(.53)	4.8(.50)
Y292 FXIDX INTWR FR AFFECT	1.9(1.0)	1.6(.80)	1.6(.78)	1.5(.67)
Y293 P1IDX INTWR PO SINCERE	5.0(1.7)	5.0(1.7)	5.1(1.7)	5.0(.15)
Y294 W1IDX INTWR WO SINCERE	4.7(.60)	4.6(.61)	4.7(.53)	4.7(.56)

MEANS AND STANDARD DEVIATIONS
OF INDICES

(continued)

INDEX	T_1 (N=784) $\bar{X}$(SD)	T_2 (N=716) $\bar{X}$(SD)	T_3 (N=686) $\bar{X}$(SD)	T_4 (N=675) $\bar{X}$(SD)
Attitudes Toward Tranquilizers (ATT VAL)				
Y401 FXIDX VALIUM HELPFUL 2I	3.4(.97)	3.4(.92)	3.4(.93)	3.4(.92)
Y402 FXIDX VALIUM HELPFUL 5I	3.4(.77)	3.4(.75)	3.5(.73)	3.5(.74)
Y403 F4IDX ATTITUDE RE TRNG	NA	NA	NA	2.4(.65)
Interview Impact (INTW)				
Y404 F4IDX INTERVIEW IMPACT	NA	NA	NA	2.2(.96)
Caffeine				
Y411 FXIDX MG CAFENE/DAY L7D	439.0(581.7)	429.2(539.4)	392.6(456.6)	406.6(488.8)
Alcohol				
Y412 FXIDX #ALC DRINKS L7D	6.2(14.9)	4.8(9.2)	4.7(8.4)	4.4(7.7)
Y413 FXIDX #ALC DRINKS LST MO	27.4(63.9)	21.6(39.5)	20.7(36.1)	20.0(33.4)

MEANS AND STANDARD DEVIATIONS
OF INDICES

(continued)

INDEX	T_1 (N=784) $\bar{X}$(SD)	T_2 (N=716) $\bar{X}$(SD)	T_3 (N=686) $\bar{X}$(SD)	T_4 (N=675) $\bar{X}$(SD)
Tobacco				
X641 FXG48AA NUMBER CIGARETTES	11.3(15.7)	10.6(15.1)	10.2(14.5)	10.1(14.6)
Selected Open-Ended Variables (OPEN)				
Y5005 FX OPEN:POSITIVE EVENTS	1.4(.82)	1.0(.62)	.98(.66)	.95(.64)
Y5007 FX OPEN:NEGATIVE EVENTS	1.9(.82)	1.4(.78)	1.2(.76)	1.2(.77)
Y5006 FX OPEN:PEOPLE-POS CNT	1.3(.82)	1.1(.88)	1.1(.90)	1.0(.91)
Y5008 FX OPEN:PEOPLE-NEG CNT	1.1(.83)	.79(.82)	.72(.82)	.68(.80)
Valium Use Measures				
X444 FXF11 MED TIMES A DAY*	1.6(.90)	1.5(.90)	1.5(.80)	1.6(.92)
X445 FXF12 MED NO A TIME*	1.1(.35)	1.1(.42)	1.0(.27)	1.0(.18)
Y501 FX DYS SINCE FIRST RX #1*	1.77** (1.65)** (4.9 years)	2.19** (1.81)** (6.0 years)	2.10** (1.55)** (5.8 years)	2.30** (1.59)** (6.3 years)
Y502 FXDYS SINCE LAST RX #1*	5.0(8.5)	4.6(9.2)	3.3(6.3)	4.5(13.4)

MEANS AND STANDARD DEVIATIONS
OF INDICES

(continued)

INDEX	T_1 (N=784) $\bar{X}$(SD)	T_2 (N=716) $\bar{X}$(SD)	T_3 (N=686) $\bar{X}$(SD)	T_4 (N=675) $\bar{X}$(SD)
Y521 FX BRAC ADJUSTED VAL L7D	1.8(1.2)	1.7(1.2)	1.7(1.2)	1.6(1.2)
Y601 FX BRAC ADJ VAL*MG L7D	7.1(9.6)	6.3(9.3)	5.9(9.3)	5.6(8.9)
Y523 FX EST #VAL PILLS L7D	4.2(7.8)	3.3(6.2)	3.0(5.6)	2.9(5.7)
Y621 FX EST #VAL P*MG L7D:B1-5	2.0(1.4)	1.8(1.4)	1.8(1.3)	1.8(1.3)
Y618 FX MG VALIUM PRESCRB/DAY	67.5(93.1)	52.9(81.9)	46.2(81.7)	44.8(78.5)
Y619 FX EST MG VAL TAKEN/DAY	48.1(90.7)	37.7(84.4)	29.2(51.1)	29.8(56.2)
Y620 FX VALIUM COMPLIANCE	43.0(104.1)	49.8(63.7)	57.5(67.0)	49.4(68.6)

* Valium users only
**Multiply by 1000

Other Medications and Substances

Y610 FX # + & +/- DRUGS 6 WKS	.93(1.2)	.96(1.2)	.90(1.1)	.85(1.1)
Y611 FX # - & +/- DRUGS 6 WKS	.35(.66)	.40(.71)	.39(.71)	.35(.68)
Y617 FX # USES STREET DRG L6W	1.3(6.8)	.90(5.3)	.91(6.0)	.92(5.9)

Appendix K

MEANS AND STANDARD DEVIATIONS
OF INDICES

(continued)

INDEX	T_1 (N=784) $\bar{X}$(SD)	T_2 (N=716) $\bar{X}$(SD)	T_3 (N=686) $\bar{X}$(SD)	T_4 (N=675) $\bar{X}$(SD)
Stress				
Y261 FX COMBINED STRESS BIG 11	1.5(.93)	1.6(.98)	1.5(1.0)	1.5(1.1)
Y262 FX COMBINED STRESS BIG 3	4.5(1.9)	4.0(1.8)	3.7(1.8)	3.6(1.9)

[1]See footnote for key to symbols on Appendix J.

[2]These means and standard deviations were computed for the entire set of respondents at each wave, not just the respondents who completed all four interviews. The "Stabilities in Means, Standard Deviations, and Relationships Over Time" section of the Results Chapter describes changes in means from Time 1 to Time 4 for the 675 respondents in all four waves of the study.

INDEX	Time 1	Females	Males	Valium	No Listed Drug	High Educ. Group	Low Educ. Group	Time 2	Time 3	Time 4
Affect										
Y277 FXIDX AFF HOP ANX	.81	.82	.81	.76	.72	.79	.83	.82	.84	.82
Y278 FXIDX AFF HOP DEP	.86	.87	.83	.86	.81	.86	.83	.83	.86	.84
Y279 FXIDX AFF HOP SOMAT	.85	.84	.86	.84	.79	.83	.86	.85	.84	.86
Y274 FXIDX AFF UM ANX-DEP	.87	.88	.84	.87	.80	.88	.88	.87	.88	.88
Y276 FXIDX AFF UM CARDVAS	.73	.69	.77	.68	.44	.71	.74	.74	.74	.75
Y271 FXIDX AFF ANGER	.85	.85	.84	.80	.81	.85	.88	.85	.82	.84
Y280 PXIDX AFF PO ANXIETY	.79	NA	NA	NA	NA	NA	NA	.75	.78	.81
Y281 PXIDX AFF PO DEPRESS	.73	NA	NA	NA	NA	NA	NA	.73	.75	.74
Quality of Life (QOL)										
Y202 FXIDX QOL SELF DT & AC	.84	.83	.85	.86	.82	.85	.84	.85	.88	.88
Y204 FXIDX QOL PL DT & AC	.85	.86	.82	.84	.82	.87	.82	.86	.85	.85
Y206 PXIDX QOL FR PL DT & AC	.84	NA	NA	NA	NA	NA	NA	.85	.85	.85
Y208 PXIDX QOL PO PL DT & AC	.85	NA	NA	NA	NA	NA	NA	.83	.86	.83
Y209 FXIDX QOL PEOPLE DT	.60	.49	.68	.69	.51	.54	.68	.60	.58	.55
Y210 FXIDX QOL MAT W-B DT	.86	.87	.86	.85	.84	.89	.86	.89	.90	.91
Y212 FXIDX QOL WL DT & AC	.84	.84	.84	.85	.84	.86	.81	.83	.83	.83
Y214 WXIDX QOL FR DT & AC	.77	NA	NA	NA	NA	NA	NA	.83	.80	.84
Y216 WXIDX QOL WO WL DT & AC	.80	NA	NA	NA	NA	NA	NA	.84	.84	.83
Y217 PXIDX QOL FR WL DT	.72	NA	NA	NA	NA	NA	NA	.72	.76	.73
Y219 FXIDX QOL HLTH 3I + AC	.91	.91	.92	.89	.87	.92	.91	.92	.92	.92
Y220 FXIDX QOL SLEEP DT	.84	.84	.84	.82	.82	.85	.84	.85	.86	.86
Y222 FXIDX QOL LAW 2I + AC	.85	.86	.84	.84	.84	.87	.80	.86	.87	.87
Y223 FXIDX QOL + A	.80	.80	.80	.80	.77	.79	.78	.82	.84	.83
Y224 FXIDX QOL - A	.78	.77	.79	.75	.73	.79	.78	.79	.79	.80
Y225 FXIDX QOL COG	.78	.76	.80	.79	.73	.80	.79	.79	.81	.82
Social Support (SS)										
Y311 FXIDX SS ACTIVE	.71	.73	.68	.71	.79	.73	.66	.76	.76	.76
Y312 FXIDX SS ESTEEM	.77	.78	.75	.77	.81	.74	.74	.80	.80	.80
Y314 FXIDX SS THERAPIST	.60	.61	.58	.63	.64	.69	.16	.52	.22	.48
Y315 FXIDX SS VAL MD	.68	.77	.50	.67	NA	.74	.61	.71	.68	.67
Y317 PXIDX SS FR ESTEEM	.76	.76	.75	.76	.82	.77	.73	.82	.83	.82
Y318 PXIDX SS FR TOTAL	.86	.86	.86	.87	.88	.88	.83	.87	.89	.89
Y319 PXIDX SS PO TO FR	.72	.72	.72	.74	.74	.77	.66	.77	.79	.80
Y320 PXIDX SS FR TO PO	.76	.75	.78	.83	.80	.78	.74	.79	.83	.80
Y322 WXIDX SS ESTEEM	.71	.70	.71	.82	.52	.72	.70	.71	.81	.80
Y323 WXIDX SS FR TOTAL	.84	.84	.84	.84	.87	.84	.88	.89	.90	.91
Y324 WXIDX SS WO TO FR	.69	.71	.66	.63	.70	.68	.69	.81	.78	.85
Y325 WXIDX SS FR TO WO	.72	.70	.74	.69	.81	.68	.80	.77	.81	.78

Appendix L

CRONBACH'S ALPHAS FOR INDICES
(continued)

INDEX	Time 1	Females	Males	Valium	No Listed Drug	High Educ. Group	Low Educ. Group	Time 2	Time 3	Time 4
Social Conflict (IC)										
Y352 FXIDX IC (PO/WO ITEMS)	.77	.78	.76	.78	.73	.78	.76	.74	.76	.78
Y353 PXIDX FR IC	.79	.79	.80	.81	.74	.80	.78	.79	.81	.80
Y354 PXIDX IC FR TOTAL	.88	.84	.90	.88	.86	.88	.86	.89	.88	.88
Y355 PXIDX IC PO TO FR	.76	.70	.78	.77	.70	.74	.75	.78	.75	.74
Y356 PXIDX IC FR TO PO	.74	.66	.79	.75	.70	.75	.69	.79	.75	.73
Y357 WXIDX FR IC	.82	.82	.83	.84	.85	.84	.77	.85	.83	.82
Y359 WXIDX IC FR TOTAL	.81	.73	.86	.80	.81	.81	.91	.83	.89	.80
Coping and Defense (C & D)										
Y301 FXIDX C&D RELIGION	.86	.86	.85	.88	.86	.88	.84	.87	.86	.86
Y302 FXIDX C&D POS APPROACH	.79	.79	.80	.76	.79	.78	.78	.82	.82	.83
Y303 FXIDX C&D REINTERPRET	.70	.67	.74	.70	.79	.72	.66	.72	.73	.75
Y304 FXIDX C&D OTHERS HELP	.62	.60	.65	.57	.63	.60	.60	.61	.56	.66
Control (CON)										
Y371 FXIDX CON HAVE INT PL	.62	.56	.68	.58	.60	.58	.62	.69	.76	.81
Y372 FXIDX CON HAVE INT EMOT	.72	.72	.74	.63	.74	.75	.63	.73	.82	.80
Y373 FXIDX CON WANT INT PL	.66	.69	.63	.65	.70	.76	.60	.70	.75	.79
Y374 FXIDX CON WANT INT EMOT	.67	.66	.68	.73	.76	.66	.67	.78	.84	.87
Y375 FXIDX CON HAVE OTH PL	.69	.66	.72	.65	.73	.68	.66	.79	.80	.82
Y376 FXIDX CON HAVE OTH EMOT	.81	.82	.81	.77	.82	.87	.80	.86	.84	.87
Y377 FXIDX CON WANT OTH PL	.55	.50	.58	.50	.65	.64	.47	.65	.78	.75
Y378 FXIDX CON WANT OTH EMOT	.70	.65	.73	.66	.73	.73	.63	.80	.79	.82
Y379 FXIDX CON HAVE CHC PL	.56	.56	.55	.42	.64	.66	.53	.70	.75	.83
Y380 FXIDX CON HAVE CHC EMOT	.74	.78	.70	.74	.83	.78	.70	.82	.86	.87
Y381 FXIDX CON WANT CHC PL	.75	.77	.72	.82	.71	.75	.71	.77	.87	.88
Y382 FXIDX CON WANT CHC EMOT	.84	.87	.81	.86	.84	.88	.79	.85	.90	.90
Y541 FXIDX INT PL S|EI-PI|	.46									
Y542 FXIDX INT EF S|EI-PI|	.56									
Y547 FXIDX OTH PL S|EI-PI|	.48									
Y548 FXIDX OTH EF S|EI-PI|	.64									
Y553 FXIDX CHA PL S|EI-PI|	.40									
Y554 FXIDX CHA EF S|EI-PI|	.62									
Role Conflict (ROLCON)										
Y241 FXIDX ROLCON WL	.84	.84	.83	.87	.82	.82	.88	.81	.82	.84

362

Appendix L

CRONBACH'S ALPHAS FOR INDICES
(continued)

INDEX	Time 1	Females	Males	Valium	No Listed Drug	High Educ. Group	Low Educ. Group	Time 2	Time 3	Time 4
Role Ambiguity (ROLAMB)										
Y242 FXIDX ROL AMB WL	.81	.81	.80	.81	.80	.83	.77	.82	.85	.87
Y243 FXIDX ROL AMB PL	.73	.75	.71	.75	.73	.76	.70	.77	.77	.81
Performance (PERF)										
Y245 FXIDX TCH PERF WL	.80	.78	.81	.77	.80	.80	.77	.85	.83	.82
Y246 FXIDX SOC PERF WL	.76	.80	.70	.81	.76	.78	.75	.75	.76	.74
Y249 WXIDX TCH PERF(ALL) FR WL	.89	.88	.90	.83	.92	.87	.84	.88	.90	.92
Y251 WXIDX SOC PERF(ALL) FR WL	.90	.89	.91	.93	.91	.89	.89	.88	.91	.92
Y253 FXIDX TCH PERF PL	.68	.65	.72	.65	.62	.69	.71	.66	.75	.71
Y254 FXIDX SOC PERF PL	.67	.69	.64	.68	.73	.68	.61	.77	.75	.72
Y257 PXIDX TCH PERF(ALL) FR PL	.82	NA	NA	NA	NA	NA	NA	.85	.85	.84
Y259 PXIDX SOC PERF(ALL) FR PL	.89	NA	NA	NA	NA	NA	NA	.90	.90	.90
Y260 PXIDX HOME PERF FR PL	.72	NA	NA	NA	NA	NA	NA	.74	.78	.77
Interviewer Ratings (INTWR)										
Y291 FXIDX INTWR FR SINCERE	.80	.82	.76	.85	.78	.83	.80	.85	.85	.83
Y292 FXIDX INTWR FR AFFECT	.67	.66	.68	.66	.54	.64	.62	.63	.62	.50
Y293 PXIDX INTWR PO SINCERE	.82	.84	.80	.88	.70	.86	.78	.85	.90	.87
Y294 WXIDX INTWR WO SINCERE	.82	.87	.79	.89	.74	.88	.88	.83	.81	.85
Attitudes Toward Tranquilizers (ATT VAL)										
Y401 FXIDX VALIUM HELPFUL 2I	.81	.82	.79	NA	NA	.77	.81	.81	.83	.87
Y402 FXIDX VALIUM HELPFUL 5I	.74	.71	.78	NA	NA	.74	.71	.78	.77	.78
Y403 F4IDX ATTITUDE RE TRNG	NA	.80	.76	NA	NA	NA	NA	NA	NA	.78
Interview Impact (INTW)										
Y404 F4IDX INTERVIEW IMPACT	NA	.69	.72	NA	NA	NA	NA	NA	NA	.70

These Cronbach alphas were computed for the entire set of respondents at each wave, not just the respondents who completed all 4 interviews. A few alphas were recomputed at Time 1 only for the 675 respondents who completed all 4 interviews. Differences were slight so it did not seem necessary to recompute all these reliability estimates.

363

APPENDIX M

EXACT PHRASINGS OF ITEMS IN INDICES AND SELECTED OTHER ITEMS'

AFFECT

Y277 FXIDX AFF HOP ANX

I am going to read you a list of problems or complaints that people sometimes have. Please tell me how much each has bothered you in the last 7 days, including today. How much were you bothered by...

X046	-nervousness or shakiness inside?
X048	-trembling?
X049	-suddenly scared for no reason?
X056	-feeling fearful?
X057	-heart pounding or racing?
X064	-having to avoid certain places or activities because they frighten you?
X067	-feeling tense or keyed up?

Y278 FXIDX AFF HOP DEP

How much were you bothered by...

X050	-a feeling of being trapped or caught?
X051	-crying easily?
X052	-blaming yourself for things?
X053	-feeling lonely?
X054	-worrying or stewing about things?
X055	-feeling no interest in things?
X059	-feeling blue?
X060	-thoughts of ending your life?
X065	-feeling hopeless about the future?
X071	-loss of sexual interest or pleasure?
X073	-poor appetite?

'See Appendix J for key to symbols

Y279 FXIDX AFF HOP SOMAT

How much were you bothered by...

X047	-pains in the heart or chest?
X058	-soreness of your muscles?
X061	-trouble getting your breath?
X062	-hot or cold spells?
X063	-numbness or tingling in parts of your body?
X066	-weakness in parts of your body?
X068	-heavy feelings in your arms and legs?
X070	-pains in the lower part of your back?
X072	-feeling low in energy or slowed down?

Y274 FXIDX AFF UM ANX-DEP

How much were you bothered by...

X050	-a feeling of being trapped or caught?
X051	-crying easily?
X053	-feeling lonely?
X059	-feeling blue?
X046	-nervousness or shakiness inside?
X054	-worrying or stewing about things?
X056	-feeling fearful?
X067	-feeling tense or keyed up?

Y276 FXIDX AFF UM CARDVAS

How much were you bothered by...

X047	-pains in the heart or chest?
X057	-heart pounding or racing?
X061	-trouble getting your breath?

Y271 FXIDX AFF ANGER

In the last 7 days, how much have you felt...

X077	-furiously angry?
X078	-mad at someone?
X079	-so angry that you felt like hitting someone?

Y280 P11DX AFF PO ANXIETY

I'm going to read you a list of symptoms. Please tell me how much each one has bothered or distressed you in the last 7 days.

X851 -nervousness or shakiness inside?
X852 -suddenly scared for no reason?
X855 -trembling?
X859 -feeling fearful?
X860 -feeling tense or keyed up?

Y281 P11DX AFF PO DEPRESS

Tell me how much each one has bothered or distressed you in the last 7 days...

X853 -a feeling of being trapped or caught?
X854 -crying easily?
X856 -blaming yourself for things?
X857 -feeling lonely?
X858 -feeling no interest in things?

365

QUALITY OF LIFE

Y202 FXIDX QOL SELF DT + AC

How do you feel about...

X270 -the way you handle problems that come up in your life?
X277 -what you are accomplishing in your life?
X281 -yourself?
X278 -your physical appearance, the way you look to others?
X284 -the extent to which you can adjust to changes in your life?

In the last 7 days, how much...

X131 -have you been the kind of person you wanted to be?
X151 -have you really enjoyed being the kind of person you've been--the way you've acted and felt?
X294 -has the kind of person you've been made you feel emotionally upset?

Y204 FXIDX QOL PL DT + AC

How do you feel about...

X273 -your (wife/husband), your marriage?
X274 -your romantic life?
X287 -your personal life?

In the last 7 days...

X130 -to what extent has your personal life been what you wanted?
X150 -how much have you really enjoyed your personal life?
X293 -how much has your personal life made you feel emotionally upset?

Y206 P1IDX QOL FR PL DT + AC

During the last 7 days/week you talked to FR, how do you think (he/she) felt about (his/her)... XX794 -personal life? By personal life I mean (his/her) relationships with people (he/she) feels close to?

X795 -(wife/husband), (his/her) marriage?
X796 -romantic life?

In the last 7 days, how much do you think...

X802 -(he/she) really enjoyed (his/her) personal life?
X803 -(his/her) personal life made (he/she) feel emotionally upset?

X804 -(FR) feels (he/she) has been doing in (his/her) personal life--how successful (he/she) has been in having (his/her) personal life be what (he/she) wanted?

Y208 P1IDX QOL PO PL DT + AC

How do you feel about...

X843 -your own personal life?
X844 -about your (wife/husband), your marriage?
X845 -your romantic life?

In the last 7 days how much...

X848 -have you really enjoyed your personal life?
X849 -has your personal life made you feel emotionally upset?

X850 -Now think about how well you've been doing in your personal life--how successful you've been in having it be what you wanted?

Y209 FXIDX QOL PEOPLE DT

How do you feel about...

X275 -your friends and acquaintances?
X276 -the people you work with--your co-workers?

Y210 FXIDX QOL MAT W-B DT

X280 -How do you feel about your (family) income?
X283 -How secure are you financially?

Y212 FXIDX QOL WL DT + AC

How do you feel about...

X271 -your work?
X286 -the work you do on the job--the work itself?

In the last 7 days...

X133 -to what extent have you achieved what you wanted in your work?
X153 -how much have you really enjoyed your work?
X296 -how much has your work made you feel emotionally upset?

Y214 W1IDX QOL FR WL DT + AC

During the last 7 days/week ago, how do you think FR felt about (his/her)...

X892 -work?
X894 -work on the job--the work itself?

X896 -(In the last 7 days/week ago) how much do you think (he/she) really enjoyed (his/her) work?

X897 -How much do you think (his/her) work has made (him/her) feel emotionally upset (in the last 7 days/weeks)?

X898 -Now think about how well (FR) feels (he/she) has been doing in (his/her) work--how successful has (he/she) been in having (his/her) work life be what (he/she) wanted?

Y216 W1IDX QOL WO WL DT + AC

How do you feel about...

X937   -your work?
X939   -the work you do on your job--the work itself?

In the last 7 days...

X941   -how much have you really enjoyed your work?
X942   -how much has your work made you feel emotionally upset?

X943   -Now think about how well you've been doing in your work. In the last 7 days, how successful have you been in having your work life be what you wanted?

Y217 P1IDX QOL FR WL DT

We would like your opinion about how FR felt about (his/her) life during the last 7 days/week you talked to (him/her). How do you think (he/she) felt about...

X798   -(his/her) work?
X800   -the work (he/she) does on the job--the work itself?

Y219 FXIDX QOL HLTH 3I + AC

X041   -How would you rate your health at present?

X044   -How much has physical health prevented you from doing the things you want to do?

X279   -How do you feel about your own health and physical condition?

X132   -To what extent have your health and physical condition been what you wanted them to be?

X152   -How much have you really enjoyed your health and physical condition?

X295   -How much has your health and physical condition made you feel emotionally upset.

Y220 FXIDX QOL SLEEP 3I

X045   -During the last 7 days, how well have you been sleeping?

X069   -In the last 7 days, how much were you bothered by a difficulty falling asleep or staying asleep?

X282   -How do you feel about the sleep you get?

Y222 FXIDX QOL LAW 2I + AC

X288   -How do you feel about your life as a whole?

X289   -Taking all these things together, how would you say things are these days?

X134   -To what extent has your life as a whole been what you wanted it to be?

X154   -How much have you really enjoyed your life as a whole?

X297   -How much has your life as a whole made you feel emotionally upset?

Y223 FXIDX QOL + A

In the last 7 days days, how much have you really enjoyed...

X150   -your personal life?
X151   -being the kind of person you've you really acted and felt?
X152   -your health and physical condition?
X153   -How much have you really enjoyed your work?
X154   -your life as a whole?

Y224 FXIDX QOL -A

X293 -How much has your personal life made you feel emotionally upset?

X294 -What about yourself? In the last 7 days, how much has the kind of person you've been made you feel emotionally upset?

X295 -How much has your health and physical condition made you feel emotionally upset?

X296 -In the last 7 days, how much has your work made you feel emotionally upset?

X297 -How much has your life as a whole made you feel emotionally upset?

Y255 FXIDX QOL COG

X130 -In the last 7 days, to what extent has your personal life been what you wanted it to be?

X131 -What about yourself--in the last 7 days how much have you been the kind of person you wanted to be?

X132 -To what extent have your health and physical condition been what you wanted them to be?

X133 -In the last 7 days, to what extent have you achieved what you wanted in your work?

X134 -To what extent has your life as a whole been what you wanted it to be?

SOCIAL SUPPORT

Y311 FXIDX SOC SUP ACTIVE

In the last 7 days, how much could you count on some one person to...

X228 -give you useful information and advice if you wanted it?
X229 -be a source of encouragement and reassurance?
X231 -listen if you wanted to confide about things that were important to you?

Y312 FXIDX SOC SUP ESTEEM

In the last 7 days, how much could you count on some one person to...

X233 -act in ways that showed he or she appreciated you?
X235 -treat you with respect?
X238 -show that he or she cared about you as a person?

Y314 FXIDX SOC SUP THERAPIST

X613 -When you visit your (KIND OF PROFESSIONAL) how much time is there to discuss with him or her all the things you want to talk about?

X615 -Would you say your (KIND OF PROFESSIONAL) is very cold towards people, somewhat cold towards people, neither cold nor warm, somewhat warm, or very warm towards people?

Y315 FXIDX SOC SUP VAL MD

X449 -When you visit your (KIND OF DOCTOR), how much time is there to discuss with him or her all the things you want to talk about?

X450 -Would you say your (KIND OF DOCTOR) is very cold towards people, somewhat cold towards people, neither cold nor warm, somewhat warm, or very warm towards people?

Y317 P1IDX SOC SUP FR ESTEEM

How much could (FR) count on some one person in (his/her) personal life to...

X823   -treat (him/her) with respect?
X825   -act in ways that show he or she appreciates what (he/she) does?
X826   -show that he or she cared about (him/her) as a person?

Y318 P1IDX SOC SUP FR TOTAL

In the last 7 (days/week) you saw or talked to FR, how much could ...

X831   -you count on (FR) to treat you with respect?
X832   -(FR) count on you to treat (him/her) with respect?
X833   -you count on (FR) to give you useful information and advice if you wanted it?
X834   -(FR) count on you to give (him/her) useful information and advice if (he/she) wanted it?
X835   -you count on (FR) to show that (he/she) cared about you as a person?
X836   -(FR) count on you to show that you cared about (him/her) as a person?

Y319 P1IDX SOC SUP PO to FR

How much could (FR) count on you to...

X832   -treat (him/her) with respect?
X834   -give (him/her) useful information and advice if (he/she) wanted it?
X836   -show that you cared about (him/her) as a person?

Y320 P1IDX SOC SUP FR to PO

How much could you count on (FR) to...

X831   -treat you with respect?
X833   -give you useful information and advice if you wanted it?
X835   -show that (he/she) cared about you as a person?

Y322 W1IDX SOC SUP ESTEEM

In the last 7 days, how much could FR count on some one person at work to...

X914   -treat (him/her) with respect?
X916   -act in ways that show he or she appreciates what (he/she) does?
X917   -show that he or she cared about (him/her) as a person?

Y323 W1IDX SOC SUP FR TOTAL

In the last 7 days/week, how much could...

X925   -you count on (FR) to treat you with respect?
X926   -FR count on you to treat (him/her) with respect?
X927   -you count on (FR) to give you useful information and advice if you wanted it?
X928   -FR count on you to give (him/her) useful information and advice if (he/she) wanted it?
X929   -you count on FR to show that (he/she) cared about you as a person?
X930   -FR count on you to show that you cared about (him/her) as a person?

Y324 W1IDX SOC SUP WO to FR

In the last 7 days/week, how much could FR count on you to...

X926   -treat (him/her) with respect?
X928   -give (him/her) useful information and advice if (he/she) wanted it?
X930   -show that you cared about (him/her) as a person?

Y325 FXIDX SOC SUP FR to WO

In the last 7 days/week, how much could you count on FR to...

X925   -treat you with respect?
X927   -give you useful information and advice if you wanted it?
X929   -show that he/she cared about you as a person?

SOCIAL CONFLICT

Y352 FXIDX IC (PO/WO items)

In the last 7 days, how much did some one person...

X230 —misunderstand the way you think and feel about things?

X236 —get on your nerves?
X237 —act in an unpleasant or angry manner toward you?
X240 —show that he or she disliked you?

Y353 P1IDX FR IC

In the last (7 days/week) you talked to (him/her), how much did someone...

X827 —get of FR's nerves?
X828 —misunderstand the way (he/she) thinks and feels about things?
X829 —in (his/her) personal life act in an unpleasant or angry manner toward (him/her)?
X830 —show that he or she disliked (him/her)?

Y354 P1IDX IC FR TOTAL

How much did...

X837 —FR get on your nerves?
X838 —you get on FR's nerves?
X839 —FR act in an unpleasant or angry manner towards you?
X840 —you act in an unpleasant or angry manner towards (him/her)?
X841 —FR show that (he/she) disliked you?
X842 —you show FR that you disliked (him/her)?

Y355 P1IDX IC PO to FR

How much did you...

X838 —get on FR's nerves?
X840 —act in an unpleasant or angry manner towards (him/her)?
X842 —show FR that you disliked (him/her)?

Y356 P1IDX IC FR to PO

How much did FR...

X837 —get on your nerves?
X839 —act in an unpleasant or angry manner towards you?
X841 —show that (he/she) disliked you?

Y357 W1IDX FR IC

In the last 7 days/week, how much did some one person...

X918 —get on FR's nerves?
X919 —misunderstand the way (he/she) thinks and feels about things?
X920 —at work act in an unpleasant or angry manner toward (him/her)?
X921 —at work show that he or she disliked (him/her)?

Y359 W1IDX IC FR TOTAL

How much did...

X931 —FR get on your nerves?
X932 —you get on FR's nerves?

COPING & DEFENSE

Y301 FXIDX C & D RELIGION

In the last 7 days, how much did you...

X090   -pray?
X105   -rely on your religious beliefs?

Y302 FXIDX C & D POS APPROACH

In the last 7 days, how much did you...

X094   -learn as much as possible about any problems you might have?
X100   -try to improve yourself so you could handle things better?
X107   -stand your ground and fight for what you wanted?
X108   -find new faith or some new truth about life?
X112   -rediscover what is important to life?
X115   -decide that you've changed or grown as a person as a result of something that might have happened?
X117   -view something that happened as a challenge?

Y303 FXIDX C & D REINTERPRET

In the last 7 days, how much did you...

X102   -try to find meaning in something that happened?
X104   -try to understand why something happened?

Y304 FXIDX C & D OTH HELP

In the last 7 days, how much did you...

X087   -talk to someone about your feelings?
X103   -ask someone you respect for advice?
X110   -get someone to help out with something?

371

CONTROL

Y371 FXIDX CON HAVE INT PL

X136   -How much has what happened in your personal life depended on what you said and did?
X142   -How much have things in your personal life been influenced or determined by you?

Y372 FXIDX CON HAVE INT EMOT

X299   -In the last 7 days how much have your feelings and emotions... depended on what you said and did?
X305   -In the last 7 days how much have your feelings and emotions been influenced or determined by yourself?

Y373 FXIDX CON WANT INT PL

X139   -How much would you like your personal life to depend on what you say and do?
X148   -How much would you personally like to be the one who influences or determines things?

Y374 FXIDX CON WANT INT EMOT

X302   -How much would you like your feeling and emotions to depend on what you say and do?
X311   -How much would you personally like to be the one who influences or determines your feelings and emotions?

Y375 FXIDX CON HAVE OTH PL

X135 —In the last 7 days, how much has what happened in your personal life depended on what other people said and did?

X141 —In the last 7 days, how much have things in your personal life been influenced or determined by other people?

Y376 FXIDX CON HAVE OTH EMOT

X298 —In the last 7 days, how much have your feelings and emotions depended on what other people said and did?

X304 —In the last 7 days, how much have your feelings and emotions been influenced or determined by other people?

Y377 FXIDX CON WANT OTH PL

X138 —How much would you like what happens in your personal life to depend on what other people say and do?

X147 —How much would you like things in your personal life to be influenced or determined by other people?

Y378 FXIDX CON WANT OTH EMOT

X301 —How much would you like your feelings and emotions to depend on what other people say and do?

X310 —How much would you like your feelings and emotions to be influenced or determined by other people?

Y379 FXIDX CON HAVE CHC PL

In the last 7 days...

X137 —how much has your personal life depended on luck, either good or bad?

X143 —How much have things in your personal life depended by chance?

Y380 FXIDX CON HAVE CHC EMOT

In the last 7 days...

X300 —how much have your feelings and emotions depended on luck, either good or bad?

X306 —how much have your feelings and emotions been influenced and determined by chance?

Y381 FXIDX CON WANT CHC PL

X140 —How much would you like your personal life to depend on luck?

X149 —How much would you like things in your personal life to be influenced or determined by chance?

Y382 FXIDX CON WANT CHC EMOT

X303 —How much would you like your feelings and emotions to depend on luck?

X312 —How much would you like your feelings and emotions to be influenced or determined by chance?

ROLE CONFLICT

Y241 FXIDX ROLE CONFLICT WL

In the last 7 days, how much did key people you work with...

X221   -ask you to do things that conflicted with your own sense of what should be done?
X222   -give you things to do that conflicted with one another?
X223   -see things about your job differently from the way you do?
X224   -give you things to do which conflicted with other work you had to do?

ROLE AMBIGUITY

Y242 FXIDX ROLE AMB WL

In the last 7 days, how sure or unsure were you about....

X209   -whether others would approve of the way you were doing your work?
X210   -whether you were doing the right things on your job?
X211   -whether you could keep up with all the responsibilities and demands of your job?
X212   -whether you were making the right decisions on your job?
X213   -what others expected of you at work?

Y243 FXIDX ROLE AMB PL

In the last 7 days, how sure or unsure have you been about whether....

X119   -the people in your personal life would approve of the way you were doing things?
X120   -you were doing the right things in your personal life?
X121   -you could keep up with all the responsibilities and demands in your personal life?
X122   -you were making the right decisions in your personal life?
X123   -about what others expected of you in your personal life?

373

PERFORMANCE

Y245 FXIDX TCH PERF WL

In the last 7 days, how well were you doing at...

X215   -handling the responsibilities and daily demands of your work?
X216   -making the right decisions?
X219   -performing without mistakes?
X220   -getting things done on time?

Y246 FXIDX SOC PERF WL

In the last 7 days, how well were you doing at...

X214   -getting along with others at work?
X217   -avoiding arguing with others?
X218   -handling disagreements by compromising and meeting other people half-way?

Y249 W1IDX TCH PERF(ALL) FR WL

How do you think FR did each of the following things at work in the last week?

X899   -working without unnecessary supervision?
X900   -performing without mistakes?
X901   -getting things done on time?
X903   -handling responsibilities and daily demands?
X904   -making the right decisions?
X908   -accepting responsibility for (his/her) actions and behaviors?
X909   -staying level headed?
X912   -doing a good job or handling all the things required of (him/her) at work?

Y251 W1IDX SOC PERF(ALL) FR WL

Tell me how well you think FR did each of the following things at work in the last 7 days...

X902   -getting along with others?
X905   -avoiding arguing with others at work?
X906   -handling disagreements by compromising and meeting people half-way?
X907   -being calm at work?
X909   -staying level headed?
X910   -giving people the time and attention they need?
X911   -being pleasant?
X913   -acting in a relaxed manner?

Y253 FXIDX TCH PERF PL

In the last 7 days, how well have you been doing the following things in your personal life?

X126   -handling responsibilities and daily demands in your personal life?
X127   -making the right decisions?

Y254 FXIDX SOC PERF PL

In the last 7 days, how well have you been doing the following things in your personal life?

X125   -getting along with others in your personal life?
X128   -avoiding arguing with others?
X129   -handling disagreements by compromising and meeting other people halfway?

Y257 P1IDX TCH PERF(ALL) FR PL

In the last 7 days, how well did FR do in...

X809   -handling responsibilities and daily demands?
X810   -making the right decisions?
X814   -accepting responsibilities for (his/her) own actions and behaviors?
X818   -doing a good job of handling all of the things required of (him/her) in (his/her) personal life?

Y259 P1IDX SOC PERF(ALL) FR PL

In the last 7 days, how well did FR do in...

X808   -getting along with others in (his/her) personal life?
X811   -avoiding arguing with others?
X812   -handling disagreements by compromising and meeting other people half way?
X813   -being calm in (his/her) personal life?
X815   -staying level-headed?
X817   -being pleasant?
X819   -acting in a relaxed manner?

Y260 P1IDX HOME PERF FR PL

In the last 7 days, how well did FR do in...

X805   -working around the house or apartment?
X806   -handling children?
X807   -being affectionate?
X816   -giving people the time and attention they need?

INTERVIEWER RATINGS

Y291 FXIDX INTWR FR SINCERE

During the interview, how much did R appear to be...

X726   -frank in (his/her) answers?
X730   -interested in providing useful answers?

Y292 FXIDX INTWR FR AFFECT

During the interview, how much did R appear to be...

X727   -tense, nervous, or jittery?
X728   -sad, blue, or depressed?

Y293 P1IDX INTWR PO SINCERE

During the interview, how much did R appear to be...

X868   -frank in (his/her) answers?
X872   -interested in providing useful answers?

Y294 W1IDX INTWR WO SINCERE

During the interview, how much did R appear to be...

X945   -frank in (his/her) answers?
X949   -interested in providing useful answers?

ATTITUDE TOWARDS TRANQUILIZERS

Y401 FXIDX VALIUM HELPFUL 2I

X454   -To what extent (does/did) (MEDICATION) make you feel better?

X455   -How helpful (do/did) you find (MEDICATION)?

Y402 FXIDX VALIUM HELPFUL 5I

X454   -To what extent (does/did) (MEDICATION) make you feel better?

X455   -How helpful (do/did) you find (MEDICATION)?

X456   -And if you (don't/didn't) take your (MEDICATION) how much discomfort (do/did) you feel?

X457   -Think about how (MEDICATION) affects your control over your emotions. Does it increase your control, decrease it, or not really affect it at all?

X458   -Think about how it affects your ability to deal with problems in your life. Does it increase your ability to deal with them, decrease it, or not really affect it at all?

Y403 F4IDX ATTITUDE RE TRNQ (at t4 only)

4695   -Based on what you know about tranquilizers, do you generally approve or generally disapprove of the present use of them, or are you undecided?

I'm going to read you some statements about tranquilizers. After I read each one, I want you to tell me how much you agree or disagree with the statement.

4697   -Using tranquilizers just prevents people from working out their problems for themselves.

4699   -Tranquilizers help people regain control over the stresses in their lives.

4700   -It is better to use willpower to solve problems than it is to use tranquilizers.

4701   -Tranquilizers cause people to lose control over what they do?

4702   -Tranquilizers are safe to take.

INTERVIEWER IMPACT

Y404 F4IDX INTERVIEW IMPACT (only at t4)

We are very interested in your opinion about what is has been like to be interviewed. We're interested in knowing both positive and negative things.

4707   -To what extent has being interviewed affected your life?

4708   -Have you done anything different in your life as a result of these interviews?

4709   -How much have you learned about yourself by participating in these interviews?

CAFFEINE

Y411 FXIDX MG CAFENE/DAY L7D

X644 —On the average, how many cups of regular coffee, by that I mean caffeinated coffee, did you drink each day during the past 7 days? (multiply times 171 mg)

X645 —On the average, how many cups of tea did you drink each day during the past 7 days? (multiply times 64 mg).

X646 —On the average, about how many cola drinks did you have each day during the past 7 days? (multiply times 47 mg).

ALCOHOL

Y412 FXIDX #ALC DRINKS L7D (X617 x X621)

X617 —I would like to ask you about alcoholic beverages—that is, wine, beer, and liquor. Again, think back over the last 7 days. On how many of those days did you drink any alcoholic beverages?

X621 —In the last 7 days, on the days that you drank alcoholic beverages, how many drinks did you usually have? By drink I mean shot or glass.

Y413 FXIDX #ALC DRNKS LST MO (X617 x X621) x 4.3 or X618 x X619)

X618 —In the last month, how many days did you have any alcoholic beverages?

X619 —When you drink alcoholic beverages, how many drinks do you usually have per day? By drink I mean a shot or a glass.

Appendix N

Codes for Open-Ended Measures'

Table of Contents

Positive Events or Conditions.................... N2

Negative Events or Conditions.................... N4

Salience of Other People: Positive Context N6

Salience of Other People: Negative Context N7

Reasons for Taking Medications .... N8(N9)

Decision Rule for Taking Medications .... N8(N9)

Health Master Code N9

Reasons for Not Filling Prescription N20

Reasons Why Tranquilizers are Used Too Much N21

'Taken directly from the coding instruction manual.

Positive Events or Conditions   (VY005)

Wave I: Refer to A4, A5, A9, B8, Thumbnail, PO B8, and events calendar
Waves II, III, and IV: Refer to A3, A4, A8, B8, Thumbnail, PO B8, and events calendar

We want to rate their current level of happiness. If it is obvious that an event or condition which R mentioned is no longer a source of happiness then it should be ignored.

When in doubt, code the lower number of the two which you might be considering.

4 = A major positive event or condition that is a source of great happiness that R might expect to last 5 or more years. Include own marriage, own engagement, birth of own child.

3 = A major positive event or condition or a combination of events (or conditions) which are a source of great happiness that R might not expect to last 5 years. Note: These events are no less positive than those coded 4, they are simply expected to last longer.

2 = (a) No major positive event or condition that is a source of great happiness but several less major positive events that add up (creating a lot of happiness) or (b) a positive event or condition of magnitude that falls between (1) & (3) which creates a lot of happiness.

1 = Some positive event(s) that is(are) not a source of great or long lasting happiness.

0 = none of the above

7 = other

Examples:

an event about which R was "ecstatic" = 3

falling in love = 3

recovering from a life threatening event which makes R very thankful to be alive = 3

recovering from a life threatening event = 2

Examples Continued

immediate family member doing very well = 2

immediate family member doing ok = 1

"I love my career" = 2

"I like my career" = 1

"A wonderful Father's day and a big anniversary celebration the kids gave us" = 2

"A wonderful Father's day and our anniversary" = 2

"Father's day and a big anniversary celebration the kids gave us" = 1

"a wonderful Father's day" =1

"Father's day and our anniversary" = 1

strong religious faith explicitly discussed by R as a source of happiness = 2

"I'm happy in my religion" = 2

family reunion = 1

"vacation in Las Vegas and son graduated preschool and I got 2 job offers" = 1

"granddaughter got married and nephew got married and twins were born to my niece and new neighbors moved in" = 1

"I feel really close to my children and this makes me very happy" = 2

"my closeness to my children" = 1

Negative Events or Conditions (VT007)

Wave I: Refer to A4, A5, A9, B8, Thumbnail, PO B8, and events calendar
Wave II, III, and IV: Refer to A3, A4, A8, B8, Thumbnail, PO B8, and events calendar

We want to rate their current level of distress. If it is obvious that an event or condition which R mentioned is no longer a source of distress then it should be ignored.

When in doubt, code the lower number of the two which you might be considering.

4 = A major problem likely to last 5 or more years.

3 = A major problem or a combination of problems which produce major negative impact but are likely to be resolved in less than 5 years. Note: These problems are no less negative than these coded 4, they are simply expected to last longer.

2 = (a) No one major problem but several non-major problems that add up (creating a lot of distress) or (b) a problem of a magnitude that falls between (1) & (3) which creates a lot of distress.

1 = Some minor problems which are not a source of major distress.

0 = none of the above

7 = other

Examples:

serious illness which is quite likely to kill R within 5 years = 4

serious illness that keeps R from working (ever or at least 5 years) and which might kill R = 4

serious illness that keeps R from working preferred job but won't kill R and R can be retrained = 3

"I had some surgery and got quite far behind in my work" = 2

"I missed a few days of work because I had the flu" = 1

chronic condition which is very bad and the evidence indicates that it will continue (e.g. horrible problems with spouse and in-laws for 12 years with no sign of plans to leave marriage) = 4

death of a spouse or other close relative or close friend = 3

traumatic loss of job = 3

divorce = 3

Examples Continued

loss of life savings = 3

loss of home and break-up of family = 3

health condition that had kept R bedridden for some time = 3

R fails exam that is crucial to career but can take the exam again = 2

PO says, "R is having horrible marriage problems and is seriously considering getting divorced" = 2

"Marital problems. I've seen an attorney. He has a drinking problem, gotten worse last couple of years. My grandmother has been seriously ill. I had bladder surgery." = 2

death of in-laws or friend = 2

"I got sued for malpractice and lost the case and my license so I'll never be able to practice medicine again" = 4

"I got laid off and I'm really depressed because I can't find another job and my debts are really piling up" = 3

laid off and this causes problems = 2

got laid off and got another job = 1

money problems but they aren't really serious = 1

81 year old with arthritis who had (successful) eye operation = 1

arrangement with brother-in-law didn't work out = 1

Salience of Other People   (VY006)

Positive Context

Wave I: Refer to A4, A5, & B8
Waves II, III, IV: Refer to A3, A4, & B8

Number of other people for whom R has some affection and/or respect whom R mentions in a positive context. R must have a personal relationship with the individual.

0 = none mentioned

1 = one mentioned

2 = 2 or more mentioned

In A4 & A5, it should be obvious if context is positive or negative by the way the questions are phrased (i.e., A4 = pleasant events, A5 = unpleasant events). For B8, however, the context can often be unclear. For example, one R stated, "I was thinking about my children and my family." In this case, you could look at R's ratings at B7. If R had rated his personal life and life as a whole as "5's" it would be clear that R had been thinking of his family in a positive context. If these ratings are ambiguous, however, then these mentions of people should be ignored in your counts.

Examples: son graduated = 1

husband got job = 1

"I enjoy being married" = 1

"I was thinking about how lovely my son's house is" = 1

"contact with doctor whom I respect and have every confidence in" = 1

"my nephew's wedding; two nieces graduated from college" = 2

family reunion = 2

"I had a fortune teller come over" = 0

"I was glad Reagan lived" = 0

Salience of Other People (VY008)

Negative Context

Wave I: Refer to A4, A5, & B8
Waves II, III, IV: Refer to A3, A4, & B8

Number of other people for whom R has some affection and/or respect whom R mentions in a negative context.

0 = none mentioned

1 = one mentioned

2 = 2 or more mentioned

In A4 & A5, it should be obvious if context is positive or negative by the way the questions are phrased (i.e., A4 = pleasant events, A5 = unpleasant events). For B8, however, the context can often be unclear. For example, one R stated, "I was thinking about my children and my family." In this case, you could look at R's ratings at B7. If R had rated his personal life and life as a whole as "5's" it would be clear that R had been thinking of his family in a positive context. If these ratings are ambiguous, however, then these mentions of people should by ignored in your counts.

Examples: "my grandchildren fight but they get over it" = 2

"a woman hit us head on and my gradson was killed" = 1

"I don't have any friends" = 0

F8. For what reason (are/were) you taking it? (VY017-VY021)

Use HEALTH MASTER CODE (see pages N9-N19)

F22. How (do/did) you decide when to take (MEDICATION)? (VY022-VY026)

Use HEALTH MASTER CODE (see pages N9-N19)

HEALTH MASTER CODE (VY009, VY010, VY011, VY012)

Several examples have been provided for each category. When R mentions a health problem which is not given in the code, refer to alphabetic ICD book. Then using the number given, find the code.
Example: deuteranomaly 368.5
code 065 includes ICD 360-389 so code this response as 065

If R mentions more than four (or 5 in F8 and F22), the "most serious" should be coded, i.e., diseases before symptoms, arthritis before a cold, high blood pressure before a tooth ache.

If R mentions 2 diseases that fall in the same category, code both. (Unless R mentions more than 4, then only use the same code once.) "I have a cold and asthma." should be coded 080 and 080.

010 Infections and parasitic diseases (ICD 001-139)
Includes diseases generally recognized as communicable or transmittable, e.g., cholera, bacterial, and protozoal intestinal diseases, TB, shingles, polio, meningitis due to virus, measles, mumps, syphilis, worms, and food poisoning (excludes influenza - see 080).

020 Neoplasms (ICD 140-239)
Include cancers and growths, both malignant and benign. If R says tumor in stomach, use this code.

030 Endocrine, nutritional and metabolic diseases and immunity disorders (ICD 240-279)
Includes thyroid, goiter, pituitary, hormones, ovaries, testes, diabetes, vitamin deficiencies, obesity, and malnutrition (excludes anemia, see 040).

040 Diseases of the blood and blood forming organs (ICD 280-289)
Includes iron deficiency, anemia, coagulation defects, aplastic anemia, and other diseases of the blood and the blood forming organs.

050 Mental Disorders (ICD 290-319 only if none of the more specific categories below apply; may also want to see 160-166).

051 tension, anxiety, nerves, "keyed up"

052 depression, blues, sadness

053 fears, phobias, apprehension

054 upset or emotional

055 alcohol withdrawal or dependence or tremors, delirium tremens, agitation or restlessness associated with alcohol withdrawal or dependence

056 withdrawal from Valium or dependence on Valium

057 withdrawal from other prescribed medication or dependence on other prescribed medication (e.g. Darvon, Tranxene)

058 withdrawal from nonprescribed drug or dependence on nonprescribed drug (e.g. heroin, PCP)

059 sleep disorders, insomnia, any problems with falling to sleep

060 Diseases of the nervous system (ICD 320-359 except as noted below) Includes bacterial meningitis, Parkinson's disease, narcolepsy, disorders of the facial nerves, muscular dystrophy, cerebral palsy, and spasticity due to neuron disorders.

061 epilepsy (ICD 345)

062 migraines (ICD 346; for headaches, see 173)

063 paraplegia & quadraplegia

065 Diseases of the sense organs (ICD 360-389) Includes glaucoma, blindness, deafness, and other disorders of the eyes and ears

070 Diseases of the circulatory system (ICD 390-459 except as noted below) Includes varicose veins, hemorrhoids, rheumatic fever, thrombosis, phlebitis, irregular heart beat, and heart murmur

071 arteriosclerosis and hardening of the arteries. (ICD 440)

072 hypertension and high blood pressure (ICD 401-405) (equivalent)

073 ischaemic heart disease, angina pectoris, myocardial infarction and heart attack. (ICD 410-414)

074 stroke, brain hemorrhage, and cerebravascular disease (ICD 430-438)

080 Diseases of the respiratory system (ICD 460-519) Includes the common cold, tonsillitis, laryngitis, bronchitis, pneumonia, influenza, and chronic obstructive pulmonary diseases like asthma and emphysema; allergies including hay fever

090 Diseases of the digestive system (ICD 520-579 except as noted below) Includes appendicitis, hernia, diseases of the intestines, liver disease, cirrhosis, and gallbladder disease

091 diseases of the tooth, jaws, and gums (ICD 520-529)

092 gastric, duodenal, and peptic ulcers and gastritis (ICD 530-535)

093 stomach disorders including indigestion, habitual vomiting (unless due to pregnancy), and acid stomach (ICD 536-537)

094 colitis, ileitis, irritable bowel, constipation, and diarrhea (ICD 555-558)

100 Diseases of the genitourinary system (ICD 580-629 except as noted below) Includes renal or kidney failure, bladder infections, disorders of the kidneys, bladder, or urethra

101 diseases of the male or female genital organs (ICD 600-626, 628-629) includes infertility, prostate problems, endometriosis, ovary, vaginal, or uterine problems

102 menopausal or post menopausal disorders or symptoms (e.g. cramps or flushing if due to these conditions) (ICD 627)

---

* USE 160-177 ONLY WHEN DISEASE CATEGORIES 100-140, 180-190 ARE INSUFFICIENT

160 Symptoms, signs, and ill-defined conditions (ICD 780-789)
Use this general code only when none of the below are relevant. This code refers to unspecified pain.

161 coma, stupor, unconsciousness

162 hallucinations

163 blackout, fainting, collapse, and syncope

164 convulsions (except epilepsy; see 061)

165 dizziness, giddiness, vertigo

166 lethargy, malaise, fatigue (code insomnia as 059)

167 shaking

170 symptoms involving nervous and musculoskeletal systems (ICD 781)

171 symptoms involving skin (ICD 782)
Includes swelling (localized), pallor, flushing, burning, numbness, tingling

172 symptoms involving nutrition, metabolism, and development (ICD 783)
Includes anorexia, abnormal gain or loss of weight, and abnormal appetite (hungry or not hungry)

173 symptoms involving head and neck (ICD 784)
Includes headache, hoarseness, and nosebleed

174 symptoms involving cardiovascular system (ICD 785)
Includes palpitations, gangrene and heart beating fast or hard

175 symptoms involving respiratory system (ICD 786)
Includes shortness of breath, cough, chest pain, and hyperventilation

176 symptoms involving digestive system (ICD 787)
Includes nausea, vomiting, heartburn, gas pain, and difficulty swallowing

177 symptoms involving urinary system (ICD 788)
Includes frequent or abnormal urination

180 Injury and poisoning (ICD 800-999)
Includes fractures, dislocations, open wounds, burns, poisoning, and radiation damage (but excludes sprains and strains of joints and muscles which are coded as 131).

190 Surgery, dialysis (ICD V50-59)
Includes any kind of surgery or dialysis treatment
Note: If the surgery "cured" the disease, code 190 only. If it did not (or if unclear) code 190 and the relevant disease. "I had open heart surgery" should be coded 190 and 073.

---

110 Complications of pregnancy, childbirth and the puerperium (ICD 630-676)
Includes abortion, normal childbirths and childbirths with complications

120 Diseases of the skin and subcutaneous tissue (ICD 680-709)
Includes skin infections, corns, skin ulcers, psoriasis, warts, acne, dermatitis, hives, and rash.

130 Diseases of the musculoskeletal system and connective tissue (ICD 710-739) except as noted below)
Includes rheumatoid arthritis, neuritis, bone and joint disorders, swelling due to arthritis

131 pulled back, sore muscles, stiff muscles, sore back, sprains and strains of muscles and joints, and muscle spasms (ICD 724)

132 bursitis, tendonitis, swelling due to either of these (ICD 727)

140 Congenital anomalies (ICD 740-759)
Includes spina bifida and congenital anomalities of the heart or any other part of the body.

Use only for F8 and F22

More Mental Disorders

501 anger, temper, "pissed off"
502 to keep calm, relax, "keep cool"
503 cry, want to cry
504 boredom
505 low self esteem, feelings of insecurity
506 unspecified discomfort; uneasy feeling

Use only for F8 and F22

Situational

601 tried other things that didn't work, so trying the medication
602 stressful situation (e.g. tragedy in family, financial problems, job stress, etc.)
603 stressed but not clear if it is due to a situation, "can't cope" but source of problem is not specified
604 used to prevent an anticipated emotional state
605 used to prevent an anticipated situation
606 to cope with anticipated situation

Use only for F8 and F22

Requested by Other

701 requested by health care professional (e.g. MD,nurse, psychiatrist counselor, psychologist)
702 requested by non-professional (e.g. spouse, friend, relative)
703 requested by unspecified other

Use only for F22

801 as prescribed; either the box is checked or R says so
802 R follows regular rules (e.g. "every night before bed"; "three times a day")
803 R takes as needed including "how I think I should take it"

850 mentions concern about addiction
860 to get high

996. no physical problems or diseases
997. Other

998. DK
999. NA

000. Inap, no further mention

383

SOME EXAMPLES OF CODING FOR F8 and F22

F8 "He (the dermatologist) wasn't sure it was allergy or nerves." This statement is not definite to qualify for coding either as allergy or nerves. It would be ignored.

F8 "I need help in sleeping if I am tense"--Code for both sleeping (059) and being tense (051).

F8 "In the past year basically to relax to sleep." Code as (502) and (059).

F8 "For my heart palpitations and in conjunction with Tedral for asthma. Take Valium to slow down heart." Code as (174) and (080).

F8 "Nervousness. I guess it's tension. She said to take it when I'm extremely tense." Code as (051) and (703).

F8 "For my shoulder. Because the muscles were tight and this would feel like a heart attack although I wasn't having a heart attack. It relaxed the muscles." Code as (131).

F8 "To control tension which triggers the stomach." Code as (051) and (176).

F8 "To keep stomach calm - hiatal hernia. If it's calm, I digest my food." Code as (090).

F8 "Nervousness. Being uptight. Nerves. Putting stress on heart. Years ago given to me for hyperthyroid condition." Code as (051) and (174), but ignore thyroid condition because that is a health condition which has not bothered R in last 6 weeks.

F22 "When I feel myself getting keyed up or great anger." Code as (051) and (501).

F22 "When I get nervous. I can feel it coming on - shaking - only lasts 5-10 minutes." Code as (051) and (167).

F22 "You feel like your head is a little loose. My head feels a little sore and I feel uneasy possibly even feel a little stress." Code as (506), (173), and (603).

F22 "When I rant and rave and cry." Code as (501) and (503).

F22 "The doctor prescribed it 3 times a day." Code as (801).

F22 "If I feel that my nervousness or anxiety will cause a problem on the job, I take half a pill." Code as (051) and (605) because the person took the medicine partly in association with an anticipated problem on the job.

F22 "Every night before bed." Code as (802) and (059) since use is associated with sleep.

F22 "I take it before I give a speech to avoid getting anxious." Code as (604).

F22 "I take it to avoid fighting with my mother-in-law." Code as (605).

F7a. **Why did you stop taking it?** (VY014, VY015, VY016)

> If more than three reasons mentioned, code first reason mentioned from each group.

NO LONGER A PROBLEM

01. R's health or somatic problem(s) went away (include being tired) and R clearly indicates that the medication was responsible for its disappearance

02. R's health or somatic problem(s) went away (include being tired) (no mention of this being due to medication)

03. Solved specified problem(s) not related to R's health

04. Problem(s) have not come up recently but could come back—may be health (e.g., stomach problems or muscle spasms) or social-psychological problem (e.g., problem at work or with other people) (If in doubt as to if the problem will come back, use code 03.)

05. Under less stress

06. Don't need any more—NEC; unspecified problem(s) went away

PROBLEM WITH USING DRUG

11. Addictive, habit-forming, dependence -- R knows this from own use

12. Addictive, habit-forming, dependence -- R knows this from experience of friends or family

13. Addictive, habit-forming, dependence -- 11 & 12 do not apply

14. Other undesirable side effects (e.g., foggy head, fatigue, loss of control)

15. Believes drug was not effective; did not work well

16. Heard negative/controversial reports in media

17. Psychopharmacological Calvinism; morally wrong to take drug; guilt; mental crutch

18. R is pregnant

F7a. Continued

REASONS RELATED TO OTHER PERSONS

21. Health professional instructed to stop

22. Non-medical person recommended stopping

23. Physician switched to a different drug for the same problem

24. No faith in physician

USING ANOTHER DRUG OR METHOD

31. Using another medicine instead (if instructed by physician code 23)

32. Using non-prescription drug instead (e.g., alcohol, street drugs)

33. Took care of problem by changing diet

34. Using other behavioral coping (except 33)

MISCELLANEOUS

81. Cost; too expensive

82. Ran out of prescription (if mention of intention to refill code 83)

83. Ran out of prescription but intend to refill

84. Too hard to remember to take

90. Didn't think it was necessary

96. No reason; "just stopped"

97. Other

98. DK

99. NA

00. InaP,   or 9
         1 in F7; no further mention

F51, F53, F55. (You said you haven't taken any (ENTER NAME OF MEDICATION) since you were last interviewed.) Why haven't you been taking it?
(VY032, VY033, VY035, VY036, VY038, VY039)

> If more than 2 reasons mentioned, code first reason mentioned from each group.

NO LONGER A PROBLEM

01. R's health or somatic problem(s) went away (include being tired) and R clearly indicates that the medication was responsible for its disappearance

02. R's health or somatic problem(s) went away (include being tired) (no mention of this being due to medication)

03. Solved specified problem(s) not related to R's health

04. Problem(s) have not come up recently but could come back—may be health (e.g., stomach problems or muscle spasms) or social-psychological problem (e.g., problem at work or with other people) (If in doubt as to if the problem will come back, use code 03.) $01, 02, 03$

05. Under less stress

06. Don't need any more—NEC; unspecified problem(s) went away

PROBLEM WITH USING DRUG

11. Addictive, habit-forming, dependence — R knows this from own use

12. Addictive, habit-forming, dependence — R knows this from experience of friends or family

13. Addictive, habit-forming, dependence — 11 & 12 do not apply

14. Other undesirable side effects (e.g., foggy head, fatigue, loss of control)

15. Believes drug was not effective, did not work well

16. Heard negative/controversial reports in media

17. Psychopharmacological Calvinism; morally wrong to take drug; guilt; mental crutch

18. R is pregnant

F51. Continued

REASONS RELATED TO OTHER PERSONS

21. Health professional instructed to stop

22. Non-medical person recommended stopping

23. Physician switched to a different drug for the same problem

24. No faith in physician

USING ANOTHER DRUG OR METHOD

31. Using another medicine instead (if instructed by physician code 23)

32. Using non-prescription drug instead (e.g., alcohol, street drugs)

33. Took care of problem by changing diet

34. Using other behavioral coping (except 33)

MISCELLANEOUS

81. Cost; too expensive

82. Ran out of prescription (if mention of intention to refill code 83)

83. Ran out of prescription but intend to refill

84. Too hard to remember to take

90. Didn't think it was necessary

96. No reason; "just stopped"

97. Other

98. DK
99. NA

00. Insp, Wave I, 1 in 14; no further mention

H6d. Why didn't you have the prescription filled for (MEDICATION)?

01. Not convenient
02. Already had some
03. Cost or too expensive
04. Didn't need or symptoms went away
05. Didn't want to take that kind of medication (except 06 or 07)
06. Addictive, habit forming or dependence
07. Afraid of side effects (except 06)
08. Don't want to take any kind of medication; anti-drug
09. Took a different medication; had a better medication
10. not effective
11. Used another technique to deal with the problem
12. Didn't trust doctor's diagnosis
13. Could be obtained without a prescription
14. Doctor changed prescription
15. Second doctor told R not to take it

97. Other
98. Don't know
99. NA
00. Inap. WaveII-III; 5, 8 or 9 in H6; no further mention

Note: If more than 6 medications are mentioned and Valium is listed beyond f, code H6d for Valium in the f. position

---

H10a. Why do you say that tranquilizers are used too much? (VY058, VY059)

Circle up to two reasons given. If more than two, choose the two most different from each other. If there are still too many choices, select the first two most different.

HEALTH CARE PRACTITIONERS

01. MD's, health care practitioners use tranquilizers to control women instead of trying to help them with their problems; use it to shut them up or to avoid spending time with them

02. MD's health care practitioners use tranquilizers to control the institutionalized instead of trying to help them with their problems; use it to shut them up or avoid spending time with them

03. MD's, health care practitioners use tranquilizers to control the elderly instead of trying to help them with their problems; use it to shut them up or to avoid spending time with them

04. MDs, health care practitioners use tranquilizers to control patients instead of trying to help their patients with their problems; use it to shut up their patients, or to avoid spending time with them (when 01-03 are not used)

05. MDs, health care practitioners prescribe too much, too freely, too easily; tranquilizers are too easy to get from MDs; MDs too often prescribe them; "Because they are easily prescribed" (Mention of easy to get but no mention of MDs, see code 90)

HEALTH EFFECTS
10. Bad for you; hurts you (NA whether physically, medically, or socially)
11. They can make you physically ill; bad for your physical health or bad for your health (where health is not specified as physical or mental)

12. They can kill you

13. People use them to commit suicide

14. Bad for your mental health; can drive you insane or crazy, make you mentally ill

15. Addictive, habit forming; foster dependence; "People get hooked on them"; "I think you can become dependent on tranquilizers"; "Can make you a junkie" (See also code 23)

16. Mention of overdose or that people take more than the prescribed amount at any one time (See also code 16)

17. People overuse them; take them too frequently, too often (See also code 15)

H10a. Continued

18. Too many people use them

19. Dangerous when combined with alcohol

20. Turns people into zombies; makes them "spaced out", "not all there", puts their "head in another place"

NEEDED VS. ALTERNATIVE

21. People take the medicine instead of using other means for dealing with their problems; better to rely on self or on other means (e.g. diet, lifestyle)

22. People take them like candy

23. People rely on them; "Everyone relies on them"

24. People don't really need them; not everyone who takes them needs them; "Some people could do without them"

25. Used as a cure-all

26. They don't work

27. Don't believe they should be used

28. It's an easy way out, people take them to avoid or escape their problems

29. Not sure tranquilizers should be used, are appropriate

30. Tranquilizers cover up or hide the real problem

31. Tranquilizers can be helpful but they are used too much
32. It's a crutch
33. They're abused; misused
LEADS TO BAD BEHAVIOR

41. Can lead to crime or other antisocial behavior

42. People take them to get high, spaced out

43. People sell them

44. Interferes with daily performance, job performance, leads to accidents

45. Sets a bad example for the young

continued next page

387

H10a Continued

I KNOW ABOUT IT FROM...

51. Own use

52. Use by people R knows

53. R heard about it on TV or radio

54. R read about it in newspaper, magazine, or other printed media

55. R heard about it from people s/he knows, but there is no mention that these individuals use tranquilizers; "From people talking"

56. Any source except those described in 51-55; "From what I hear about it.

90. Tranquilizers are too easy to get; "They're too easy for kids to get hold of"
91. Too many tranquilizers are available
97. OTHER
92. The structure of our society makes them necessary
95. DK
99. NA
00. Inap, WaveII-III; 2, 3, 8 or 9 in H10, no further mention

Examples for H10a coding

1) "Because I hear overdose, overdose from friends winding up in the hospital" -- 16 and 52

2) "I think it's detrimental to their health, minds, and so forth. I wouldn't have them. They get to using them and then think they have to have them" -- 11, 14, 15

3) "Just from what I've heard and read" -- 56, 54

Appendix O

Common Therapeutic Uses and Drug Effects for
Drugs on Interview Follow-up List at Wave I[1]

	Similar to Valium	Opposite to Valium	Both Similar and Opposite to Valium	TOTALS
Antihistamines	27	0	24	51
Anticholinergics	26	0	1	27
Muscle Relaxants	5	0	1	6
Antiarrythmics	53	0	0	53
Antihypertensives	95	0	0	95
Opiate Alkaloids & Synthetic Derivatives	134	0	0	134
Non-opiate Analgesics	10	0	0	10
Anticonvulsants	13	0	0	13
Antidepressants	36	0	0	36
Anti-psychotics Phenothiazine	17	0	1	18
Others	7	0	0	7
Stimulants	0	12	0	12
Benzodiazepines	477 (406 Valium)	0	0	477
Barbiturates	24	0	0	24
Other anti-anxiety/ sedative hypnotics	11	0	0	11
Diuretics	14	0	0	14
Anti-diarrheal	10	0	0	10
Other gastro-intestinal (including Cimetidine)	20	0	1	21
Antitussives	19	0	3	22
Expectorants	3	1	0	4
Oral Decongestants	0	2	27	29
TOTALS	1,001	15	58	1074
% OF ALL MENTIONS OF DRUGS	82% (72% excluding Valium)	9%	30%	67% (59% excluding Valium)

1These frequencies represent the numbers of mentions of drugs having the various therapeutic uses and drug effects—not the numbers of respondents. Thus, while the 784 respondents mentioned barbiturates 24 times, fewer than 24 respondents may account for the mentions (i.e., if some respondents took more than one barbiturate).

APPENDIX P

ESTIMATING THE NUMBER OF PILLS OF VALIUM TAKEN DURING
"THE LAST 7 DAYS" PRIOR TO EACH INTERVIEW

Retrospecive calendar measures for the "week" prior to the inteview were based on different numbers of days for respondents who were inteviewed on different days of the week (see calendar section of the interview and discussion below). Thus, we had no direct measure of the number of Valium pills taken during the period of "the last 7 days" which matched the time frame used for most other primary variables (e.g. anxiety, quality of life, social support, etc.). We therefore examined possible transformations of the data to see which measure provided the best estimation of the amount of Valium taken during the week prior to the interview. The purpose of this appendix is to summarize our thinking about the problem and the analyses done to produce the desired estimate of Valium use.

The only place in the interview where respondents estimated the number of Valium pills taken during a specific time period was in the calendar. Respondents selected a code (1-5) indicating a range which represented the number of Valium pills taken each week over the last six weeks, where each week began on Sunday. Depending on the day of the week on which a person was interviewed, the first "week" prior to the interview could have consisted of 2-8 days. For example, respondents interviewed on a Monday supposedly estimated the number of pills taken over two days (Sunday to "today" [Monday]); whereas, respondents interviewed on Sunday were supposed to estimate the number of pills taken over the last eight days (last Sunday to "today" [this Sunday]).

(Note that this variability in "week" length was not a problem in the estimates for the previous 2-6 weeks of the calendar because each of those ranged from "Sunday to Saturday." Only respondents interviewed on Saturday provided an estimate of the number of Valium pills taken during the same time frame of "the last 7 days" for which they were directed to answer other questions (e.g. anxiety, quality of life). It therefore seemed apparent that some sort of adjustment needed to be made to respondents' estimates of Valium taken the first "week" prior to the interview.

As explained above, respondents' reports of the amount of Valium taken "this week" should have been biased according to the day of the week the interview was held. On the average, reported Valium use should have been higher for respondents interviewed later in the week because they were reporting on more days. To get an idea of the extent of the bias in the estimates of Valium taken the first "week" prior to the interview, several preliminary analyses were done. First, the dates of all interviews were recoded from 2-8 to represent the number of days since the previous Sunday, where 2=(a Monday interview) and 8=(a Sunday interview). This recode indicated the following numbers of interviews taken on a given day of the week for the 406 Time 1 Valium users:

```
Mondays:     83 Interviews
Tuesdays:    75 Interviews
Wednesdays:  80 Interviews
Thursdays:   76 Interviews
Fridays:     62 Interviews
Saturdays:   21 Interviews
Sundays:      9 Interviews
```

Thus, only 21 respondents (Saturday interviews) should have given estimates for number of Valium pills taken over the same 7-day period that they estimated anxiety, quality of life, etc.

Next, this "day of the week of interview" variable was correlated

with the calendar estimates of Valium taken each of the six weeks prior to the interview. If respondents had reported their Valium intake according to calendar instructions, we would have expected a positive correlation between the "day of the week" variable and the estimate of amount of Valium taken during the "week" prior to the interview. That is, on the average, respondents interviewed later in the week should have indicated higher amounts of Valium because they were reporting on more days "this week" than those interviewed early in the week. No correlation was expected between the "day of the week of interview" and reported amounts of Valium taken during the previous 2-6 weeks.

Although the expected positive association between "day of the week of interview" and amount of Valium taken "this week" was found, it was much weaker than expected (r=.09, .04, .11, .18 for Waves 1-4, respectively). At each of the four waves these were the largest positive correlations between the "day of the week" and the six weekly estimates of Valium use prior to the interview. Correlations for the 2-6 week reports tended to be closer to zero or negative. The magnitude of some of the negative correlations was greater than expected, although they were still small (the largest was -.10). These findings suggested that only a small percent of variance in Valium use "this week" was due to the day of the week on which respondents were interviewed. Even though this small effect would probably have no effect on subsequent findings, we still wanted to make the best adjustment possible given the importance of this variable in the study.

Logically, it seemed necessary to apply a transformation to the reports of Valium taken "this week" which would adjust for the number of days supposedly reported on "this week." The most straightforward transformation was to adjust all reports to reflect a 7-day consumption period based on the quantity of Valium taken so far "this week." This first transformed variable was computed as follows:

R300 = vX770: $\dfrac{\text{Reported \# of Valium pills taken "This Week"}}{\text{\# of Days in "This Week" of Interview}} \times 7$

If respondents had made their calendar reports of Valium use according to instructions, this transformation should have reduced any correlation between "day of the week of interview" and amount taken "this week" to zero. However, this transformation appeared to over-adjust the report of Valium taken "this week" as indicated by relatively large negative correlations between "day of week of interview" and amount of Valium taken "this week" adjusted to a 7-day period (r=-.24, -.29,-.27,-.17 for Waves 1-4, respectively).

The apparent over-adjustment indicated by these correlations along with the small positive correlations between "day of week" and the untransformed reports of Valium taken "this week" seemed to indicate that some respondents failed to follow calendar instructions for reporting Valium taken on the specific days "this week" of the interview. One interpretation of these results was that some respondents actually were indicating Valium consumption for a 7-day period for the week of the interview, even when the number of days from Sunday to the day of the interview was less than seven. This seemed like a reasonable interpretation considering that many of our questions prior to the calendar items asking about medications had asked about "the last 7 days" and the calendar focused on weekly reports for the six

¹Note: vX770 was originally coded as ranges of pills (e.g., 1-4, 5-9); for this transformation, vX770 was recoded to reflect the median number of pills in each interval before it was entered into this equation.

weeks prior to the interview. Some respondents might have assumed that a week-long estimate for the first "week" prior to the interview was the desired response.

The next step was to identify a subset of individuals who seemed likely to be reporting Valium use for a 7-day period irrespective of the actual number of days "this week" of the interview. For such a group, no adjustment would be made to their report of Valium taken "this week." For all other respondents, reported amount of Valium taken "this week" would be adjusted to an equivalent 7-day amount.

To identify respondents who reported a 7-day amount of Valium taken "this week," other questions regarding Valium intake (cf., F10, F11, and F12) were used to estimate the amount of Valium usually consumed in a 7-day period. This information was used to construct an estimate of the person's likely number of Valium pills taken during "this week" of the interview (under the assumption that "this week" was a usual week) which could then be compared with the respondent's calendar report. If the respondent's report was greater than our computed estimate, we would assume that the respondent was reporting Valium use for a 7-day period rather than only for the number of days "this week." These people would not have their reports of Valium taken "this week" adjusted and their calendar report would be used.

If our estimate for Valium taken during "this week" matched or was greater than the respondent's calendar report, we would assume the person was following instructions and reporting Valium taken only on the days from "[previous] Sunday to [day of interview]." For these respondents, calendar reports for Valium taken "this week" would be adjusted (as in the equation for R300 above) to represent amounts equivalent to a 7-day period.

The computational steps for identifying the groups to be adjusted versus not adjusted were as follows:

(a) Compute the number of days during "this week" that the respondent could potentially have taken Valium

(b) Multiply (a) by # of Valium pills usually taken per day to estimate the # pills person was likely to have taken during "this week" of the interview

(c) Bracket the estimate in (b) to coincide with interval ranges for calendar report of # of pills taken "this week"

(d) Match our estimate (c) with respondent's calendar report for "this week"

i. If respondent's calendar report of # Valium pills taken was greater than our estimate, use calendar report as estimate of amount of Valium taken during "the last 7 days" (these respondents were assumed to have reported on a 7-day period rather than following interviewer instructions)

ii. If respondent's calendar report for "this week" was equal to or less than our estimate, adjust calendar report to get equivalent amount of Valium taken during "the last 7 days" with the following transformation (these respondents were assumed to have followed interviewer instructions):

$$vY521^2 = vX770: \frac{\text{Reported \# of Valium pills taken "This Week"}}{\text{\# of Days in "This Week" of Interview}} \times 7$$

Following the procedure outlined above, calendar reports of amount of Valium taken "this week" were adjusted to estimate use over "the last 7 days" for 74%, 72%, 73%, and 79% of the samples at Waves 1-4, respectively. "This week" calendar reports were not adjusted for the other 26%, 28%, 27%, and 21% of respondents at Waves 1-4 whose calendar reports.

²Note: This variable was then bracketed so that the estimated # of pills falls into the interval ranges equivalent to those of calendar reports.

³Note: vX770 was originally coded as ranges of pills (e.g., 1-4, 5-9); for this transformation, vX770 was recoded to reflect the median number of pills in each interval before it was entered into this equation.

391

reports were presumed to reflect the amount of Valium consumed in a 7-day period. The adjustment procedure appeared to provide a good estimate of Valium use during "the last 7 days" judging from two general findings of additional analyses. First, means and standard deviations of the "adjusted Week 1" estimate of Valium use (vY521) were much more similar to reports of use during Weeks 2-6 prior to the interview (vX771-X775) than the unadjusted Week 1 report (vX770). Second, correlations for "adjusted Week 1" Valium use with the "day of the week of the interview" variable were much closer to zero than the unadjusted report (n's were -.03, -.07, .02, and .01 for Waves 1-4, respectively). Both of these results were the desired goals of the transformation to provide a good estimate of the amount of Valium consumed during "the last 7 days" prior to each interview.

APPENDIX Q

AN EXPLANATION OF THE CODING SCHEMES OF COMMON
THERAPEUTIC CATEGORIES AND EFFECT CODES OF MEDICATIONS

The coding scheme of common therapeutic uses of medications developed for this study is a modification of the American Hospital Formulary Service (AHFS), a collection of drug monographs for the health care community that is kept current by periodic (quarterly) supplements. The Formulary Service is a tested and proven source of comparative unbiased and evaluative drug information and contains a monograph on virtually every drug entity in the United States. Its monographs are prepared with the expert advice of leading medical scientists, clinicians, pharmacists, pharmacologists and other professionally qualified persons. Each monograph is reviewed prior to publication by consultants in the specific field of drug therapy under consideration and by the appropriate manufacturer(s), (AHFS, 1982).

The Coding scheme used for AMA's Drug Evaluations was considered for use in the study, but it was rejected primarily because we did not feel that many of the major categories used in the scheme were specific enough for use in this study. Also, many of the drugs from the study had not yet been included in the latest edition of the publication. AMA's Drug Evaluations is published approximately every three years (1971, 1973, 1977, and 1980).

While retaining the basic AHFS framework, the therapeutic categories were modified to meet the specific needs of the study. This modification involved both expanding and condensing, as well as the adding of new categories. For example, AHFS divides anti-infectives into twelve major categories. However, we divided anti-infectives into only five categories including an "Other Anti-Infective" category. Not only did this action

eliminate categories in which there were few or no agents (e.g., plasmodicides and treponenicides); it allowed us to group agents into categories more relevant to this study. Another example is that we had very few "Diagnostic Agents", so we included them in the "Ingredients Unclassified" category. In other instances we expanded the coding scheme, e.g., we separated "Opiate Alkalouds and Synthetic Derivatives" from "Non-Opiate Analgesics." AHFS lists all analgesics under the "Analgesics and Antipyretics" category.

Because some single entity drugs have more than one therapeutic effect, it was sometimes necessary to include a drug in more than one therapeutic category. Relatively few of the drugs in this study had this characteristic, however, so most single entity drugs were classified according to the therapeutic effect for which they are most commonly used. Many combination products (i.e., drugs with more than one active ingredient) were placed into more than one category, e.g., Actifed (R), Bellabarb(R), because each active ingredient often has a different therapeutic effect.

After selecting the therapeutic categories needed and placing drugs in their respective categories, we developed a system to determine the potential for each drug to produce effects additive or opposite to diazepam. Drugs are usually described by their most prominent effects or by the actions thought to be the basis of those effects. However, such descriptions should not obscure the fact that no drug produces only a single effect. Drugs are adequately characterized only in terms of their full spectrum of effects (Goodman and Gilman, 1980). Some of the drugs in the study may produce an effect similar to diazepam due to their expected therapeutic action. These drugs were defined as having a primary effect like that of diazepam. Other drugs in the study may produce side effects similar to the effects of diazepam. These drugs were considered to have a secondary effect similar to diazepam. With this in mind,

392

the following system was used to show this possible
relationship:

(+)   Drugs containing active ingredient(s) that could be
       expected to primarily or secondarily produce an
       effect similar to that of diazepam.

(-)   Drugs containing active ingredient(s) that could be
       expected to primarily or secondarily produce an
       effect opposite to that of diazepam.

(+/-) Drugs containing active ingredients that could be
       expected to primarily or secondarily produce both an
       effect similar <u>and</u> opposite to that of diazepam
       (e.g., combination products).

(0)   Drugs whose active ingredient(s) cause effects which
       are neither similar to nor opposite from that of
       diazepam.

(?)   Drugs containing unknown or unspecified active
       ingredients(s).

       No attempt was made to determine the degree of effect
within the (+) and (-) categories because in many instances
the effect of the same drug on two individuals may be as
variable as the effects of two drugs on the same individual.
It cannot be stated with certainty that every person taking
a (+) drug will have a response which is similar to a
diazepam effect because of individual variability. However,
a significant potential for the occurrence of an effect
similar or additive to diazepam does exist.

       To supplement clinical judgments regarding the (+) and
(-) effects of the drugs, a variety of references were used
including: Facts and Comparisons, American Hospital
Formulary Services, AMA's Drug Evaluation, Physician's Desk
Reference, The Pharmaceutical Basis of Therapeutics, Side
Effects of Drugs, United States Pharmacopeia National
Formulary.

NUMBER OF RESPONDENTS AT EACH TIMEPOINT TAKING
MEDICATIONS CLASSIFIED BY COMMON THERAPEUTIC USE
(Total N=675)

Common Therapeutic Use	Time 1	Time 2	Time 3	Time 4
Antihistamines (100)	66	75	73	65
Antiinfectives (200)				
Antibiotics (210)	53	51	63	63
Sulfonamides (230)	11	13	9	17
Urinary Germicides (240)	7	4	6	5
Other Anti-infectives (250)	6	10	14	18
Anti neoplastics (300)	2	1	2	2
Autonomic Drugs (400)				
Anti cholinergics (410)	38	35	35	34
Skeletal Muscle Relaxants (420)	22	16	22	21
Cerebral Vasodilators (430)	0	1	0	0
Others (440)	2	2	2	2
Anticoagulants (500)	8	7	6	6

Appendix R

NUMBER OF RESPONDENTS AT EACH TIMEPOINT TAKING
MEDICATIONS CLASSIFIED BY COMMON THERAPEUTIC USE
(continued)

Common Therapeutic Use	Time 1	Time 2	Time 3	Time 4
Cardiovascular Drugs (600)				
Anti-arrythmias (610)	62	59	66	60
Cardiac glycosides (620)	35	36	35	38
Anti-hypertensives (630)	122	125	123	122
Vasodilators (640)				
Coronary Vasoldilators (641)	55	53	55	55
Peripheral Vasodilators (642)	22	24	23	22
Other Cardiovascular Drugs (650)	19	24	23	19
Central Nervous System Drugs (700)				
Analgesics (710)				
Synth. Derivatives & Opiate Alkaloids (711)	111	102	93	92
Non-Opiate Analgesics (712)	50	55	57	47
Non-Steroidal Anti-inflam. Drugs (720)	54	72	69	58

NUMBER OF RESPONDENTS AT EACH TIMEPOINT TAKING
MEDICATIONS CLASSIFIED BY COMMON THERAPEUTIC USE
(continued)

Common Therapeutic Use	Time 1	Time 2	Time 3	Time 4
Anti-Gout Agents (730)				
Uricosurics (731)	0	1	1	1
Others (732)	9	10	8	10
Anti-convulsants (740)	13	11	9	11
Anti-depressants (750)	33	33	33	27
Anti-psychotics (760)				
Phenothiazine (761)	19	19	16	21
Others (762)	6	10	11	12
Stimulants (770)	11	15	10	7
Anti-anxiety agents/Sedative hypnotics (780)				
Benzodiazepines (781)	374	330	277	265
Barbiturates (782)	34	37	34	29
Others (783)	17	14	13	12

Appendix R

NUMBER OF RESPONDENTS AT EACH TIMEPOINT TAKING
MEDICATIONS CLASSIFIED BY COMMON THERAPEUTIC USE
(continued)

Common Therapeutic Use	Time 1	Time 2	Time 3	Time 4
Other CNS Drugs (790)	2	2	2	2
Electrolytic & Water Balance (800)				
Potassium (810)	32	33	39	45
Diuretics (820)	158	160	157	158
Otic & Ophthalmic Preparations (900)				
Anti-infective (910)	4	1	7	4
Anti-inflammatory drugs (920)	1	1	3	3
Miotic & Mydratics (930)	3	3	3	2
Vasoconstrictors (940)	2	0	1	0
Others (950)	3	4	5	3
Gastrointestinal Drugs (1000)				
Antacids, Adsorbents, & Antiflatulants (1010)	3	3	2	4
Anti-diarrheal Agents (1020)	11	15	14	8

NUMBER OF RESPONDENTS AT EACH TIMEPOINT TAKING
MEDICATIONS CLASSIFIED BY COMMON THERAPEUTIC USE
(continued)

Common Therapeutic Use	Time 1	Time 2	Time 3	Time 4
Laxatives (1030)	2	2	2	3
Others (including Cimetidine) (1040)	33	37	40	40
Hormones and Synthetic Substitutes (1100)				
Androgens (1110)	2	1	1	1
Contraceptives (1120)	9	10	11	9
Corticosteroids (1130)	16	15	9	14
Estrogens (1140)	23	24	24	22
Anti-diabetic Agents (1150)				
Insulins (1151)	13	16	16	16
Oral agents (1152)	10	12	13	12
Thyroid Drugs (1160)	43	44	42	43
Others (1170)	4	5	4	4
Skin & Mucous Membranes Preparations (1200)				

Appendix R

NUMBER OF RESPONDENTS AT EACH TIMEPOINT TAKING
MEDICATIONS CLASSIFIED BY COMMON THERAPEUTIC USE
(continued)

Common Therapeutic Use	Time 1	Time 2	Time 3	Time 4
Anti-infectives (1210)	6	6	2	4
Anti-inflammatory agents (1220)	6	5	1	6
Anti pruritics & local anesthetics (1230)	5	5	5	4
Others (1240)	1	0	1	1
Vitamins and Minerals (1300)				
Single ingredient vitamins (1310)	10	10	9	9
Multiple vitamins with or without minerals (1320)	18	21	24	19
Iron preparations (1330)	8	9	8	6
Others (1340)	1	1	0	1
Respiratory Drugs (1400)				
Bronchodialators (1410)				
Methylxanthines derivatives (1411)	23	27	29	23
Sympathomimetic (1412)	8	10	12	12

NUMBER OF RESPONDENTS AT EACH TIMEPOINT TAKING
MEDICATIONS CLASSIFIED BY COMMON THERAPEUTIC USE
(continued)

Common Therapeutic Use	Time 1	Time 2	Time 3	Time 4
Antitussives and Expectorants (1420)				
Antitussives (1421)	19	11	16	19
Expectorants (1422)	9	17	12	15
Decongestants (1430)				
Oral (1431)	46	58	57	49
Topical (1432)	0	1	1	0
Others (1440)	1	1	1	1
Ingredients unclassified (1500)	3	2	3	4
Miscellaneous (1600)				
Ingredients unknown (unspecific) (1610)	42	16	18	10
Ingredients not stated (1620)	21	32	30	36

APPENDIX S

CODING SCHEME FOR "MULTIPLE STRESS" MEASURE (VY262)

Step Number	If	Interpersonal Conflict Equals:	and	Role Ambiguity Equals:	and	Negative Events Equals:	then	Multiple Stress Equals:
1		1.0-1.9		1.0-1.9		0-1		1
2		1.0-1.9		2.0-2.5		0-1		2
4		2.0-5.0		2.6-5.0		2-4		7
5		2.0-5.0		2.0-2.5		2-4		6

Step Number	If	Interpersonal Conflict Equals:	and	Multiple Stress Does Not Already Equal:			then	Multiple Stress Equals:
3		1.0-1.9		1-2				3
6		2.6-5.0		6-7				5
7		2.0-2.5		6-7				4

APPENDIX T

DETAILED DESCRIPTION OF MODERATOR ANALYSES

In the text which follows, a rationale is provided for the major categories of moderator variables which were examined. Following each discussion of expected hypotheses, the relevant findings are reviewed. Overall, few moderator effects were found which were consistent enough or strong enough to necessitate further subgroup analyses. Therefore, discussion of the implications of these findings was intentionally avoided. Further replication of these findings is necessary before such discussion is warranted. Furthermore, it should be noted that the causal ordering of the three variables examined in any one moderator analysis cannot be determined definitively through this type of analysis. Although causal directions are posited in the hypotheses which are presented, further analyses are necessary to confirm them.

Demographic variables. Sex, age, race, and socio-economic status were chosen as demographic moderators. Although it is possible that respondents in some of these subgroups (e.g., sex and age) might metabolize diazepam differently, any moderating effects found in this study would more likely be related to the experience of anxiety, depression, or stress for these subgroups. For example, females are more likely to score high on negative affective symptoms than are males (e.g., review by Warheit, et al., 1975). Investigators have suggested a number of reasons for these differences. They include:

(a) biological differences

(b) differences in awareness of symptoms (e.g., Padesky & Hammen, 1981; Broverman, et al., 1970)

(c) greater social exposure to stressors among females (e.g., Weissman & Klerman, 1977; Kessler, 1979b; Dohrenwend & Dohrenwend, 1976; Aneshensal, et al.,

1981) and greater social vulnerability (Kessler, 1979b)

(d) methodological artifacts such as bias in the psychiatric judgments made by raters (Broverman, et al., 1970) and in the inclusion of symptoms whose expression and willingness to report (e.g., crying) varies according to social norms (Newman, 1981; Kessler, 1979a).

The debate about the validity of each of the above explanations continues. Nevertheless, some of these possible explanations could introduce interaction effects, so gender was included as a moderator. For example, differences in symptom awareness could mean that measures of anxiety would be more sensitive for one sex than for the other.

Results in this study indicated a trend for the magnitude of the correlations between Valium use and outcome variables to be stronger for females than for males. There was a stronger positive relationship between Valium use and depression for females than for males. Similarly, there was a stronger negative relationship between Valium use and perceptions of quality of life in the self, personal life, and work domains for females than for males (differences in r's ranged from .13 to .21). Conversely, for males there was a strong positive relationship between Valium use and perceiving Valium as being helpful while there was no such relationship for females (difference in r's about .45).

With regard to age as a moderator, previous research has indicated that the elderly appear to require less Valium (cf., Hoffmann-La Roche, Inc., 1982) and are more likely to exhibit adverse drug reactions for all classes of drugs. This may be the result of failing health and the likelihood of drug interactions due to the use of multiple medications for a variety of health problems (e.g., Hurwitz, 1969). Consequently, age was examined as a potentially important moderator.

Results in this study indicated that for older respondents (ages 60-85) Valium use was somewhat more strongly correlated with low quality of life in the self domain than it was for younger respondents (ages 17-29; difference in r's about .15). Conversely, Valium use was associated with better and somewhat poorer social performance for older respondents and somewhat poorer social performance for younger respondents (difference in r's about .30) Overall, age did not appear to have many moderator effects in these analyses.

With regard to race, previous research has shown that nonwhites, like women, are overrepresented among those with negative affective symptomatology (Dohrenwend & Dohrenwend, 1976). Although nonwhites have been found to have a higher rate of such symptoms because of overexposure to stressors, there has been no evidence that race influences the effects of diazepam or other tranquilizers on anxiety or that race influences the effects of stress on mental well-being (Kessler, 1979b). Nevertheless, race and education were included as potential moderators because of their central importance to sociological study and to explore their role as moderators given this unique opportunity.

Results in this study showed a modest trend for Valium use to be more strongly associated with negative outcomes for black respondents than for white respondents. The negative relationships between Valium use and quality of life in the self, personal life, work life, and positive affect domains were stronger for black respondents than for white respondents (differences in r's ranged from .10 to .21). There was also a fairly strong negative relationship between Valium use and esteem social support for black respondents but not for white respondents (difference in r's about .40). Valium use was also positively associated with misfit on control by chance for black respondents but not for white respondents (difference in r's about .25).

Social support and social conflict. As reviewed in Chapter 1, minor tranquilizers may be most effective when used as an adjunct to counseling or related therapy (Rickels, et al., 1971; Persson, 1976; Uhlenhuth, et al., 1966). Extension of this theory suggests the hypothesis that social support from lay people may have similar effects as a moderator of the effects of diazepam use. The current study is the first to examine the extent to which lay support (e.g., from family, or friends) has similar effects, and the extent to which social conflict with significant others might have undermining effects.

Results in this study indicated that neither social support nor social conflict appeared to moderate the relationship between Valium use and a broad range of outcome variables. Neither social support from significant others nor from the physician who prescribed Valium affected these relationships. One should not conclude, however, that social support has no moderating effects in this study. Other analyses which have been conducted with these data indicated that social support did moderate the relationship between stress and these outcome variables, but not the relationship between Valium use and these same outcomes (Abbey, 1983).

Performance. Performance may moderate the effects of diazepam on various outcomes to the extent that such performance represents a skill or ability resource upon which the person can draw. The person with poor social performance skills in relating to others may be at a relative disadvantage even with the help of anxiety-reducing interventions. This is because, although anxiety may interfere with performance, skills are still a necessary component of gaining mastery over one's life. This theory is best reflected in the classic formula for performance: Performance = Motivation X Ability; as ability decreases, so does the effect of motivation.

In the present study, social performance appeared to have a modest impact on the relationship between Valium use and various outcomes. Respondents whose social performance was poor showed a stronger positive relationship between Valium use and depression than did respondents whose social performance was good (difference in r's about .25). Similarly, the negative relationship between Valium use and quality of life regarding one's health and negative affect was stronger for poor performers than for good performers (difference in r's about .15).

Attitudes about using tranquilizers. National sample surveys of Americans' attitudes towards the use of minor tranquilizers (e.g., Manheimer, et al., 1973) showed that most people believe it is better to use will power than medicines to control one's emotions. No study has ever examined the consequences of taking a medication for control of one's emotions when the patient has strong beliefs that this is the wrong strategy. Such a belief may weaken Valium's effects. Previous studies have suggested that expectancy accounts for a statistically significant portion of the variance in anxiety in double-blind placebo group trials (e.g., review by Ross & Olson, 1981; Persson, 1976). Hypotheses such as these led us to include measures of attitudes toward tranquilizers as potential moderators.

Results in this study indicated that attitudes about tranquilizers did not appear to moderate the relationship between Valium use and outcomes. Respondents with positive attitudes about tranquilizer use did show a stronger relationship between Valium-taking at one timepoint and Valium-taking at a later timepoint than did respondents with more negative attitudes about tranquilizer use (differences in r's range from .15 to .35). This suggests (not surprisingly) that positive attitudes foster continued use of Valium. Similar findings have appeared previously in numerous studies of the relationship between expecting

benefits and subsequent health-seeking behavior (e.g., Becker, et al., 1977).

Control over emotions. This study measured both the amount of control people perceived themselves as having as well as the amount which they wanted. From these two sets of measures indices of person-environment misfit were derived (absolute discrepancies between the amount the person wants [P] and the amount the person has [E]; see Chapter 4 for details regarding the construction of these indices). Because misfit on control over one's emotions was considered potentially relevant to Valium use, this P-E fit measure was examined as a moderator of the effects of diazepam use on various outcomes.

Similar arguments can be made with regard to perceived control over one's personal life. Persons who believe that their personal lives are controlled excessively by others or by chance may view anxiolytic medications as a path to restoring some of that control to themselves. Or they may view dependence on medication as a loss of control.

Results in this study indicated that perceptions of control misfit affected very few of the relationships between Valium use and other variables. Only, the positive relationships between Valium use and anxiety and depression were somewhat larger for individuals who felt chance was strongly controlling their personal lives than for individuals who felt that chance had little control over their personal lives (differences in r's about .20).

Potential stressors. Ambiguity is one of the key concomitants of anxiety (Archer, 1979). Role ambiguity refers specifically to uncertainty about how one is supposed to perform in a certain role in either work or some other domain of life (e.g., parenting, being a spouse). Role conflict refers not to a lack of clarity, but rather to the presence of conflicting messages about how a role should be performed (Kahn, et al., 1964). For example, a supervisor may receive one set of demands from subordinates and another set of demands from superiors, and the two sets may be in conflict ("we want less work" versus "we want more output"). It was hypothesized that the relationships between Valium use, affect, and life quality might be heightened for individuals experiencing high levels of these stresses.

A somewhat different type of stressor which might serve as a moderator is health. Persons taking Valium primarily as a muscle relaxant rather than for anxiety may show little psychotherapeutic effect of the drug partly because that was not the indication for taking it. Persons who have serious physical illnesses of a chronic nature which significantly interfere with their social and task performance and who take Valium might also be unlikely to show marked changes in performance outcomes as a result of anxiolytic therapy. For these reasons, perceived physical health was included as a stressor. Negative life events, a stressor frequently examined in the social psychological literature (e.g., Dohrenwend & Dohrenwend, 1974), was also examined.

Results in this study indicated that role ambiguity, role conflict, and negative life events did not appear to moderate the relationship between Valium use and outcome variables. Quality of life regarding one's health had a modest moderating effect on the relationship between Valium use and other quality of life measures. For individuals with poor health life quality there was a small, negative relationship between Valium use and quality of life regarding the self, work life, positive affect, and cognition, while the relationship was virtually zero for individuals with good health life quality (differences between r's ranged from .20 to .26).

Coping and defense. Some previous research has suggested that coping and defense can modify the effects of stressors on strains (e.g., Caplan, et al., 1982; Billings & Moos, 1981). A random sample of Chicago households, for

example, found that the more coping responses people used, the weaker the positive association between stressors and strains (Pearlin & Schooler, 1978). This reduction or buffering was more likely to occur for stressors that were potentially controllable (for example, the economy is less controllable than one's relationships with family members).

Such findings led us to include measures of coping and defense in this study. There have been no prior studies, however, of the relationship of coping and defense to the use of minor tranquilizers. Nor have there been any studies of the extent to which coping and defense might influence the effects of anxiolytic therapy on outcomes of interest such as anxiety, quality of life, and performance. No predictions were made as to whether certain coping and defensive responses might enhance, interfere with, or have no effect upon anxiolytic therapy because not enough is known about the conditions under which coping and defense do and do not promote well-being. So these analyses must be viewed as exploratory.

As an example of potential effects, some defenses might allow the person to approach stressful situations successfully once anxiety is reduced; other defenses, if they persist, might prevent the person from taking needed action (e.g., from taking steps to diagnose a potentially serious, treatable illness). A good discussion of some of the costs and benefits of coping and defense can be found elsewhere (e.g., Lazarus, in press; Brickman, et al., 1982).

Of the four coping and defense measures examined in this study (maintaining a positive approach, reinterpretation of negative events, seeking help from others, and relying on religious beliefs), only religious beliefs appeared to moderate the relationship between Valium use and outcome variables. The negative relationship between Valium use and quality of life was consistently stronger for individuals who frequently defended against problems by relying on religious beliefs than it was for individuals who infrequently used this defensive technique. Use of religion as a defense moderated the relationship between Valium use and quality of life in the self, health, and life as a whole domains and the positive affect, negative affect, and cognitive dimensions of quality of life (differences between r's ranged from .25 to .37). The effects of religious beliefs might be an inherent result of such beliefs and/or the effects of social support derived from participating in church or synagogue-related activities (e.g., Comstock, 1972). The effects did not appear to be due to a general negative attitude toward tranquilizers, as there was virtually no correlation between religious beliefs and general attitudes toward tranquilizers.

Use of other drugs. The use of other drugs with CNS depressant effects, such as alcohol, other minor tranquilizers, and antihistamines, may confound the effects of diazepam by producing similar effects. Similarly, CNS stimulants, such as amphetamines, may also have confounding effects, but in the opposite direction. These effects can be taken into account by examining the joint direct effects of diazepam and other substances with CNS effects in additive, multivariate analyses.[1] It is also possible for other substances (e.g., alcohol, Cimetidine) to interact with diazepam. Thus, potential moderator effects of stimulant and sedative substances were examined because such relationships seemed plausible.

Results in this study indicated that CNS depressant-like drugs ("+" effect drugs--i.e., similar to Valium's effect)[2] did not appear to moderate the relationship

---

[1]None of the analyses conducted thus far indicated any substantial main effects of the use of CNS stimulants or depressants on variables of primary interest in this study.

[2]See Appendix M for a detailed description of "+" and "-" drugs.

between Valium use and outcome variables. This was true for alcohol as well as for prescribed medications. The use of CNS stimulant-like drugs ("-" effect drugs--i.e., opposite to Valium's effect) did, however, moderate the relationship between Valium use and outcome variables. The positive relationship between Valium use and depression was stronger for respondents taking CNS stimulant-like drugs than for respondents not taking these medications (difference in r's about .30). Similarly, the negative relationship between Valium use and quality of life was stronger for respondents not taking CNS stimulant-like drugs than for respondents taking these drugs. Use of CNS stimulant-like drugs moderated the relationship between Valium use and quality of life in the self, personal life, work life, and life-as-a-whole domains and positive affect, negative affect, and cognitive aspects of quality of life (differences in r's ranged from .16 to .22). The mixture of Valium use and stimulant-like drugs appeared to have a negative impact on depression and quality of life.

Method of diazepam use. Several variations in how individuals take Valium were thought to potentially moderate the relationship between Valium use and outcome measures. According to some research, Valium use might be more beneficial for individuals also receiving psychotherapy than for individuals not receiving such therapy (Rickels, et al., 1971). It was also hypothesized that individuals taking a "therapeutic dose" of Valium (defined as 30-280 mg a week in this study) might receive more benefits from Valium use than individuals taking a less-than-therapeutic dose. Similarly, it was hypothesized that respondents who followed the physician's recommendations and took the prescribed dose might receive more beneficial effects from Valium use than might patients who took either more or less than the physician prescribed.³

In the present study, all three of these variables had some moderating effects. For individuals in psychotherapy there was a slight negative relationship between Valium use and social support, while there was no effect for individuals not in such therapy (difference between r's about .12). The relationship between Valium use and several indicators of stress (e.g., role conflict, role ambiguity, misfit on control) were also moderated by therapy. For example, for individuals in psychotherapy there was a moderate positive relationship between Valium use and perceptions of misfit in the amount of control they had over their emotions and the control others had over their personal lives, while this relationship did not exist for individuals not in such therapy (difference between r's about .20).

For individuals in this study taking a therapeutic dose of Valium there was a moderately positive relationship between Valium use and anxiety and depression while the relationship was slightly negative for individuals not taking a therapeutic dose (differences between r's about .35). Similarly, there were moderately negative relationships between Valium use and quality of life in the self, personal life, and health domains for respondents taking a therapeutic dose of Valium but not for other respondents (differences in r's ranged from about .25 to .40).

Compliance showed effects opposite to those for therapeutic dose. For individuals taking less Valium than their physician prescribed there was a moderately positive

³So few respondents (15 or 4.5% of users at Time 1) took more Valium than was prescribed that only two levels of this variable could be considered: compliance and under use.

relationship between Valium use and anxiety and depression, while the relationship was slightly negative for individuals who took Valium in the amount prescribed (difference between r's about .35). Similarly, there was a moderately negative relationship between Valium use and quality of life in the self, personal life, and work life domains and positive affective dimension of quality of life for respondents taking less than the prescribed amount, while the relationship was slightly positive for compliant respondents (difference in r's about .30).

Reason for taking diazepam. It was hypothesized that Valium might influence affect and life quality only for individuals taking Valium for reasons related to anxiety. Individuals taking Valium for purely physical reasons such as epilepsy, tremors, or muscle problems may not be psychologically affected by Valium use in the same way that anxious individuals are. Also individuals' levels of anxiety may have an effect. Individuals who are not anxious may receive less benefits from Valium use. Similarly, individuals whose levels of depression are higher than their levels of anxiety may show less beneficial effects of Valium use, even if they are relatively anxious, because Valium is not recommended for depression (Hollister, 1977).

Results in this study indicated that these variables did not exert many moderating effects on the relationship between Valium use and outcome variables. The negative relationship between Valium use and positive affect and cognitive quality of life was slightly stronger for highly anxious respondents than it was for nonanxious respondents (difference in r's about .20). Not surprisingly, the positive relationship between Valium use and anxiety was somewhat higher for individuals who reported taking Valium for anxiety rather than for other reasons (difference between r's about .10).

References

Abbey, A. The effects of social support on emotional well-being. Paper presented at the First International Symposium on Behavioral Health, Nag's Head Conference Center, June, 1983.

Abbey, A., Abramis, D. J., & Caplan, R. D. Measuring social support: The effects of frame of reference on the relationship between social support and strain. Paper presented at the American Psychological Association, Los Angeles, CA, 1981.

Abbey, A., Holland, A. E., & Wortman, C. B. The misguided helper: An analysis of people's responses to their loved ones' crises. In D. G. McGuigan (Ed.), Women's lives: New theory, research and policy. Ann Arbor: University of Michigan, 1980.

Abramson, L. Y., Seligman, M. E. P., & Teasdale, J. D. Learned helplessness in humans: Critique and reformulation. Journal of Abnormal Psychology, 1978, 87, 49-74.

American Hospital Formulary Service, Bethesda, MD., American Society of Hospital Pharmacists, 1983.

Andrews, F. M., Morgan, I. N., Sonquist, J. A., & Klem, L. Multiple classification analysis. A report on a computer program for multiple regression using categorical predictors. Ann Arbor, MI: The Institute for Social Research, 1973.

Andrews, F. M., & Withey, S. B. Social indicators of well-being: Americans' perceptions of life quality. New York: Plenum, 1976.

Aneshensel, C. S., Frerichs, R. R., & Clark, V. A. Family roles and sex differences in depression. Journal of Health and Social Behavior, 1981, 22 (December), 379-393.

Archer, R. P. Relationships between locus of control and anxiety. Journal of Personality Assessment, 1979, 43, 617-626.

Arieti, S. Cognition and feeling. In M. Arnold (Ed.), Feelings and Emotions. New York: Academic Press, 1970, 135-144.

Armitage, K. J., Schneiderman, L. J., & Bass, R. A. Response of physicians to medical complaints in men and women. International Journal of Women's Studies, 1980, 3, 111-116.

Arnold, H. J. Moderator variables: A clarification of conceptual, analytic, and psychometric issues. Organizational Behavior and Human Performance, 1982, 29, 143-174.

Avorn, J., Chen, m., & Hartley, R. Scientific versus commercial sources of influence on the prescribing behavior of physicians. The American Journal of Medicine, 1982, 73, 4-8.

Bales, R. F. Interaction process analysis. Cambridge, MA: Addison-Wesley, 1950.

Barrett, J. E., & DiMascio, A. Comparative effects on anxiety of the "minor tranquilizers" in "high" and "low" anxious student volunteers. Diseases of the Nervous System, 1966, 27, 483-486.

Bazerman, M. H. Impact of personal control on performance: Is added control always beneficial? Journal of Applied Psychology, 1982, 67 (4), 472-479.

Becker, M. H., Maiman, L. A., Kirscht, J. P., Haefner, D. P., & Drachman, R. H. The health belief model and prediction of dietary compliance: A field experiment. Journal of Health and Social Behavior, 1977, 18, 348-366.

Bentler, P. M. Multivariate analysis with latent variables: Causal modeling. Annual review of psychology, 1980, 31, 419-456.

Bibliographic Retrieval Services, Inc. Offline bibliography search (double-blind studies of diazepam; 1979-May, 1983). Latham, New York, April 7, 1983.

Billings, A. G. & Moos, R. H. The role of coping responses and social resources in attenuating the stress of life events. Journal of Behavioral Medicine, 1981, 4, 139-157.

Blake, R. R., & Mouton, J. S. The managerial grid: Key orientations for achieving production through people. Houston: Gulf Publishing, 1964.

Bodendorfer, T. W., Briggs, G. G., & Gunning, J. E. Obtaining drug exposure histories during pregnancy. American Journal of Obstetrics and Gynecology, 1979, 135, 490.

Boffey, P. M. Worldwide use of Valium draws new scrutiny. The New York Times, October 1981, pp. C1-C2.

Bowers, D. G., & Seashore, S. E. Predicting organizational effectiveness with a four-factor theory of leadership. Administrative Science Quarterly, 1966, 11, 238-263.

Bradburn, N. M. The structure of psychological well-being. Chicago: Aldine, 1969.

Brickman, P., & Campbell, D. T. Hedonic relativism and planning the good society. In M. H. Appley (Ed.), Adaptation level theory. New York: Academic Press, 1971, 287-304.

Brickman, P., Rabinowitz, V. C., Karuza, J., Jr., Coates, D., Cohn, E., Kidder, L. Models of Helping and Coping. American Psychologists, April 1982, 37(4), 368-384.

Broverman, I., Broverman, D., Clarkson, F., Rosenkrantz, P., & Vogel, S. Sex roles stereo-types and clinical judgements of mental health. Journal of Consulting and Clinical Psychology, 1970, 34, 1-7.

Bruner, J. S., & Tagiuri, R. Person perception. In G. Lindzey (Ed.), Handbook of social psychology (Vol. 2). Reading, MA: Addison-Wesley, 1954.

Bunker, M. L., & Williams, M. Caffeine content of common beverages. Journal of the American Dietetic Association, 74, 1979.

Burger, J. M., & cooper H. M. The desirability of control. Motivation and Emotion, 1979, 3, 381-393.

Cahalan, D., Cisin, I. H., & Crossley, H. M. American drinking practices. New Brunswick, NJ: Rutgers Center of Alcohol Studies, 1969.

Campbell, A., converse, P. F., & Rodgers, W. L. Quality of American Life: Perceptions, evaluations, and satisfactions. New York: Russell-Sage, 1976.

Cannell, C. F., & Fowler, F. J. Interviewing and interviewing techniques. From the National Center for Health Services Research Proceedings, Proceedings of a National Invitational Conference, Airlie House, Airlie, VA, 1975.

Caplan, R. D. Patient, provider and organization: Hypothesized determinants of adherence. In S. J. Cohen (Ed.), New directions in patient compliance. Lexington, MA: D. C. Heath, 1972, 75-110.

Caplan, R. D. Person-environment fit: Past, present, and future. In C. Cooper (Ed.), Stress research: Directions for the 1980s. London: Wiley, 1983.

Caplan, R. D. Organizational stress and individual strain: A social-psychological study of risk factors in coronary heart disease among administrators, engineers, and scientists. Doctoral dissertation, University of Michigan, Ann Arbor, MI: University Microfilms, 1971, No. 72-14822.

Caplan, R. D., Cobb, S., French, J. R. P., Jr., Harrison, R. V., & Pinneau, S. R., Jr. Job demands and worker health: Main effects and occupational differences. Ann Arbor: Institute for Social Research, 1980a (originally published as HEW Publication No. (NIOSH) 75-160, 1975).

407

Caplan, R. D., Harrison, R. V., Wellons, R. V., & French, J. R. P., Jr. Social support and patient adherence: Experimental and survey findings. Research Report Series, Ann Arbor: Institute for Social Research, 1980.

Caplan, R. D., & Jones, K. W. Effects of work load, role ambiguity, & Type A personality on anxiety, depression, and heart rate. Journal of Applied Psychology, 1975, 60, 713-719.

Caplan, R. D., Naidu, R. K, & Tripathi, R. C. Coping and defense: Constellations vs. components. University of Michigan, unpublished manuscript, 1982.

Caplan, R. D., Robinson, E. A. R., French, J. R. P., Jr., Caldwell, J. R., & Shinn, M. Adhering to medical regimens: Pilot experiments in patient education and social support. Ann Arbor: Institute for Social Research, 1976.

Cattell, R. B. Factor analysis. New York: Harper, 1952.

Cobb, S. Social support and health through the life course. In M. W. Riley (Ed.), Aging from birth to death: Interdisciplinary perspectives. Washington, D. C.: American Association for the Advancement of Science, 1979.

Cobb, S. Social support as a moderator of life stress. Psychosomatic Medicine, 1976, 38, 300-314.

Comstock, G. W., & Partridge, K. B. Church attendance and health. Journal of Chronic Disease, 1972, 25, 665-672.

Conway, T. L., Abbey, A., & French, J. R. P., Jr. Beliefs about control in different life domains. Paper presented at the American Psychological Association, Anaheim, CA, 1983.

Conway, T. L., Vickers, R. R., Jr., Ward, H. W., & Rahe, R. H. Occupational stress and variation in cigarette, coffee, and alcohol consumption. Journal of Health and Social Behavior, 1981, 22, 155-165.

Cooperstock, R., & Hill, J. The effects of tranquillization: Benzodiazepine Use in Canada. Canada: National Health and Welfare, 1982.

Cooperstock, R., & Parnell, P. Research on psychotropic drug use. Social Science and Medicine, 1982, 16, 1179-1196.

Coyne, J. C., Aldwin, C., & Lazarus, R. S. Depression and coping in stressful episodes. Journal of Abnormal Psychology, 1981, 90, 439-447.

Cypress, B. K. Drug utilization in office visits to primary care physicians: National Ambulatory Medical Care Survey, 1980. National Center for Health Statistics Advance Data, October 1982, 86, 1-16.

Depue, R. A., & Monroe, S. M. Learned helplessness in the perspective of the depressive disorders: Conceptual and definitional issues. Journal of Abnormal Psychology, 1978, 87, 3-20.

Derogatis, L. R., Lipman, R. S., Rickels, K., Uhlenhuth, E. h., & Covi, L. The Hopkins Symptom Checklist (HSCL): A measure of primary symptom dimensions. In P. Pichot (Ed.), Psychological measurements in Psychopharmacology. Modern problems in pharmacopsychiatry, Vol. 7, Karger, Basel, 1974, 79-110.

DiMascio, A., & Barrett, J. Comparative effects of Oxazepam in "high" and "low" anxious student volunteers. Psychosomatics, 1965, 6, 298-302.

Dohrenwend, B. P., & Dohrenwend, B. S. Sex differences and psychiatric disorder. American Journal of Sociology, 1976, 81, 1147-1454.

Dohrenwend, B. S., & Dohrenwend, B. P. (Eds.). Stressful life events: Their nature and effects. New York: Wiley, 1974.

Douglas, S. P., & Wind, Y. Examining family role and authority patterns: Two methodological issues. Journal of Marriage and the Family, 1978, 40, 35-47.

Dunbar, J. Issues in assessment. In Stuart J. Cohen (Ed.), New directions in patient compliance. Lexington, MA: Lexington, 1979, 41-58.

Eaton, W. W. Life events, social supports, and psychiatric symptoms: A re-analysis of the New Haven data. Journal of Health and Social Behavior, 1978, 19, 230-234.

Ericcson, K. A., & Simon, H. A. Verbal reports as data. Psychological Review, 1980, 87, 215-251.

Falk, J. L., Schuster, C. R., Bigelow, G. E., & Woods, J. H. Progress and needs in experimental analysis of drug and alcohol dependence. American Psychologist, 1982, 37, 1124-1127.

Felton, B. J., Revenson, T. A., & Hinrichsen, G. A. Stress, coping, and psychological adjustment among chronically ill adults. Department of Psychology, New York University, unpublished manuscript, 1981.

Fishburne, P. M., Abelson, H. I., & Cisin, I. National survey on drug abuse: Main findings: 1979. Rockville, MD: National Institute on Drug Abuse, 1979. Contract No. 271-78-3508.

Fisher, J. D., Nadler, A., & Whitcher-Alagna, S. Recipient reactions to aid. Psychological Bulletin, 1982, 91, 27-54.

Frankenhaeuser, M. Psychoendocrine approaches to the study of
stressful person-environment transactions. In Selye,
H. (Ed.), Selye's guide to stress research (Vol. 1).
New York: Van Nostrand, 1980.

French, J. R. P., Jr. Person role fit. Occupational Mental
Health, 1974, 3, 15-20.

French, J. R. P., Jr., & Caplan, R. D. Organizational stress
and individual strain. In A. J. Marrow (Ed.), The
failure of success. New York: AMACOM, 1973.

French, J. R. P., Jr., Caplan, R. D., & Harrison, R. V. The
mechanisms of job stress and strain. London: Wiley,
1982.

French, J. R. P., Jr., & Kahn, R. L. A programmatic approach
to studying the industrial environment and mental
health. Journal of Social Issues, 1962, 18, 1-47.

French, J. R. P., Jr., Rodgers, W., & Cobb, S. Adjustment as
person-environment fit. In G. V. Coelho, D. A. Hamburg
& J. E. Adams (Eds.), Coping and adaptation. New York:
Basic Books, 1974, pp. 316-333.

Freud, S.   (1926) Inhibitions, symptoms, and anxiety (Standard
Edition). London: Hogarth Press, Vol. 20, 1959.

Frydman, M. I. Social support, life events and psychiatric
symptoms: A study of direct, conditional and interaction effects. Social Psychiatry, 1981, 16, 69-78.

Gibson, J. L., Ivancevich, J. M., & Donnelly, J. H., Jr. Organizations: Behavior, structure, processes. Dallas:
Business Publications, Inc., 1979.

Goldberg, S. C., Schooler, N. R., Hogarty, G. E., and Roper, m.
Prediction of relapse in schizophrenic outpatients
treated by drug and sociotherapy. Archives in General
Psychiatry, 1977, 34 (Feb.), 171-184.

Goodman, A.G. and Gilman, L.S. (ed.), Goodman and Gilman's The
Pharmacological Basis of Therapeutics, (6th ed.), New
York: Macmillian Publishing Co, Inc., 1980, p.38.

Gottschalk, L. A. Effects of certain benzodiazepine derivatives on disorganization of thought as manifested in
speech. Current Therapeutic Research, 1977, 21,
192-206.

Gove, W. R. Sex differences in mental illness among adult men
and women: An evaluation of four questions raised
regarding the evidence on the higher rates of women.
Social Science and Medicine, 1978, 12B, 187-198.

Greenblatt, D. J., & Shader, R. I. Benzodiazepines in clinical
practice. New York: Raven Press, 1974.

Gurin, G., Veroff, J., & Feld, S. c. Americans view their mental health. New York: Basic Books, 1960.

Harrison, R. V. Person-environment fit and job stress. In C. L. Cooper & R. Payne (Eds.), Stress at work. New York: Wiley, 1978.

Harrison, R. V., Caplan, R. D., French, J. R. P., Jr., & Wellons, R. V. Combining field experiments with longitudinal surveys: Social research on patient adherence. Applied Social Psychology Annual, 1982, 3, 119-150.

Haynes, R. B., Sackett, D. L., Gibson, E. S., Taylor, D. W., Hackett, B. C., Roberts, R. S., & Johnson, A. L. Improvement of medication compliance in uncontrolled hypertension. Lancet, 1976, 1, 1265-1268.

Hays, W. L. Statistics for the social sciences (2nd ed.). New York: Holt, Rinehart and Winston, Inc., 1973.

Hesbacher, P., Stepansky, P., Stepansky, W., & Rickels, K. Psychotropic drug use in family practice. Pharmakopsychiatrie. Neuropsychopharmakologie, 1976, 9, 50-60.

Hirsch, B. J. Natural support systems and coping with major life changes. American Journal of Community Psychology, 1980, 8, 159-171.

Hoffmann-La Roche, Inc. Valium (diazepam/Roche) tablets [package insert]. Manati, Puerto Rico: Roche Products Inc., 1982.

Hollister, L. E. Clinical use of psychotherapeutic drugs. Springfield, IL: Charles C. Thomas, 1974.

Hollister, L. E. Prudent use of antianxiety drugs in medical practice. In B. S. Brown (Ed.), Clinical anxiety/tension in primary medicine. Amsterdam: Excepta Medica, 1977, 51-65.

Holmes, T. H., & Rahe, R. H. The social readjustment scale. Journal of Psychosomatic Research, 1967, 11, 213-218.

House, J. S. Work stress and social support. Reading, MA: Addison-Wesley, 1981.

Hulka, B. S., Cassel, J. C., Kupper, L. L., & Burdette, J. A. Communication, compliance, and concordance between physicians and patients with prescribed medication. American Journal of Public Health< 1976, 66, 847-853.

Hurwitz, N. Predisposing factors in adverse reactions to drugs. British Medical Journal, 1969, 1 (5643), 536-539.

411

Ilfeld, F. W., Jr. Psychologic status of community residents along major demographic dimensions. _Archives of General Psychiatry_, 1978, _35_, 716-724.

Janis, I. L. _Psychological stress: Psycho-analytic and behavioral studies of surgical patients_. New York: Academic Press, 1974.

Janoff-Bulman, R., & Brickman, P. Expectations and what people learn from failure. In N. T. Feather (Ed.), _Expectations and actions_. Hillsdale, NJ: Lawrence Erlbaum Associates, 1982.

Johnson, L. C., & Chernick, D. A. Sedative-hypnotics and human performance. _Psychopharmacology_, 1982, _76_, 101-113.

Joreskog, K. G. & Sorbom, D. Lisrel IV users guide. Chicago: National Educational Resources, 1978.

Joreskog, K. G., & Sorbom, D. Statistical models and methods for the analysis of longitudinal data. In d. J. Aigner & A. S. Goldberger (Eds.), _Latent variables in socioeconomic models_. Amsterdam: North-Holland, 1977.

Kadushin, C. Long term stress reactions: some causes, consequences, and naturally occurring support systems. In _Legacies of Vietnam: Comparative adjustment of veterans and their peers_ (Vol. 4) 97th Congress, 1st Session, House Committee Print No. 14, Washington D.C.: U.S. Government Printing Office, 1981.

Kahn, R. L. & Quinn, R. P. Role stress: A framework for analysis. In A. McLean (Ed.), _Mental health and work organizations_. Chicago: Rand McNally, 1970.

Kahn, R. L., Wolfe, D. M., Quinn, R. P., Snoek, J. D., & Rosenthal, R. A. _Organizational stress: Studies in role conflict and ambiguity_. New York: Wiley, 1964.

Kanner, A. D., Coyne, J. C., Schaefer, C., & Lazarus, R. S. Comparisons of two modes of stress measurement: Daily hassles and uplifts versus major life events. _Journal of Behavioral Medicine_, 1981, _1_, 1-38.

Kaplan, B. H., Cassel, J. C., & Gore, S. Social support and health. _Care_, 1977, _15_ (supplement), 47-58.

Katz, D., & Kahn, R. L. _Social psychology of organizations_. New York: Wiley, 1978.

Kessler, R. C. A strategy for studying differential vulnerability to the psychological consequences of stress. _Journal of Health and Social Behavior_, 1979a, _20_, 100-108.

Kessler, R. C. Stress, social status, and psychological distress. _Journal of Health and Social Behavior_, 1979b, _20_ (September), 259-272.
412

Kessler, R. C., Brown, R. L., & Broman, C. L. Sex difference in psychiatric help-seeking: Evidence from four large-scale surveys. Journal of Health and Social Behavior, 1981, 22, 49-64.

Kessler, R. C., & Greenberg, D. F. Linear panel analysis. New York: Academic Press, 1981.

Kleinknecht, R. A., & Donaldson, D. A review of the effects of Diazepam on cognitive and psychomotor performance. The Journal of Nervous and Mental Disease, 1975, 161 399-411.

Klerman, G. L. Psychotropic hedonism vs. pharmacological Calvinism. Hastings Center Report, 1972, 2 (4), 1-3.

Koch, H. Drugs most frequently used in office-based practice: National Ambulatory Medical Care Survey, 1980. National Center for Health Statistics Advance Data, May 1982a, 78, 1-12.

Koch, H. Drug utilization in office practice by age and sex of the patient: National Ambulatory Medical Care Survey, 1980. National Center for Health Statistics Advance Data, July 1982b, 81, 1-12.

Koch, H., & Campbell, W. H. Utilization of psychotropic drugs in office-based ambulatory care: National Ambulatory Medical Care Survey, 1980 and 1981. NCHS Advancedata, 1983, (90).

Koumjian, K. The use of Valium as a form of social control. Social Science and Medicine, 1981, 15E, 245-249.

Kraut, A. The study of role conflicts and their relationships to job satisfaction, tension, and performance (Doctoral dissertation, University of Michigan). Dissertation Abstracts, 1965, 26, 7476.

Kulka, R. A. Interaction as person-environment fit. New Directions for Methodology of Behavioral Science, 1979, 2, 55-71.

Labovitz, S. The assignment of numbers to rank order categories. American Sociological Review, 1970, 35(3), 515-524.

LaRocco, J. M., House, J. S., & French, J. R. P., Jr. Social support, occupational stress, and health. Journal of health and Social Behavior, 1980, 21, 202-218.

Lazarus, R. S. The costs and benefits of denial. In S. Breznitz (Ed.), Denial of stress. New York: International Universities Press, 1982.

Lazarus, R. S. The stress and coping paradigm. In C. Eisdorfer, D. Cohen, A. Kleinman, & P. Maxim (Eds.),

Theoretical bases for psychopathology. New York: Spectrum, 1981.

Lefcourt, H. M. Locus of control: Current trends in theory and research (2nd ed.). Hillsdale, NJ: Lawrence Erlbaum Associates, 1982.

Leff, J., & Tarrier, N. The home environments of schizophrenic patients, and their response to treatment. In M. J. Christie & P. G. Mellett (Eds.), Foundations of psychosomatics. London: Wiley, 1981, 407-420.

Lennard, H. L., Epstein, L. J., Berstein, A., & Ransom, D. C. Mystification and Drug Misuse. San Francisco: Jossey-Bass, 1971.

Levenson, H. Activism and powerful others: Distinctions within the concept of internal-external control. Journal of Personality Assessment, 1974, 38, 377-383.

Levenson, H. Multidimensional locus of control in psychiatric patients. Journal of Consulting and Clinical Psychology, 1973, 41, 397-404.

Levi, L. (Ed.). Stress and distress in response to psychosocial stimuli. Oxford: Pergamon Press, 1972.

Lundberg, U., & Frankenhaeuser, M. Psychophysiological reactions to noise as modified by personal control over noise density. Biological Psychiatry, 1978, 6, 51-59.

Maier, N. R. F. Frustration: The study of behavior without a goal. New York: McGraw-Hill, 1949.

Manheimer, D. I., Davidson, S. T., Balter, M. B., Mellinger, G. D., Cisin, I. H., & Parry, H. J. Popular attitudes and beliefs about tranquilizers. American Journal of Psychiatry, November 1973, 130(11), 1246-1253.

Manual of the International Statistical Classification of diseases, injuries, and causes of death. Geneva: World Health organization, 1977.

Maruyama, G., & McGarvey, B. Evaluating causal models: An application of maximum-likelihood analysis of structural equations. Psychological Bulletin, 1980, 87, 502-512.

McGrath, J. E. Stress and behavior in organizations. In M. D. Dunnette (Ed.), Handbook of industrial and organizational psychology. Chicago: Rand McNally, 1976, 1353-1396.

McKennell, A. C., & Andrews, F. M. Models of cognition and affect in perceptions of well-being. Social Indicators Research, 1980, 8, 257-298.

Mcree, C. Corder, B. F., & Haizlip, T. Psychiatrists' responses to sexual bias in pharmaceutical advertising.
414

American Journal of Psychiatry, November 1974, 131(11), 1273-1275.

Mellinger, G. D., Balter, M. B., Manheimer, D. I., Cisin, I. H., & Parry, H. J. Psychic distress, life crisis, and use of psychotherapeutic medications. Archives of General Psychiatry, 1978, 35, 1045-1052.

Miles, R. H. & Perreault, W. D., Jr. Organizational role conflict: Its antecedents and consequences. In D. Katz, R. Kahn, and J. S. Adams (Eds.), The Study of Organizations, San Francisco, CA: Jossey-Bass Limited, 1980.

National Disease and Therapeutic Index of 1978. Ambler, PA: IMS America Limited, 1978.

Nesbitt, P. D. Smoking, physiological arousal, and emotional response. Journal of Personality and Social Psychology, 1973, 25, 137-144.

Newmann, J. P. Sex differences in depression: An assessment of sources of measurement error. Paper presented at meeting of the American Sociological Association, Toronto, August 1981.

Nunnally, J. C. Psychometric theory. New York: McGraw-Hill, 1967.

O'Hanlon, J. F., Haak, T. W., Blaauw, G. J., & Riemersma, J. B. J. Diazepam impairs lateral position control in highway driving. Science, 1982, 217(2), 79-81.

Oksenberg, L., Vinokur, A., & Cannell, C. F. The effects of commitment to being a good respondent on interview performance. In C. F. Cannell, L. Oksenberg, & J. M. Converse (Eds.), Experiments in health reporting, 1971-1977. Ann Arbor: Institute for Social Research, University of Michigan, 1979.

Opinion Research Corporation, unpublished data, Princeton, NJ, 1983.

Owen, R. T. & Tyrer, P. Benzodiazepine dependence: A review of the evidence. Drugs, 1983, 25, 385-398.

Padesky, C. A., & Hammen, C. L. Sex differences in depressive symptom expression and help-seeking among college students. Sex Roles, 1981, 7, 309-320.

Paganini-Hill, A., & Ross, R. K. Reliability of recall of drug usage and other health related information. American Journal of Epidemiology, 1982, 116, 114.

Park, L. C., & Lipman, R. S. A comparison of patient dosage deviation reports with pill counts. Psychopharmacologia, 1964, 6, 299-302.

Parry, H. J., Balter, M., & Cisin, I. H. Primary levels of underreporting psychotropic drug use. Public Opinion Quarterly, 1970-71, 34, 582.

Parry, H. J., Balter, M. B., Mellinger, G. D., Cisin, I. H., & Manheimer, D. I. National patterns of psychotherapeutic drug use. Archives of General Psychiatry, 1973, 28, 769-783.

Pearlin, L. I., & Schooler, C. The structure of coping. Journal of Health and Social Behavior, 1978, 19, 2-21.

Persson, G. Non-pharmacological factors in drug treatment of anxiety states. Acta Psychiatrica Scandinavica, 1976, 54, 238-247.

Pevnick, J. S., Jasinski, D. R., & Haertzen, C. A. Abrupt withdrawal from therapeutically administered diazepam. Archives of General Psychiatry, 1978, 35, 995-998.

Pinneau, S. R., Jr. Effects of social support on psychological and physiological strains. (Doctoral dissertation, University of Michigan) Ann Arbor, MI: University Microfilms, 1975, No. 76-9491.

Prather, J., & Fidell, L. S. Sex differences in the content and style of medical advertisements. Social Science and Medicine, 1975, 9, 23-26.

Prusoff, B. A., & Klerman, G. L. Differentiating depressed from anxious neurotic outpatients. Archives of General Psychiatry, 1974, 30, 302-309.

Quarm, D. Random measurement error as a source of discrepancies between the reports of wives and husbands concerning marital power and task allocation. Journal of Marriage and the Family, 1981, 521-535.

Quinn, R. P., & Cobb, W., Jr. What workers want: Factor analyses of importance ratings of job facets. In R. P. Quinn, et al., The 1972-73 Quality of Employment Survey. Ann Arbor: Survey Research Center, University of Michigan, 1977.

Quinn, R. P., & Shepard, L. The 1972-1973 quality of employment survey. Ann Arbor: Survey Research Center, University of Michigan, 1974.

Rabkin, J. G., & Streuning, E. I. Life events, stress, and illness. Science, 1976, 194, 1013-1020.

Rickels, K. Benzodiazepines: Use and misuse. In D. F. Klein & J. G. Radkin (Eds.), New research and changing concepts. New York: Raven Press, 1981.

Rickels, K. Use of antianxiety agents in anxious outpatients. Psychopharmacology, 1978, 58, 1-17.

Rickels, K., Hesbacher, P., Fisher, E., & Norstad, N. The private research group (PPRG): A working model from psychopharmacology for clinical research in family practice. Clinical Pharmacology, 1977a, 17, 541-554.

Rickels, K., Lipman, R. S., Park, L. C., Covi, L., Uhlenhuth, E. H., & Mock, J. E. Drug, doctor warmth, and clinic setting in the symptomatic response to minor tranquilizers. Psychopharmacologia (Berl.),1971 20, 128-152.

Rickels, K., Pereira-Ogan, J., Csanalosi, I., Morris, R. J., Rosenfeld, H., Sablosky, L., Schless, A., & Werblowsky, J. H. Halazepam and Diazepam in neurotic anxiety: A double-blind study. Psychopharmacology, 1977b, 52, 129-136.

Rodin, J., Rennert, K., & Solomon, S. K. Intrinsic motivation for control: Fact or fiction. In A. Baum & J. E. Singer (Eds.), Advances in environmental psychology (Vol.2). Applications of personal control. Hillsdale, NJ: Lawrence Erlbaum Associates, 1980.

Ross, M., & Olson, J. M. An expectancy-attribution model of the effects of placebos. Psychological Review, 1981, 88, 408-437.

Roth, H. P., & Caron, H. S. Accuracy of doctors' estimates and patients' statements on adherence to a drug regimen. Clinical Pharmacology and Therapeutics, 1978, 23, 361-370.

Rotter, J. B. Generalized expectancies for internal versus external control of reinforcement. Psychological Monographs: General and Applied, 1966, 80, Whole no. 609, 1-28.

Schaefer, C., Coyne, J. C., & Lazarus, R. S. The health-related functions of social support. Journal of Behavioral Medicine, 1981, 4, p. 381-406.

Schubert, D. S. Arousal seeking as a central factor in tobacco smoking among college students. The International Journal of Social Psychiatry, 1965, 11, 221-225.

Schubert, D. S. Arousal seeking as a motivation for volunteering: MMPI scores and central-nervous-system-stimulant use as suggestive of a trait. Journal of projective techniques and personality assessment, 1964, 28, 337-340.

Schulz, R., & Hanusa, B. H. Long-term effects of control and predictability-enhancing interventions. Findings and ethical issues. Journal of Personality and Social Psychology. 1978, 36, 1194-1201.

Seligman, M. E. P. Helplessness. On depression, development, and death. San Francisco: W. H. Freeman & Co., 1975.

Silver, R. L., & Wortman, C. B. In J. Garber and M. E. P. Seligman (Eds.), Human Helplessness. New York: Academic Press, 1980.

Statistical Abstract of the United States: 1980 (101st edition). Washington, D. C.: U.S. Bureau of the Census, 1980.

Survey Research Center. Interviewer's Manual (Revised Edition). Ann Arbor: Survey Research Center, Institute for Social Research, University of Michigan, 1976.

Thoits, P. A. Undesirable life events and psychophysiological distress. A problem of operational confounding. American Sociological Review, 1981, 46, 97-109.

Uhlenhuth, E. H., Balter, M. B., & Lipman, R. S. Minor tranquilizers. Archives of General Psychiatry, 1978, 35, 650-655.

Uhlenhuth, E. H., Rickels, K., Fisher, S., Park, L. C., Lipman, R. S., & Mock, J. Drug, doctor's verbal attitude and clinic setting in the symptomatic response to pharmacotherapy. Psychopharmacologia, 1966, 9, 392-418.

United States Senate Committee on Labor and Human Resources. Use and misuse of Benzodiazepines. Washington, D.C.: U.S. Government Printing Office, 1980.

Vanfossen, B. E. Sex differences in the mental health effects of social support and equity. Journal of health and Social Behavior, 1981, 22, 130-143.

Verbrugge, L. Female illness rates and illness behavior: Testing hypotheses about sex differences in health. Women and Health, 1979, 4, 61-79.

Vinokur, A., & Selzer, M. L. Desirable versus undesirable life events: Their relationship to stress and mental distress. Journal of Personality and Social Psychology, 1975, 32, 329-337.

Waldron, I. Increased prescribing of Valium, Librium and other drugs--An example of the influence of economic and social factors on the practice of medicine. International Journal of Health Services, 1977, 7, 37-62.

Ware, J. E., Davies-Avery, A., & Donald, C. A. The conceptualization and measurement of health for adults in the Health Insurance Study: Volume V, general health perceptions. Santa Monica, CA: The Rand Corporation, 1978.

Warheit, G. J., Holzer, C. E., III, & Arey, S. A. Race and mental illness: An epidemiologic update. Journal of Health and Social Behavior, 1975, 16, 243-256.

Weissman, M. M., & Klerman, G. L. Sex differences and the epidemiology of depression. _Archives of General Psychiatry_, 1977, <u>34</u>, 98-111.

Winokur, A., Rickels, K., Greenblatt, D. J., Snyder, P. J., & Schatz, N. J. Withdrawal reaction from long-term, low-dosage administration of Diazepam. _Archives of General Psychiatry_, January 1980, <u>37</u>, 101-105.

Wittenborn, J. R. Effects of benzodiazepines on psychomotor performance. _British Journal of Clinical Pharmacology, Supplement 1_, 1979, <u>7</u>, 61-67.

Wolcott, D. L., Wellisch, D. K., Robertson, C. R., & Arthur, R. J. Serum Gastrin and the family environment in Duodenal Ulcer Disease. _Psychosomatic Medicine_, December 1981, <u>43</u>(6), 501-507.

Woods, J. H., Katz, J. L., & Winger, G. _Abuse and dependence liabilities of benzodiazepines._ University of Michigan, 1982.

World Health Organization. _Manual of the international statistical classification of diseases, injuries, and causes of death._ Geneva: World Health Organization, 1977.

Wortman, C. B. Impact and measurement of social support of the cancer patient. _Cancer_, in press.

Yerkes, R. M., & Dodson, J. D. The relation of strength of stimulus to rapidity of habit-formation. _Journal of Comparative and Neurological Psychology_, 1908, <u>18</u>, 459-482.

ISR RESEARCH REPORTS

The following Research Reports have been published by ISR. They are available in paperbound editions only. For information on prices and availability, write to the ISR Publishing Division, P.O. Box 1248, Ann Arbor, Michigan 48106.

Career Change in Midlife: Stress, Social Support, and Adjustment. John R. P. French, Jr., Steven R. Doehrman, Mary Lou Davis-Sacks, and Amiram Vinokur. 1983. 152 pp.

Compensating for Missing Survey Data. Graham Kalton. 1983. 164 pp.

Residential Displacement in the U.S., 1970-1977. Sandra J. Newman and Michael S. Owen. 1982. 98 pp.

Sex Role Attitudes among High School Seniors: Views about Work and Family Life. A. Regula Herzog and Jerald G. Bachman. 1982. 272 pp.

Subjective Well-Being among Different Age Groups. A. Regula Herzog, Willard L. Rodgers, and Joseph Woodworth. 1982. 115 pp.

Employee Ownership. Michael Conte, Arnold S. Tannenbaum, and Donna McCulloch. 1981. 70 pp.

Recreation and Quality of Urban Life: Recreational Resources, Behaviors, and Evaluations of People in the Detroit Region. Robert W. Marans and J. Mark Fly. 1981. 240 pp.

A Comparative Study of the Organization and Performance of Hospital Emergency Services. Basil S. Georgopoulos and Robert A. Cooke. 1980. 512 pp.

An Evaluation of "Freestyle": A Television Series to Reduce Sex-Role Stereotypes. Jerome Johnston, James Ettema, and Terrence Davidson. 1980. 308 pp.

Occupational Stress and the Mental and Physical Health of Factory Workers. James S. House. 1980. 356 pp.

Job Demands and Worker Health: Main Effects and Occupational Differences. Robert D. Caplan, Sidney Cobb, John R. P. French, Jr., R. Van Harrison, and S. R. Pineau, Jr. 1980. 342 pp.

Perceptions of Life Quality in Rural America: An Analysis of Survey Data from Four Studies. Robert W. Marans and Donald A. Dillman, with the assistance of Janet Keller. 1980. 118 pp.

Social Support and Patient Adherence: Experimental and Survey Findings. Robert D. Caplan, R. Van Harrison, Retha V. Wellons, and John R. P. French, Jr. 1980. 283 pp.

Working Together: A Study of Cooperation among Producers, Educators, and Researchers to Create Educational Television. James S. Ettema. 1980. 220 pp.

Experiments in Interviewing Techniques: Field Experiments in Health Reporting, 1971-1977. Edited by Charles F. Cannell, Lois Oksenberg, and Jean M. Converse. 1979. 446 pp.

The 1977 Quality of Employment Survey: Descriptive Statistics, with Comparison Data from the 1969-70 and 1972-73 Surveys. Robert P. Quinn and Graham L. Staines. 1979. 364 pp.

The Physical Environment and the Learning Process: A Survey of Recent Research. Jonathan King, Robert W. Marans, and associates. 1979. 92 pp.

Results of Two National Surveys of Philanthropic Activity. James N. Morgan, Richard F. Dye, and Judith H. Hybels. 1979. 204 pp.

A Survey of American Gambling Attitudes and Behavior. Maureen Kallick, Daniel Suits, Ted Dielman, and Judith Hybels. 1979. 560 pp.